Cavernous Malformations

Edited by
Issam A. Awad, MD,
and Daniel L. Barrow, MD

AANS Publications Committee

American Association of Neurological Surgeons
Park Ridge, Illinois

ISBN: 1-879284-07-3

Daniel L. Barrow, MD, Chairman
AANS Publications Committee

Linda S. Miller, AANS Staff Editor

AANS 1M393

Contents

List of Contributors

Issam A. Awad, MD, MSc, FACS
Head, Section of Cerebrovascular Surgery
Vice-Chairman, Department of Neurological
  Surgery
Cleveland Clinic Foundation
Cleveland, Ohio

Deepak Awasthi, MD
Chief Resident
Department of Neurosurgery
Louisiana State University School of Medicine
New Orleans, Louisiana

Daniel L. Barrow, MD
Associate Professor and Deputy Chief
Division of Neurosurgery
Emory Clinic
Atlanta, Georgia

James E. Baumgartner, MD
Assistant Professor of Neurosurgery
The University of Texas Medical Branch
  at Houston
Houston, Texas

Robert J. Coffey, MD
Assistant Professor
Department of Neurologic Surgery
Mayo Clinic
Rochester, Minnesota

Michael S.B. Edwards, MD
Director, Division of Pediatric Neurosurgery
Professor of Neurosurgery and Pediatrics
University of California
San Francisco, California

John Golfinos, MD
Resident in Neurosurgery
Barrow Neurological Institute
Phoenix, Arizona

Roberto C. Heros, MD
Professor and Chairman, Department of
  Neurological Surgery
University of Minnesota School of Medicine
Minneapolis, Minnesota

Frank P.K. Hsu, BS
University of Maryland Medical System
Baltimore, Maryland

Stephen L. Huhn, MD
Chief Resident
Division of Neurosurgery
University of Maryland Medical System
Baltimore, Maryland

Peter C. Johnson, MD
Chairman, Division of Neuropathology
Barrow Neurological Institute
Phoenix, Arizona

Ali Krisht, MD
Resident, Division of Neurosurgery
The Emory Clinic
Atlanta, Georgia

L. Dade Lunsford, MD
Professor, Department of Neurological Surgery,
  Radiology and Radiation Oncology
University of Pittsburgh School of Medicine
  and Specialized Neurosurgery Center
Pittsburgh, Pennsylvania

Michael P. Marks, MD
Assistant Professor and Director,
  Cerebrovascular Neuroradiology
Department of Radiology
Stanford University School of Medicine
Stanford, California

Paul C. McCormick, MD
Assistant Professor of Neurosurgery
Columbia Presbyterian Medical Center
New York, New York

W. Jost Michelsen, MD
Division of Neurological Surgery
St. Luke-Roosevelt Hospital
New York, New York

John Perl, MD
Assistant Staff, Section of Neuroradiology
Cleveland Clinic Foundation
Cleveland, Ohio

Daniele Rigamonti, MD, FACS
Associate Professor of Neurosurgery
Division of Neurosurgery
University of Maryland Medical System
Baltimore, Maryland

John R. Robinson, MD
Resident in Neurologic Surgery
Cleveland Clinic Foundation
Cleveland, Ohio

Jeffrey S. Ross, MD
Head of MRI
Section of Neuroradiology
Cleveland Clinic Foundation
Cleveland, Ohio

Mitesh V. Shah, MD
Resident in Neurosurgery
Department of Neurosurgery
University of Minnesota
Minneapolis, Minnesota

Robert F. Spetzler, MD, FACS
Director, Barrow Neurological Institute
Chairman, Division of Neurosurgery
Phoenix, Arizona

Bennett M. Stein, MD
Professor and Chairman, Department of
   Neurological Surgery
Columbia Presbyterian Medical Center
New York, New York

Gary K. Steinberg, MD, PhD
Assistant Professor and Head, Cerebrovascular
   Surgery
Stanford University School of Medicine
Stanford, California

Thomas M. Wascher, MD
Neuroscience Group
Appleton, Wisconsin

Charles B. Wilson, MD
Chairman, Department of Neurologic Surgery
Professor of Neurosurgery
University of California - SF
San Francisco, California

Joseph M. Zabramski, MD
Assistant Professor of Surgery, University of
   Arizona
Head of Cerebrovascular Laboratory, Barrow
   Neurological Institute
Phoenix, Arizona

AANS Publications Committee

Inspirational Dedication

"The moderns are, in relation to the ancients, as a
dwarf placed on the shoulder of a giant; he sees all
that the giant perceives plus a little bit more."
Henri De Mondeville
Thirteenth Century French Surgeon

"They do certainly give strange and new-fangled names
to diseases."
Plato

L.K. was 40 years old when she suffered her stroke. She had complained of headaches for some time, but none were as bad as that day when she could no longer move her left arm and leg. She also felt numbness throughout her body and experienced double vision. She always feared that she might suffer a stroke at a young age, especially since strokes seemed to run in her family.

L.K.'s grandfather always suffered from severe headaches; he had died at a young age. Her father and two paternal uncles also complained of headaches and "pressure in the head," but they never had any other problem. Their children, however, seemed to have a strange disease. Four of L.K.'s cousins (two males and two females) suffered strokes in their thirties. One cousin was severely debilitated by multiple strokes and underwent several brain operations for cerebral hemorrhage. Finally, he had to be placed in a nursing home where he died at the age of 38. The two female cousins' teenage children have been diagnoised with epilepsy. L.K.'s own brother had suffered a small stroke with double vision and difficulty walking a few weeks before her own stroke. Her sister was diagnosed as harboring a "brain lesion," and she, too, suffered from severe headaches.

L.K. thought that the "worst was happening to her" when she could not move her left side. She recalled her young cousin who was in a nursing home following numerous strokes. The doctors seemed to know that members of the family were suffering cerebral hemorrhages, and they seemed to indicate that all the patients harbored cerebral vascular malformations. No member of the family was ever told about the possible familial or genetic transmission of this disease. The doctors always seemed to be surprised that the lesions hemorrhaged despite normal angiograms.

L.K. finally underwent magnetic resonance imaging and the diagnosis of familial cavernous malformations was made (shown in Figure 1). In all, she harbored no less than 6 lesions which were visible on the imaging study. Yet, 2 lesions had hemorrhaged simultaneously—the left sylvian lesion and the right pontine lesion. The latter was likely the cause of her neurologic deficit. The right pontine lesion was excised via a transpetrous transtentorial anterolateral pontine route. Two months later, she underwent trans-sylvian resection of the left cerebral lesion, which had shown evidence of hemorrhage into adjacent eloquent brain.

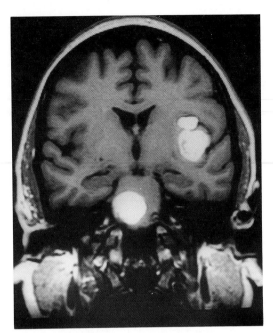

Figure 1. Magnetic resonance imaging of the brain showing 2 cavernous malformations that have recently hemorrhaged.

Two years following surgery, the 2 excised lesions have not recurred and the other smaller lesions, which have been followed conservatively, have not shown detectable change. L.K. is now leading a full and productive life (see Figure 2).

L.K.'s courage is exemplary. Other members of her family have not fared so well. As noted, 2 relatives were severely disabled, 1 died, 2 others underwent brain surgeries, and the rest have remained gripped with fear and uncertainty.

L.K. and her family have been a source of inspiration to us. As we have cared for several members of the family, we have learned together and taught each other about many aspects of this disease. We have learned that some lesions can be debilitating, while others can remain for years without change or symptoms. We have learned that surgery should not be performed on most lesions, but also that surgery should not be held back from lesions that are progressing toward serious disability and death.

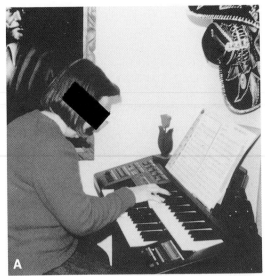

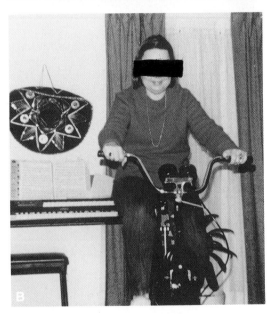

Figure 2. L.K. six months following brain operations for resection of the two cavernous malformations which had hemorrhaged. She is now neurologically intact, able to play the organ (**A**) and ride her exercise bicycle (**B**). She spends much of her time caring for and counseling numerous relatives with cavernous malformations.

The plight of this family has raised many other questions. Which lesions bleed, and why? Is there a period in life when lesions behave more aggressively than at other times? Do aggressive lesions continue to behave aggressively until the patient is disabled or dies? What is the likelihood that a newly diagnosed lesion will remain quiescent? How is the disease inherited? With so many cousins overtly affected, why did L.K.'s father and uncles remain symptom free? Some of the female members of the family appeared to worsen following pregnancy and delivery; how should they be counseled about childbearing? The teenage relatives with epilepsy know that they harbor the lesions; will they be disabled like their parents and uncles in midlife?

These and numerous other questions are highly personal. A decade ago, the field of medicine could not even begin to answer them. Cavernous malformations were not well recognized, and their multiplicity and familial nature were thought to be rare. Many patients with these lesions have eluded diagnosis, while others have lived and died under false diagnoses, which have included multiple sclerosis, brain stem glioma, and idiopathic cerebral hemorrhage.

Much has been learned in recent years about this disease and much remains to be learned.

—*The Editors*

Preface

The cavernous malformation (CM) is a hamartomatous hemorrhagic lesion. It consists of cavernous spaces lined by endothelial cells and collagen. It is void of any smooth muscle. The caverns contain blood at various stages of stasis, thrombosis, organization, and calcification. There are minute feeding and draining vessels, but no evidence of high flow or arteriovenous shunting within the lesion. There is no brain tissue between caverns in the core of the lesion itself.

This pathologic entity was thought to be very rare, and reports of its clinical significance were highly sporadic prior to the era of magnetic resonance imaging (MRI). The early literature was heavily biased toward larger lesions with advanced clinical symptomatology. This lesion was not easily detected by computed tomography (CT) unless it was very large and contained substantial calcification. The lesion also generally was occult on angiography.

Since the advent of MRI, the lesion has been recognized increasingly as an incidental or asymptomatic entity and also associated with a variety of neurologic symptoms including seizures, focal neurologic deficits, and headache. Catastrophic and apoplectic hemorrhages are exceedingly rare in the setting of a carefully characterized CM. However, focal hemorrhage is invariably present and is a histopathologic *sine qua non* of the lesion. In carefully performed autopsy studies, the lesion is found in approximately 0.4% of unselected consecutive postmortem examinations. A similar high case prevalence has been confirmed in consecutive MR examinations of the brain performed for all indications.

With the realization of the high prevalence of this lesion and its increased detection in the clinical setting, a clinical-radiologic-pathologic profile has evolved. Much data has accumulated in recent years about the clinical natural history, symptomatic associations, radiologic features, and detailed histopathologic characteristics of this entity.

Other unique features of the CM have been elucidated. There is a frequent incidence of lesion multiplicity in contrast to other vascular malformations of the brain. Also, there is familial clustering of cases with multiple lesions, consistent with an autosomal dominant pattern of inheritance with incomplete expression. This is akin to other phakomatoses also associated with vascular malformations. There is also a peculiar association with another totally different lesion, the venous malformation (an abnormal coalescence of draining veins to a region of the brain). In other instances, the brain of patients with CMs is found to harbor islands of capillary malformations, some of which appear to be coalescing so as to form "baby" CMs. These curious associations have stimulated numerous hypotheses about lesion etiogenesis.

The clinical manifestations of the CM have been attributed to focal microhemorrhages, to lesion expansion, or less commonly to frank exsanguination from the lesion. Factors predisposing to these events and to particular clinical sequelae (including seizures and focal neurologic deficits) are being sought in careful clinical studies and institutional registries.

The massive convergence of information on CMs has been presented at numerous scientific meetings and in the neuroscience literature in the past decade. Few textbooks have included chapters dedicated to this lesion that incorporate some of this recent information. To date, there has not been a textbook or monograph that compiles, integrates, and synthesizes such information. Upon recommendation of the Publications Committee of the American Association of Neurological Surgeons, the editors have embarked on just such a task. Experts in the fields of pathology, neuroradiology, and neurosurgery have been invited to contribute respective chapters related to various facets of this topic.

As with any multi-authored textbook addressing a focused topic with rapidly evolving information, the following chapters will include some overlap of data and some divergence of views. The integrated information from the following pages represents, however, state-of-the-art knowledge about this lesion and the spectrum of opinions about its nature, clinical behavior, and management strategies. We hope that this textbook will be of use to residents and to neurosurgeons at all levels who may be called upon to manage CMs. It also hopefully will be used by workers in related disciplines as a reference for these lesions.

The editors are indebted to numerous teachers and mentors and to members of the Publications Committee of the American Association of Neurological Surgeons for guidance and advice. We are also indebted to Ms. Linda Miller and Mr. Jeremy Longhurst from the American Association of Neurological Surgeons staff for expert assistance throughout stages of manuscript preparation and book production. Ms. Shirley McDaniel and Ms. Wendy Barringer also have admirably performed a multitude of tasks related to the editorial process. Lastly, we thank our families, our colleagues, our students, and above all the patients with cavernous malformations for their endless inspiration and support.

Issam A. Awad, MD
Daniel L. Barrow, MD

Chapter 1

Definition and Pathologic Features

Peter C. Johnson, MD, Thomas M. Wascher, MD, John Golfinos, MD, and Robert F. Spetzler, MD

Cerebral vascular malformations occur in approximately 0.1% to 4.0% of the general population.[11,29,30,50] Of the four classically described types of vascular malformations, cavernous malformations (CMs) are thought to account for 8% to 15% of both intracranial and spinal cases.[23,27,32,42,50] The true incidence of CMs is difficult to estimate because the features of these lesions appear to overlap with some other types of cerebral vascular malformations.[43,50] Most CMs are asymptomatic. When symptomatic, they typically present with seizures, hemorrhage, and focal mass effects.[13,24,27,56,59,62] Hydrocephalus, cranial neuropathies, papilledema, hypothalamic disturbances, and progressive or transient neurologic deficits occur less frequently.[13,36,50,52] Symptomatic lesions have been described in all age groups; most series indicate that the onset of symptoms is primarily between the third and the fifth decades without a sex predominance.[24,27,40,63] CMs may comprise a significant percentage of angiographically occult cerebral vascular malformations.*

CMs occur sporadically and in a familial setting, with up to 50% of CM patients having a strong family history that is usually autosomal dominant with incomplete penetrance. CMs may be particularly prominent in families of Hispanic descent.** These lesions have been reported throughout the brain, spinal cord, and cauda equina. They have been described to occur most often in the brain stem or in a subcortical location near the rolandic fissure and basal ganglia; the majority are located supratentorially.*** Although usually solitary, multiple lesions also occur, especially in the familial cases.[11,40,63] Extra-axial lesions that involve the cavernous sinus and dura of the middle cranial fossa have been described.[19,35,44,48,54] The cranial nerves, especially the optic nerve and chiasm, may also be involved.[22] Their natural history of growth and hemorrhage is being elucidated more clearly with the widespread use of magnetic resonance imaging (MRI).

This chapter focuses on the gross and microscopic pathologic features of CMs, contrasting them with arteriovenous malformations (AVMs), venous malformations, and capillary telangiectases. It also con-

---

*References 4,7,8,10,11,14,21,33,34,55,58,64

**References 2,3,5,11,15,18,25,41,42,51
***References 3,20,27,33,37,40,47,61,63,66,67

siders the relationship of CMs to other vascular anomalies and discusses transitional forms of vascular malformations.

Pathology of Vascular Malformations

Various classification schemes have been proposed to categorize vascular malformations of the central nervous system. The most widely accepted schema was devised by McCormick.[29-32] Vascular malformations have been divided into four groups based on the nature of their component vessels and on the character of the intervening brain as: AVMs, venous malformations, capillary telangiectases, and CMs (see Table 1).[32,50]

Arteriovenous Malformations

AVMs have a direct shunt between the arterial and venous systems without an intervening capillary bed. Their gross appearance is a tangle of dilated arteries and arterialized veins, destroying and replacing intervening brain (Figure 1). By microscopy, arteries are typically normal while veins are variably dilated with irregular fibromuscular thickening of their walls (Figure 2).[32] Venous channels contain no well-defined elastica.[23] AVMs lack a normal intervening capillary bed; brain parenchyma within the lesion is gliotic and may show residua of previous hemorrhage and collagenous scarring. Surrounding brain may show thin-walled vascular channels, perhaps representing recently recruited venous drainage. AVMs may be partly or completely situated in the subarachnoid space; this feature differentiates them from other forms of vascular malformations. Thrombi of varying ages and mineralization are common.

Venous Malformations

Venous malformations are characterized by the presence of one or more anomalous veins, often located in the deep white matter. Macroscopically, a radially arranged configuration of medullary veins separated by normal brain parenchyma drains into one or more central dilated draining veins, which may empty into the deep or superficial venous systems (Figure 3).[32] Microscopically, component veins may appear normal or, less commonly, show degenerative changes characterized by thickening and hyalinization. No arteries are found intimately associated with the lesion.[23,32,46] Calcification, hemorrhage, and spontaneous thrombosis are rare.[32] A varix may be a variant of the venous malformation that involves a single dilated vein, again surrounded by normal parenchyma, that often demonstrates a fibrotic, thickened hyalinized wall.[32]

Capillary Telangiectases

Capillary telangiectases are punctate lesions composed of small, dilated capillaries (Figures 4 and 5). These malformations are clusters of dilated capillaries devoid of smooth muscle or elastic fibers. The intervening brain may be normal, or less commonly, show residua of previous hemorrhage and/or gliosis. These lesions may drain into an abnormally large central venous channel.[32]

Cavernous Malformations

On gross examination, CMs are discrete, lobulated, well-circumscribed, red-to-purple, raspberrylike lesions. They vary from punctate to several centimeters in size (Figure 6). Giant lesions involving an entire lobe or lobes of the brain have been described, primarily in infants and children.[50]

Microscopically, CMs are composed of dilated, thin-walled capillaries that have a simple endothelial lining with variably thin fibrous adventitia indistinguishable from the lining of a capillary telangiectasia.[32,43] The typical CM has no brain parenchyma between the centrally placed vascular channels—a feature that has been said to typically distinguish CMs from capillary

Table 1. **Epidemiologic and Pathologic Characteristics of Cerebrovascular Malformations**

Type	Incidence at Autopsy	Topography	Family History	Multiplicity	Gross Pathology	Histopathology	Clinical Presentation
Arteriovenous malformation	1%	Distribution of the middle cerebral artery Intra-axial and subarachnoid	Rare	Rare	Tangle of vessels Thickness of vessel wall varies Luminal diameter varies Hemosiderin staining of surrounding brain	Arteries and arterialized thick-walled veins Thrombosis, recanalization Gliotic intervening parenchyma Hemosiderin	Spontaneous hemorrhage Seizures Headaches Progressive neurologic deficit Hydrocephalus Increased intracranial pressure Bruit High output cardiac failure
Cavernous malformation	0.4%	Anywhere, usually parenchymal	Common, especially in patients of Hispanic descent	Familial Form—50% Sporadic Form—rare	Lobulated Well-circumscribed Non-encapsulated Raspberry-like	Large, rounded vascular channels with thin walls lined by endothelium No smooth muscle or elastic fibers Evidence of prior hemorrhage No central intervening normal brain parenchyma	Seizures Headache Mass effect Hemorrhage Hydrocephalus Incidental finding on MRI Progressive or transient neurologic deficits
Venous malformation and varix	2%	Cerebral hemispheres	Unknown	10%–15%	Radial rearrangement of veins draining into a larger vein Intervening normal parenchyma	Venous wall No elastica Hyalinization Calcification, hemorrhage, and thrombosis (rare)	Almost always asymptomatic Headache Hemorrhage Associated lesions common
Capillary telangiectasia	0.7%	Pons Middle cerebellar peduncle Dentate nucleus of the cerebellum	Common	Common	Punctate Small, capillary-type vessels	Saccular, dilated capillaries No smooth muscle or elastic fibers Interspersed in normal parenchyma	Asymptomatic Hemorrhage (rare)

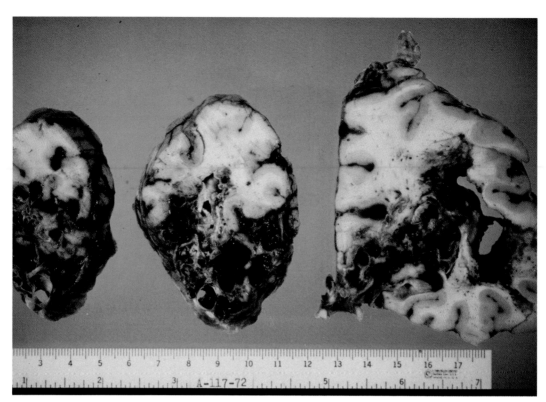

Figure 1. Gross specimen of a parieto-occipital giant AVM demonstrating massively dilated vascular spaces separated by brain with evidence of surrounding recent and old hemorrhage. Considerable brain has been destroyed by bleeding and mass effect.

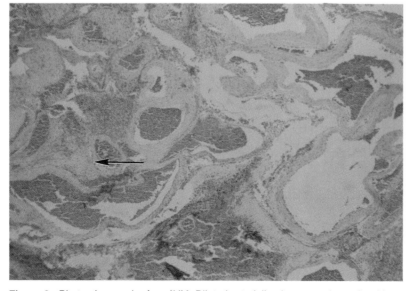

Figure 2. Photomicrograph of an AVM. Dilated arterialized venous channels with irregularly thickened walls are seen with accompanying arterial channels. Small areas of intervening gliotic brain are also present (arrow). Hematoxylin and eosin.

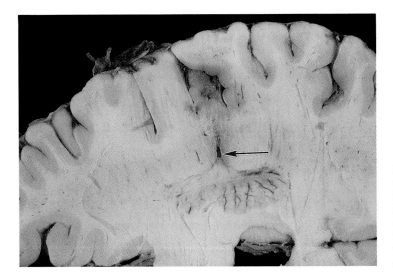

Figure 3. Gross specimen of a venous malformation. The lesion is in the periventricular white matter as a radial array of dilated medullary veins draining into a dilated central vein (arrow) that, in turn, drains toward the cortex. There is no hemosiderin.

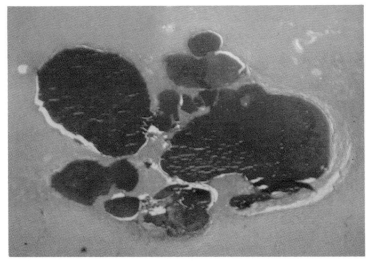

Figure 4. Photomicrograph of capillary telangiectasis from frontal lobe white matter of same patient as shown in Figure 5. Note the absence of hemosiderin and the presence of intervening brain among the thin-walled, dilated capillaries. Hematoxylin and eosin.

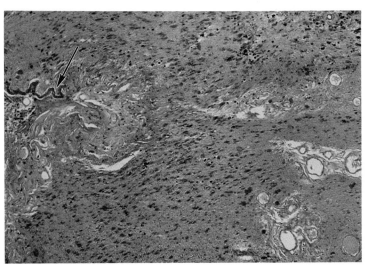

Figure 5. Photomicrograph of periventricular, sclerotic capillary telangiectasis. Widespread deposition of brown hemosiderin indicates previous hemorrhage that likely obliterated some of the vascular channels (arrow). Hematoxylin and eosin. The gross appearance is shown in Figure 6.

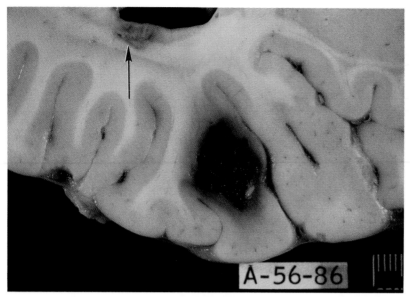

Figure 6. Autopsy specimen demonstrating typical appearance of a CM. The lesion is a lobulated, small mass sharply demarcated from the surrounding brain which is slightly edematous and has hemosiderin staining. A coincidental capillary telangiectasis (see Figure 5), is also adjacent to the atrium of the ventricle (arrow). The telangiectasis contains small vascular spaces with surrounding hemosiderin.

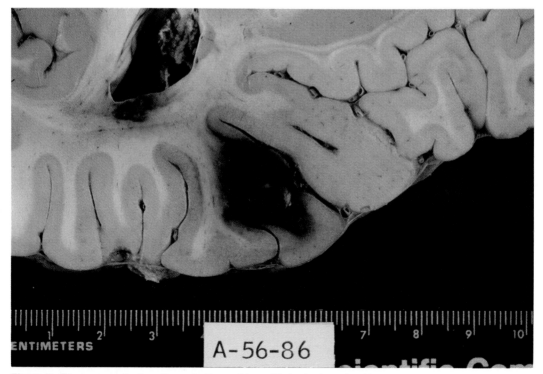

Figure 7. The same patient as shown in Figure 1 but with the brain stained by the Perl's method to reveal hemosiderin (blue) deposition around both the CM and the accompanying capillary telangiectasis.

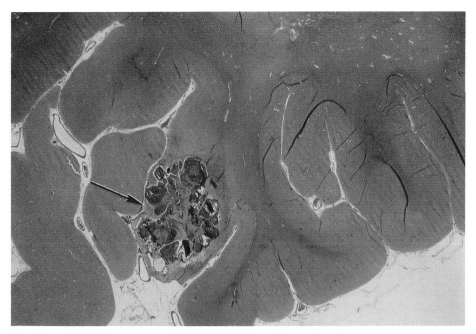

Figure 8. Photomicrograph of the CM seen in the previous gross sections. Brain is seen between vascular channels (arrow). Hematoxylin and eosin.

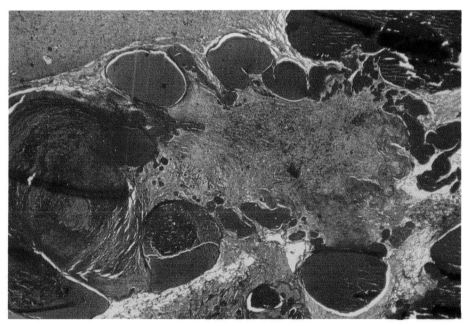

Figure 9. Photomicrograph of the same lesion at a higher power demonstrating the characteristic thin-walled, dilated capillary spaces. Gliotic and fibrotic tissues are in the center of the lesion along with brown hemosiderin deposits. Note the uniformly thin-walled vascular channels. There is intervening brain between these channels at the periphery. The large vessel on the left contains a laminated thrombus. Hematoxylin and eosin.

telangiectases.[32,50] However, at the periphery of CMs, dilated capillaries will be found in the surrounding brain (Figures 8 and 9).[43] Elastic fibers in the walls of the vascular spaces are absent.[30,50,56] Residua of previous hemorrhages, including fibrous scarring and collections of hemosiderin-laden macrophages, may be present (see Figures 7 and 9).[26,57] The lesion is surrounded by a variable degree of gliosis with increased tissue water. Inflammation, calcification, and even ossification may occur, particularly in larger lesions.[3,30,49,50] Vascular channels can be thrombosed (Figure 9) with various stages of reorganization.[50] The surrounding vasculature is normal; and the arterial supply is rarely visualized.

Three rare variants of CMs have been described: (1) a cystic form; (2) the dural-based malformation; (3) and the so-called *hemangioma calcificans*.[27] The cystic CM is characterized by a cyst with surrounding edema and a tendency to continuous growth with progressive neurologic deficit from recurrent hemorrhages.[1,39,57] Cystic malformations are more common in the posterior fossa.[1,39]

Hemangioma calcificans are densely calcified lesions that may represent a calcified CM (although this is unproven because of a lack of histopathologic confirmation).[9,17,27,38,49,50,53] They are commonly reported to be located in the temporal lobe and to cause seizures and only rarely hemorrhage. They are associated with bony metaplasia and abnormal vascular channels.

Dural-based CMs represent the third variant and are histologically composed of dilated cavernous channels lacking mural smooth muscle, which usually arises from the middle cranial fossa near the midline or parasellar regions involving the cavernous sinus; although entirely intracavernous lesions have also been described.[19,27,48,54] Dural CMs are prone to bleed massively at surgery and have a more aggressive clinical course.[19,35,44,54]

Cavernous Malformations and Other Associated Lesions

An association between intracranial CMs, especially when multiple lesions are present, and similar vascular anomalies of other organ systems have been described. Familial cases of *multiple hemangiomatosis* involving symptomatic central nervous system CMs and angiomatous hamartomas of the brain, retina, liver, kidneys, heart, and skin have suggested that CMs can be a feature of the constellation of phacomatoses (neuroectodermoses).[13,27] CMs of the cerebral hemispheres have been described in patients with hereditary hemorrhagic telangiectasis (Rendu-Osler-Weber syndrome).[65] Two cases of concurrent cavernous lesions and gliomas have been described.[12]

Mixed and Transitional Vascular Malformations

CMs, especially of the familial variety, may coexist in combination with AVMs, venous malformations, and capillary telangiectases.[10,16,20,45,46,60] A spectrum of transitional forms, especially with regard to CMs and capillary telangiectases, also exists (see Figures 4, 5, and 6). The essential differences between capillary telangiectases and CMs are the presence of brain tissue centrally, the size of the lesions, and the size of the composite vascular channels. Telangiectatic vessels with intervening brain are often seen in the periphery of CMs.[43,50] CMs and capillary telangiectases share other similarities: multiplicity, frequent pontine involvement, familial variety, and the association with vascular lesions elsewhere in the body.[50] These similarities suggest capillary telangiectases may be precursors of CMs.[43,46] According to this theory, capillary telangiectases and CMs represent two extremes within the same spectrum of vascular malformation and should be grouped as a single category called *cerebral capillary malformations*.[43] Transitional forms between the two extremes may represent stages in the evolution from telangiectasia to CM,[46,50] and may be present in the same brain.[43] Capillary telangiectases have also been shown to exist in association with venous malformations; in cases associated with hemorrhage, the telangiectatic portion of the malformation is most likely responsible for the hemorrhage.[28]

Cavernous Malformations and Cryptic/Occult Cerebrovascular Malformations

The terminology applied to symptomatic intracranial vascular anomalies, which are not readily imaged radiographically, includes the ill-defined term *cryptic/occult cerebrovascular malformation*, which refers to small or otherwise indiscernible vascular anomalies that have ruptured.[7] This term has since come to refer to vascular malformations that cannot be demonstrated on high-quality four-vessel cerebral angiography, including subtraction and magnification, angiotomography, and rapid serial angiography.[6,34,55] Although sometimes used interchangeably with the term *cryptic malformation*, the terms *occult*, or *angiographically occult*, or *thrombosed vascular malformation* have been applied to vascular hamartomas that are not visualized by serial angiography but are seen on computed tomography (CT) or MRI.[14,21,64] Histopathologically, these lesions have been found to be AVMs, CMs, venous malformations, capillary telangiectases, and transitional forms. Thrombosed, cryptic, and occult vascular malformations are therefore radiographic terms, not distinct clinicopathologic entities.

Conclusion

CMs account for 8% to 15% of the four generally recognized forms of cerebrovascular malformations. Grossly, the lesions are lobulated, well-circumscribed, raspberry-like lesions. Microscopically, there is a mass of irregularly dilated, blood-filled spaces lined by endothelium. There is no elastic or smooth muscle. Complicating hemorrhages, recent and old, as well as fibrous scarring, are seen. There is variable gliosis in the surrounding brain. Histopathologic keys to differentiating a CM from an AVM are the absence of elastic fibers and smooth muscle fibers, and the presence of intervening brain and accompanying arteries. Unlike venous malformations and capillary telangiectases, CMs have no intervening brain in the center of the mass. Special stains for smooth muscle and elastin may be useful in establishing the diagnosis. Thrombosis, organization, inflammatory changes, calcification, collagen deposition, and, especially, evidence of a prior hemorrhage with hemosiderin may be seen in the typical CM and AVM.

A relationship between multiple or familial CMs with or without vascular malformations elsewhere in the body as a form of a phacomatosis has been suggested. A histopathologic spectrum of transitional cerebrovascular malformations has been described, especially between CMs and capillary telangiectases. CMs may account for a significant proportion of "cryptic," "thrombosed," or "occult" vascular malformations.

References

1. Bellotti C, Medina M, Oliveri G, et al. Cystic cavernous angiomas of the posterior fossa: report of three cases. *J Neurosurg.* 1985;63:797–799.
2. Bicknell JM. Familial cavernous angioma of the brain stem dominantly inherited in Hispanics. *Neurosurgery.* 1989;24:102–105.
3. Bicknell JM, Carlow TJ, Kornfeld M, et al. Familial cavernous angiomas. *Arch Neurol.* 1978;35:746–749.
4. Chin D, Harper C. Angiographically occult cerebral vascular malformations with abnormal computed tomography. *Surg Neurol.* 1983;20:138–142.
5. Clark JV. Familial occurrence of cavernous angiomata of the brain. *J Neurol Neurosurg Psychiatry.* 1970;33:871–876.
6. Cohen HCM, Tucker WS, Humphreys RP, et al. Angiographically cryptic histologically verified cerebrovascular malformations. *Neurosurgery.* 1982;10:704–714.

7. Crawford JM, Russell DS. Cryptic arteriovenous and venous hamartomas of the brain. *J Neurol Neurosurg Psychiatry.* 1956;19:1–11.

8. Davis DH, Kelly PJ. Stereotactic resection of occult vascular malformations. *J Neurosurg.* 1990;72:698–702.

9. DiTullio MV Jr, Stern WE. Hemangioma calcificans: case report of an intraparenchymatous calcified vascular hematoma with epileptogenic potential. *J Neurosurg.* 1979;50:110–114.

10. Ebeling JD, Tranmer BI, Davis KA, et al. Thrombosed arteriovenous malformations: a type of occult vascular malformation. Magnetic resonance imaging and histopathological correlations. *Neurosurgery.* 1988;23:605–610.

11. El-Gohary EM, Tomita T, Gutierrez FA, et al. Angiographically occult vascular malformations in childhood. *Neurosurgery.* 1987;20:759–766.

12. Fischer EG, Sotrel A, Welch K. Cerebral hemangioma with glial neoplasia (angioglioma?): report of two cases. *J Neurosurg.* 1982;56:430–434.

13. Giombini S, Morello G. Cavernous angiomas of the brain: account of fourteen personal cases and review of the literature. *Acta Neurochir (Wien).* 1978;40:61–82.

14. Gomori JM, Grossman RI, Goldberg HI, et al. Occult cerebral vascular malformations: high-field MR imaging. *Radiology.* 1986;158:707–713.

15. Hayman LA, Evans RA, Ferrell RE, et al. Familial cavernous angiomas: natural history and genetic study over a 5-year period. *Am J Med Genet.* 1982;11:147–160.

16. Hirsh LF. Combined cavernous-arteriovenous malformation. *Surg Neurol.* 1981;16:135–139.

17. Kasantikul V, Wirt TC, Allen VA, et al. Identification of a brain stone as calcified hemangioma: case report. *J Neurosurg.* 1980;52:862–866.

18. Kidd HA, Cumings JN. Cerebral angiomata in an Icelandic family. *Lancet.* 1947;1:747–748.

19. Kudo T, Ueki S, Kobayashi H, et al. Experience with the ultrasonic surgical aspirator in a cavernous hemangioma of the cavernous sinus. *Neurosurgery.* 1989;24:628–631.

20. Lee KS, Spetzler RF. Spinal cord cavernous malformation in a patient with familial intracranial cavernous malformations. *Neurosurgery.* 1990;26:877–880.

21. Lobato RD, Perez C, Rivas JJ, et al. Clinical, radiological, and pathological spectrum of angiographically occult intracranial vascular malformations: analysis of 21 cases and review of the literature. *J Neurosurg.* 1988;68:518–531.

22. Manz HJ, Klein LH, Fermaglich J, et al. Cavernous hemangioma of the optic chiasm, optic nerves, and right optic tract: case report and review of the literature. *Virchows Archiv A Pathol Anat Histol.* 1979;383:225–232.

23. Martin N, Vinters H. Pathology and grading of intracranial vascular malformations. In: Barrow DL, ed. *Intracranial Vascular Malformations.* Park Ridge, Ill: American Association of Neurological Surgeons; 1990:1–30.

24. Martin NA, Wilson CB, Stein BM. Venous and cavernous malformations. In: Wilson CB, Stein BM, eds. *Intracranial Arteriovenous Malformations.* Baltimore, Md: Williams & Wilkins; 1984:234–245.

25. Mason I, Aase JM, Orrison WW, et al. Familial cavernous angiomas of the brain in an Hispanic family. *Neurology.* 1988;38:324–326.

26. McConnell TH, Leonard JS. Microangiomatous malformations with intraventricular hemorrhage: report of two unusual cases. *Neurology.* 1967;17:618–620.

27. McCormick PC, Michelsen WJ. Management of intracranial cavernous and venous malformations. In: Barrow DL, ed. *Intracranial Vascular Malformations.* Park Ridge, Ill: American Association of Neurological Surgeons; 1990:197–217.

28. McCormick PW, Spetzler RF, Johnson PC. Cerebellar hemorrhage associated with capillary telangiectasia and venous angioma: a case report. *Surg Neurol.* In press, 1992.

29. McCormick WF. Classification, pathology, and natural history of angiomas of the central nervous system. *Weekly Update: Neurol Neurosurg.* 1975;1.

30. McCormick WF. The pathology of vascular ("arteriovenous") malformations. *J Neurosurg.* 1966;24:807–816.

31. McCormick WF. Vascular disorders of nervous tissue: anomalies, malformations, and aneurysms. In: Bourne GH, ed. *The Structure and Function of Nervous Tissue. Vol III. Biochemistry and Disease.* Orlando, Fla: Academic Press, Inc; 1969:537–596.

32. McCormick WF. Pathology of vascular malformations of the brain. In: Wilson CB, Stein BM, eds. *Intracranial Arteriovenous Malformations.* Baltimore, Md: Williams & Wilkins; 1984:44–63.

33. McCormick WF, Hardman JM, Boulter TR. Vascular malformations ("angiomas") of the brain, with special reference to those occurring in the posterior fossa. *J Neurosurg.* 1968;28:241–251.

34. McCormick WF, Nofzinger JD. "Cryptic" vascular malformations of the central nervous system. *J Neurosurg.* 1966;24:865–875.

35. Meyer FB, Lombardi D, Scheithauer B, et al. Extra-axial cavernous hemangiomas involving the dural sinuses. *J Neurosurg.* 1990;73:187–192.

36. Mizutani T, Goldberg HI, Kerson IA, et al. Cavernous hemangioma in the diencephalon. *Arch Neurol.* 1981;38:379–382.

37. Pagni CA, Canavero S, Forni M. Report of a cavernoma of the cauda equina and review of the literature. *Surg Neurol.* 1990;33:124–133.

38. Penfield W, Ward A. Calcifying epileptogenic lesions: hemangioma calcificans; report of a case. *Arch Neurol Psychiatr.* 1948;60:20–36.

39. Pozzati E, Gaist G, Poppi M, et al. Microsurgical removal of paraventricular cavernous angiomas: report of two cases. *J Neurosurg.* 1981;55:308–311.

40. Rigamonti D. Natural history of cavernous malformations, capillary malformations (telangiectases), and venous malformations. In: Barrow DL, ed. *Intracranial Vascular Malformations.*

Park Ridge, Ill: American Association of Neurological Surgeons; 1990:45–51.

41. Rigamonti D, Drayer BP, Johnson PC, et al. The MRI appearance of cavernous malformations (angiomas). *J Neurosurg.* 1987;67:518–524.

42. Rigamonti D, Hadley MN, Drayer BP, et al. Cerebral cavernous malformations. Incidence and familial occurrence. *N Engl J Med.* 1988;319:343–347.

43. Rigamonti D, Johnson PC, Spetzler RF, et al. Cavernous malformations and capillary telangiectasia: a spectrum within a single pathological entity. *Neurosurgery.* 1991;28:60–64.

44. Rigamonti D, Pappas CTE, Spetzler RF, et al. Extracerebral cavernous angiomas of the middle fossa. *Neurosurgery.* 1990;27:306–310.

45. Rigamonti D, Spetzler RF. The association of venous and cavernous malformations: report of four cases and discussion of the pathophysiological, diagnostic, and therapeutic implications. *Acta Neurochir (Wien).* 1988;92:100–105.

46. Rigamonti D, Spetzler RF, Johnson PC, et al. Cerebral vascular malformations. *BNI Quart.* 1987; 3:18–28.

47. Roda JM, Alvarez F, Isla A, et al. Thalamic cavernous malformation: case report. *J Neurosurg.* 1990;72:647–649.

48. Rosenblum B, Rothman AS, Lanzieri C, et al. A cavernous sinus hemangioma: case report. *J Neurosurg.* 1986;65:716–718.

49. Runnels JB, Gifford DB, Forsberg PL, et al. Dense calcification in a large cavernous angioma: case report. *J Neurosurg.* 1969;30:293–298.

50. Russell DS, Rubinstein LJ. *Pathology of Tumours of the Nervous System.* 5th ed. Baltimore, Md: Williams & Wilkins; 1989:727–790.

51. Rutka JT, Brant-Zawadzki M, Wilson CB, et al. Familial cavernous malformations: diagnostic potential of magnetic resonance imaging. *Surg Neurol.* 1988;29:467–474.

52. Saito N, Yamakawa K, Sasaki T, et al. Intramedullary cavernous angioma with trigeminal neuralgia: a case report and review of the literature. *Neurosurgery.* 1989;25:97–101.

53. Shafey S, Gargano F, Mackey E. Angiomatous malformation as a cause of cerebral calculus: case report. *J Neurosurg.* 1966;24:898–900.

54. Shibata S, Mori K. Effect of radiation therapy on extracerebral cavernous hemangioma in the middle fossa: report of three cases. *J Neurosurg.* 1987;67:919–922.

55. Shuey HM Jr, Day AL, Quisling RG, et al. Angiographically cryptic cerebrovascular malformations. *Neurosurgery.* 1979;5:476–479.

56. Simard JM, Garcia-Bengochea F, Ballinger WE Jr, et al. Cavernous angioma: a review of 126 collected and 12 new clinical cases. *Neurosurgery.* 1986;18:162–172.

57. Steiger HJ, Markwalder TM, Reulen H-J. Clinicopathological relations of cerebral cavernous angiomas: observations in eleven cases. *Neurosurgery.* 1987;21:879–884.

58. Steiger HJ, Tew JM Jr. Hemorrhage and epilepsy in cryptic cerebrovascular malformations. *Arch Neurol.* 1984;41:722–724.

59. Tagle P, Huete I, Mendez J, et al. Intracranial cavernous angioma: presentation and management. *J Neurosurg.* 1986;64:720–723.

60. Takamiya Y, Takayama H, Kobayashi K, et al. Familial occurrence of multiple vascular malformations of the brain. *Neurol Med Chir (Tokyo).* 1984;24:271–277.

61. Vaquero J, Carrillo R, Cabezudo J, et al. Cavernous angiomas of the pineal region: report of two cases. *J Neurosurg.* 1980;53:833–835.

62. Vaquero J, Leunda G, Martinez R, et al. Cavernomas of the brain. *Neurosurgery.* 1983;12:208–210.

63. Voigt K, Yasargil MG. Cerebral cavernous haemangiomas or cavernomas: incidence, pathology, localization, diagnosis, clinical features and treatment: review of the literature and report of an unusual case. *Neurochirurgia.* 1976;19:59–68.

64. Wakai S, Ueda Y, Inoh S, et al. Angiographically occult angiomas: a report of thirteen cases with analysis of the cases documented in the literature. *Neurosurgery.* 1985;17:549–556.

65. Wilkins RH. Natural history of intracranial vascular malformations: a review. *Neurosurgery.* 1985;16:421–430.

66. Yamasaki T, Handa H, Moritake K. Cavernous angioma in the fourth ventricle. *Surg Neurol.* 1985;23:249–254.

67. Zentner J, Hassler W, Gawehn J, et al. Intramedullary cavernous angiomas. *Surg Neurol.* 1989;31:64–68.

Chapter 2

Epidemiology of Cavernous Malformations

Frank P.K. Hsu, BS, Daniele Rigamonti, MD, FACS,
and Stephen L. Huhn, MD

Cavernous malformations (CMs), also known as angiomas, cavernous hemangiomas, or cavernomas, are a type of vascular malformation or vascular hamartoma of the central nervous system. The classification of such vascular lesions has undergone numerous revisions over the years, and a continuous reappraisal of these entities occurs with the acquisition of new knowledge.

Pathologically, CMs vary in size—from almost microscopic to very large. Lesions are usually well defined, lobulated, and dark red in color. Structure consists of a honeycomb of vascular spaces of varying sizes filled with blood and separated by fine fibrous strands. Thrombosis and hemorrhage are more common than calcification and ossification. The surrounding tissue usually is discolored by the presence of hemosiderin due to old hemorrhage. Abnormally increased vascularity is not typically found around the lesion,[25,37] except in unusual instances of associated venous malformation.[31,33,35]

A lesion microscopically appears to be a collection of large vascular spaces, without a capsule, adjacent to the brain. The vascular walls are composed of endothelium, without smooth muscle or elastic fibers. Hemosiderin-laden macrophages are a constant feature. Brain parenchyma usually is not found in the center of the lesion, where the dilated vascular channels are contiguous with one another. An enlarged vein can be encountered in association with this lesion, but no abnormal arterial structure is found. Occasionally, associated lesions of similar histology have been described in other organs. The extent of this association between central and peripheral lesions is not known to date. A familial incidence of this malformation has been described.[4,6,7,11,18,23,26,34]

Incidence of Cavernous Malformations in Pathologic Series

The overall incidence of cerebrovascular malformations in autopsy material ranges from 0.1% to 4.0% in different series.[2,37,38] Unfortunately, scant information is available regarding the incidence of CMs. They did not appear in the first large consecutive autopsy series of Courville, where the incidence of all vascular malformations was reported at 0.1%, with arteriovenous malformations (AVMs) in less than 0.01%.[8] The earliest of the more informative studies is that of Berry et al in 1966, who reported data from 6,686 consecutive autopsies performed over a 21-year period. They found the incidence of CM to be 0.02% (compared to 0.03% for AVMs and 0.4% for telangiectases).[2]

In a prospective autopsy study of 4,069 consecutive brains, McCormick found that 165 brains (4.05%) harbored one or more angiomas. Venous malformations accounted for 2.6% of the cases, telangiectases for 0.7%, AVM for 0.6%, and CMs for 0.4% of the cases.[25]

A wide discrepancy, by a factor of 20, exists in the incidence of AVMs and CMs in the two studies. Noteworthy is that the proportion between the two types of lesions is the same in the two studies (i.e. 3 AVMs:2 CMs). In a very recent autopsy series of 24,535 consecutive autopsies performed between 1957 and 1986, there were 131 cases of CMs for an incidence of 0.53%.[29]

Incidence of Cavernous Malformations in Clinical Series

The clinical knowledge about this entity has accrued in a saltatory fashion over the years, in parallel with the development of more sophisticated diagnostic modalities. We think it helps the understanding of this condition to maintain an artificial division of the literature, based on historic periods denoting the availability of particular diagnostic tools: pre-angiography, angiography, computed tomography (CT), and magnetic resonance imaging (MRI).

Pre-angiography

In 1928, Walter Dandy reported 44 cases of CMs—39 from the literature and 5 of his own.[10] In 1936, Bergstrand et al reviewed the same literature and stated that in many cases Dandy was mistaken. Bergstrand et al counted 20 sure cases published up to 1936, to which they added 2 personal cases.[1]

Angiography

In 1957, Krayenbuhl and Yasargil described 82 cerebral cavernous angiomas.[22] By 1971, fewer than 100 clinical cases were reported, according to Jonutis;[20] while Voigt and Yasargil found a total of 164 cases, with special reference to incidence, localization, diagnosis, and clinical findings.[45]

In 1978, Giombini and Morello reviewed their 27 years of experience with 285 vascular malformations of the brain diagnosed angiographically and histologically. Their 14 CM cases represented 4.7% of all cases.[17]

CMs accounted for approximately 5% of all cerebral vascular malformations encountered by Pool and Potts.[30] In these two large clinical series collected just prior to the advent of CT scanning, the relative incidence of CMs, compared to the incidence of AVMs, was that of 1 CM to every 20 AVMs.

Computed Tomography

An excellent review of the pertinent literature—with detailed discussion of histopathologic, clinical, and radiologic features of CMs—was conducted by Simard et al in 1986. However, the information regarding incidence and epidemiology was not available. The only epidemiologic data inferred from this excellent study is that the authors encountered 12 cases in about 10 years (or 1.2 cases/year).[40] A slightly higher yearly occurrence (1.5 cases/year) of CMs was reported in 1986 by Yamasaki et al from Kyoto University. They reported their experience with 30 cases treated at their institution between 1965 and 1984.[48]

Also in 1986, Tagle et al reported their experience of 13 cases over a 6-year period, giving a yearly incidence even higher than preceding reports (i.e. 2.2 cases/year).[42] Unfortunately, these data cannot be used for epidemiologic information, because of the lack of information regarding yearly total admissions at each institution, or the number of AVMs diagnosed at the same institution over the same period.

Magnetic Resonance Imaging

Two very recent series dealing with the natural history of CMs, have provided useful information regarding the incidence of these lesions since the advent of MRI.

The first series analyzed 8,131 MRIs performed over a 4-year period at North Carolina Baptist Hospital. Thirty-two CM cases were found for a case incidence rate of 0.39% and an occurrence of 8 cases per year.[9] The second series reviewed 14,035 MRIs performed during a 5-year period at the Cleveland Clinic Foundation. The 66 CM cases that were encountered represented a case incidence rate of 0.47% and a yearly occurrence of 13 cases.[36]

The apparent increase in the number of cases being diagnosed every year at different institutions does not reflect the beginning of an epidemic of such lesions, but may illustrate the fact that CT and MRI have allowed the diagnosis of **(1)** previously angiographically occult lesions, **(2)** lesions that may be moderately or mildly symptomatic, or **(3)** asymptomatic lesions incidentally found in the course of workup of other problems. This hypothesis is strengthened by the fact that the case incidence rate of the most recent MRI series (0.39% at North Carolina Baptist Hospital and 0.47% at Cleveland Clinic)[9,36] is almost the same as that of the most recent, large consecutive autopsy series (0.4% Sarwar and McCormick, and 0.53% Otten).[29,38]

How many cases of CMs exist in the United States? Michelsen calculated, based on the assumption that intracranial aneurysms are about seven times more frequent than AVMs, that approximately 280,000 cases of AVM exist in the United States.[28] This would bring the expected cases of CMs to about 185,000. According to the Berry study, however, aneurysms are 53 times more frequent than AVMs; this assumption would lead to a calculated number of 37,000 AVMs and 24,500 CMs in the United States.[2] These estimates provide an approximate range of prevalence of this lesion.

Familiality

Cerebral CMs are, for the majority of cases, sporadic lesions. However, familial incidences have been documented for quite some time. In 1928, Kufs reported two cases: an 81-year-old man who presented with "multiple intracranial nodular telangiectases," and his daughter, suspected of harboring a lesion in the pons.[23] In 1936, Michael and Levin reported a family in which a 34-year-old man harbored a histologically verified lesion and whose sister, mother, and uncle suffered from seizures. The sister's skull radiograph showed multiple calcifications.[26] In 1947, Kidd and Cumings reported the occurrence of intracranial hemorrhage in two siblings, one in whom the histologic examination suggested the diagnosis of hemangioma.[21] In 1970, Clark reported a family in which the histology of the lesion was initially out of the question.[6]

In 1977, Houtteville and colleagues, in a personal communication, mentioned a familial character in two of their seven cases. In 1978, Bicknell reported two families.[4] It was the landmark work of Hayman et al in 1982 that confirmed the existence of the familial form—the autosomal dominant transmission proven by the study of a 122-member Mexican family.[18] In 1983, Combelles et al reported two more families.[7] In 1988, Rigamonti et al reported six families affected by this condition, suggesting that the familial is more prevalent than previously expected, with a high incidence of multiple lesions best seen on MRI.[32] A neuro-oculo-cutaneous syndrome, first described by Weskamp and Cotlier in 1940,[47] was established by Gass in 1971.[16] To date, at least 18 families with CMs of the central nervous system and retina, with inconsistent cutaneous manifestations, have been reported.

The incidence of familial CMs, compared to the incidence of sporadic occurrences of CMs, is not known thus far. MRI will help identify asymptomatic carriers; thus the relative proportion of familial cases should continue to rise. We can conservatively state that from available information, the incidence of the familial form is 36 per 600(6%).

Multiplicity

Frequency of cases with multiple lesions varies greatly between the sporadic and familial forms. Giombini and Morello reported an incidence of 6% in their series.[17] In their review of the literature, Voigt and Yasargil reported a multiple lesion incidence of 13.4%.[45] A lower incidence (9.9%) was described in a prospective series of 24,535 autopsies.[29]

In a series of 8,131 MRIs, the incidence of multiple lesions was reported at 18.7%.[9] This is not unexpected, considering the fact that MRIs may identify more asymptomatic or mildly symptomatic patients. As far as the familial form is concerned, recent familial studies suggest that as many as 50% to 73% of patients with familial CMs have multiple lesions.[11,32]

Sex Incidence

Voigt and Yasargil reported an equal sex incidence in a review of the literature.[45] A female predominance was reported by Simard et al (1.1 female: 1 male),[40] Yamasaki et al (1.1 female: 1 male),[48] and Vaquero et al (1.5 female: 1 male).[48] A male predominance was reported by Giombini and Morello (1.7 male: 1 female)[17] and Otten et al (1.5 male: 1 female).[29] In our own recent compilation of 634 patients with lesions verified pathologically or by MRI, there is no sex predominance (Table 1).

Age

Giombini and Morello reported 27% CMs in the pediatric population, with the majority (61%) of the patients presenting be-

Table 1. Sex Incidence in the Present Series Collected from Literature

Sex		Total	Percent
Male		318	50.16%
Female		304	47.95%
Unspecified		12	1.89%
	Total	634	100.00%

Note: Patient cases for this table were obtained from the following references: 3, 5, 7, 9, 13, 14, 15, 19, 24, 28, 29, 32, 36, 39, 40, 41, 42, 43, 44, 46, 49, 50, 51.

tween 20 and 40 years of age.[17] Voigt and Yasargil did not specify the incidence of pediatric cases but stated that CMs usually are diagnosed between ages 20 and 50, with the highest incidence occurring in the fourth decade.[45] Simard reported a pediatric incidence of 23%,[40] and normal distribution over the decades. In the most recent literature, the incidence of pediatric cases has been reported at about a fourth of the total: 28% (Robinson et al),[36] 26% (Yamasaki et al).[49] In our present compilation, the pediatric cases amount to 27% of the total 464 patients in whom information about the age is available (Table 2).

Localization

In the Giombini and Morello series, supratentorial lesions were most common (90%).[17] Supratentorial lesions amounted to 76.8% of the total in the Voigt and Yasargil review.[45] Approximately the same incidence was described by Simard et al,[40] Otten et al (76.6%),[29] and Robinson et al (77%).[36] A higher incidence of supratentorial lesions has been reported by Curling et al (84%); however in their series, 12.5% of all patients had multiple lesions.[9] A lower incidence of supratentorial lesions was reported by Bertalanffy et al (64%), though this may represent a referral pattern.[3]

Many authors have stated that supratentorial CMs tend to be located cortically and subcortically in the rolandic area or in the basal ganglia.[37] In the Voigt and Yasargil

Table 2. **Age Distribution in the Present Series**

	Total	Percent
Unspecified	151	23.82%
Adult	339	53.47%
Pediatric	144	22.71%

Note: Patient cases for this table were obtained from the following references: 3, 5, 7, 9, 13, 14, 15, 19, 24, 28, 32, 36, 39, 40, 41, 42, 43, 44, 46, 49, 50, 51.

review,[45] it has been noted that the pons is another area of preferred localization, in 14.6% of all CMs and 70.6% of those in the posterior fossa. In Simard et al, these statements could not be supported: the most common supratentorial location was the temporal lobe (19.2%) and the pons represented 7.2% of all CMs (and 41% of those in the posterior fossa).[40] In the single largest pathologic review of literature, it was found that: **(1)** there is no difference in lateralization, **(2)** 53.3% of the lesions are located in the white matter, and **(3)** 31.8% are subcortical.[29] In our compilation of 634 patients, we were able to find 455 supratentorial lesions (74%) and 163 infratentorial lesions (26%). There were 58 lesions whose location was not specified, mostly in patients with multiple lesions. The frontal lesions were most common supratentorial, the pontine location most common infratentorial (Table 3).

Size

Data regarding the size of lesions is not always readily available. In the Giombini and Morello surgical series, the size of the CM varied from 3 mm to 9 cm, with a mean size of 3.5 cm. If a hematoma was present, the size of the mass was obviously larger than the CM alone.[17] In Yasargil's most recent surgical series, the size of the CM varied between 1 cm and 6 cm, with a mean of 2.2 cm.[50] In a recent MRI series in which 14% of the patients were asymptomatic, the lesion ranged in size between 3

mm and 4 cm, with a mean size of 1.7 cm.[36] In a very recent autopsy series, the size of the lesion varied between 1 mm and 27 mm, with a mean size of 4.9 mm $\pm$ 0.3 mm in these series. Only 6 of 131 (4.5%) cases were symptomatic with the symptomatic lesions being statistically larger ($P < .005$).[30] These data seem to suggest that there is a correlation between size and clinical relevance of CMs.

Symptomatology

In the Giombini and Morello series, the most common symptom was seizures (38%), followed by headache (28%), hemorrhage (23.5%), and focal neurologic findings (12%).[17] Voigt and Yasargil stated that a specific clinical syndrome—resulting from cerebral CMs—has not been defined.[45] In their review of the previous literature, Simard et al were able to find a slight predominance of seizures as the presenting symptom (39%), followed by hemorrhage (32%) and mass effect (29%).[40] Rigamonti et al, reviewing the symptoms of members of six different families with CMs proven histologically or documented on MRI, suggested that CMs can be asymptomatic even when multiple in a significant percentage of cases (11%). They confirmed seizures as the most common symptom (55%), followed by progressive neurologic symptoms (15%), headache (15%), and hemorrhage (4%).[32] The two most recent MRI series also confirmed the existence of a substantial number of asymptomatic cases and a slightly more benign natural history than previously feared.[9,36]

Curling et al reported the predominance of seizures as the major symptom (50% of the cases) and headache as the second most common complaint (34%). Six of their 32 patients (18.7%) were asymptomatic.[9] Robinson et al confirmed seizures as the most common symptom (51%), followed by neurologic deficits (45%) and headache

Table 3. **Location of Cavernous Malformations in the Present Series Collected from Literature**

Supratentorial	455	73.62%
Frontal	99	21.76%
Temporal	68	14.95%
Parietal	72	15.82%
Occipital	16	3.52%
Thalamus	7	1.54%
Basal Ganglia	22	4.84%
Lateral Ventricle	13	2.86%
Paraventricular	2	0.44%
Hypothalamus	2	0.44%
Third Ventricle	5	1.10%
Chiasm	1	0.22%
Pineal	2	0.44%
Supra Sellar	1	0.22%
Holohemispheric	1	0.22%
Infratentorial	163	26.38%
Midbrain	20	12.27%
Cerebellum	28	17.18%
Pons	43	26.38%
Medulla	13	7.98%
Fourth Ventricle	3	1.84%
Pineal	3	1.84%
CPA	6	3.68%
Pontomedullary	6	3.68%
Cord	2	0.68%
Unspecified	58	

Note: Patient cases for this table were obtained from the following references: 3, 5, 7, 12, 13, 14, 15, 19, 24, 28, 29, 32, 36, 39, 40, 41, 42, 43, 44, 46, 49, 50, 51.

(30%). They confirmed a high occurrence of asymptomatic patients (14%).[36]

In our present compilation of patients, we confirmed the predominance of seizures as the main symptom (31%), followed by neurologic deficit (25%), hemorrhage (13%), and headache (6%). Asymptomatic patients, however, are more common than previously reported (21%) (Table 4).

The data regarding the incidence of bleeding and recurrent bleeding have the most clinical relevance because they affect the decision regarding surgery. The mean age of hemorrhage was 30 years of age in the Simard et al series,[40] 26.3 years in the Curling et al study,[9] and 30.4 years in the Robinson et al study.[36] In Robinson's series, there was a female predominance in regard to bleeding (5 females: 1 male). An oppo-site tendency was reported by Curling et al (1 female: 2 males).[9] In the first natural-history study of this condition, Hayman et al followed 7 patients, with CT, over 5 years. Two patients developed new lesions, bleeding occurred in 2 patients, and 4 patients showed no changes. The 7 patients that were followed harbored 15 initial lesions. According to this very limited study the bleeding rate was 5.7% per person per year, or 6.6% per lesion per year (2.6% symptomatic and 4% asymptomatic but documented on CT).[18]

Two recent MRI studies suggested, however, a lower incidence of bleeding. The risk is expressed in percentage bleeding rate per person-year of exposure and bleeding rate per lesion per year of exposure.

Curling et al estimated the bleeding risk at 0.25% per person-year of exposure and

Table 4. Incidence of Symptoms in the Present Series Collected from the Literature

Symptoms	664	100.00%
Asymptomatic	137	20.63%
Seizure	207	31.17%
Hemorrhage	89	13.40%
Recurrent Hemorrhage	10	1.51%
Tumor (Mass Effect)	169	25.45%
Headache	40	6.02%
Vertigo	1	0.15%
Increased ICP	3	0.45%
Vomiting	1	0.15%
Macrocephalic	4	0.60%
Microcephalic	1	0.15%
Irritability	1	0.15%
Autopsy	1	0.15%

Note: Patient cases for this table were obtained from the following references: 3, 5, 9, 12, 13, 14, 15, 19, 24, 28, 29, 32, 36, 39, 40, 41, 42, 43, 44, 46, 49, 50, 51.

0.1% per lesion per year of exposure.[9] By doing similar calculations on the data provided by Robinson et al, it is possible to estimate the bleeding rate at approximately 0.3% per person-year of exposure and at 0.2% per lesion per year of exposure. These authors, however, provided information on the bleeding rate during a 26-month period of followup at 0.8% per person-year of followup and at 0.7% per lesion per year of followup.[36]

Summary

The above information can be recapitulated as follows:

1. Autopsy series have found the incidence of CMs to be:

- 0.02% (Berry et al, 1966)[2]
- 0.49% (Sarwar and McCormick, 1978)[38]
- 0.53% (Otten, 1989)[29]

2. The relative incidence of CMs compared to AVMs is 1:1.5 in two large autopsy series:

- Berry et al, 1966[2]
- Sarwar and McCormick, 1978[38]

3. The relative incidence of CMs compared to AVMs is approximately 1:20(5%) in two large clinical series in the pre-CT period:

- Pool and Potts, 1965[30]
- Giombini and Morello, 1978[17]

4. The case incidence of CMs in two large MRI series was:

- 0.39% (Curling et al, 1991)[9]
- 0.47% (Robinson et al, 1991)[36]

5. CMs occur in sporadic and in familial forms. The incidence of the hereditary form is as yet undefined, but:

- Thought to be very rare (Russell and Rubenstein, 1989)[37]
- Thought to be as high as 50%, at least in some ethnic groups (Rigamonti, 1988)[32]

6. Solitary lesions are more common than multiple lesions. The incidence of multiple lesions is reported at:

- 6% (Giombini and Morello, 1978)[17]

- 9% (Otten, 1989)[29]
- 13.4% (Voigt and Yasargil, 1976)[45]
- 18.7% (Curling et al, 1991)[9]

7. The familial form has multiple lesions in as high as:

- 50% of the cases (Dobyns et al, 1987)[11]
- 73% of the cases (Rigamonti et al, 1988)[32]

8. There is no sex prevalence:

- Present compilation of 634 patients (see Table 1)

9. The age of presentation is reported as:

- Between 20–40 (Giombini and Morello, 1978)[17]
- Between 20–50 (Voigt and Yasargil, 1976)[45]
- Normal distribution over the decades (Simard et al, 1986,[40] present review, see Table 2)

10. Localization is supratentorial in:

- 90% (Giombini and Morello, 1978)[17]
- 76.8% (Voigt and Yasargil, 1976)[45]
- 76.6% (Otten et al, 1989)[29]
- 64% (Bertalanffy et al, 1991)[3]
- 77% (Robinson et al, 1991)[36]
- 84% (Curling et al, 1991)[9]
- 74% (present review, see Table 3)

11. The size of CMs varies from millimeters to centimeters. The mean size was reported as:

- 5 mm (Otten et al, 1989)[29] [4.5% symptomatic]

- 1.7 cm (Robinson et al, 1991)[36] [86% symptomatic]
- 2.2 cm (Yasargil, 1988)[50] [100% symptomatic]
- 3.5 cm (Giombini and Morello, 1978)[17] [100% symptomatic]

The symptomatic cases were statistically larger than the asymptomatic:

- $P < 0.005$ (Otten et al, 1989)[29]

12. Symptoms are not always present—autopsy series and MRI series point to a various percentage of asymptomatic cases reported as:

- 95.5% (Otten et al, 1989)[29]
- 18.7% (Curling et al, 1991)[9]
- 14% (Robinson et al, 1991)[36]
- 11% (Rigamonti et al, 1988)[32]
- 21% (present review, see Table 4)

13. When symptoms are present, seizures tend to be predominant in:

- 38% (Giombini and Morello, 1978)[17]
- 39% (Simard et al, 1986)[40]
- 50% (Curling et al, 1991)[9]
- 51% (Robinson et al, 1991)[36]
- 55% (Rigamonti et al, 1988)[32]
- 31% (present review, see Table 4)

Focal neurologic deficits were reported at:

- 12% (Giombini and Morello, 1978)[17]
- 29% (Simard et al, 1986)[40]
- 15% (Rigamonti et al, 1988)[32]
- 45% (Robinson et al, 1991)[36]
- 25% (present review, see Table 4)

Hemorrhage occurred in:

- 23.5% (Giombini and Morello, 1978)[17]

- 32% (Simard et al, 1986)[40]
- 4% (Rigamonti et al, 1988)[32]
- 10.9% (Robinson et al, 1991)[36]
- 13% (present review, see Table 4)

Headache occurred in:

- 28% (Giombini and Morello, 1978)[17]
- 15% (Rigamonti et al, 1988)[32]
- 34% (Curling et al, 1991)[9]
- 30% (Robinson et al, 1991)[36]
- 6% (present review, see Table 4)

14. Risk of bleeding through lifetime is estimated at:

- 0.25% per person-year of exposure (Curling et al, 1991)[9]
- 0.3% per person-year of exposure (obtained from Robinson et al data through our own calculations, 1991)[36]

Risk of bleeding during a followup is reported at:

- 0.8% per person-year of followup (Robinson et al, 1991)[36]
- 0.7% per lesion per year of followup (Robinson et al, 1991)[36]

Additional Comments

It is interesting to note that new MRI series suggest the same case incidence (0.4% to 0.5%) of CMs already found in two large prospective-consecutive autopsy series.[29,38] The discrepancy between the relative incidence of CMs and AVMs in autopsy series (1:1.5) and old clinical series (1:20) reflects that AVMs are more symptomatic. The apparent "epidemic" of CMs in recent years is actually due to the advent of MRI, which, with its greater diagnostic sensitivity, allows the detection of mildly symptomatic or even asymptomatic cases.

CMs usually are sporadic, though the familial cases are more common than previously thought. Multiple lesions are very common in the familial form (50% to 73%).[11,32]

Cerebral CMs do not have a sex prevalence and can occur at any age. They do not have a predilection for a specific location.

The size of a CM is strongly related to its clinical symptomatology. In the majority of cases, symptomatic lesions are greater than 1 cm in diameter.

Seizures (30%) are more common than progressive neurologic deficits (25%) and hemorrhage (13%). The risk of bleeding amounts to 0.25% to 0.30% per person per year of exposure.[9,36] However, once the lesion has been diagnosed and later becomes symptomatic, for the majority (80% to 85%) of the patients, the risk of rebleeding appears higher.

References

1. Bergstrand A, Olivecrona H, Tonnis W. Gefassmissbildungen und Gefassgeschwulste des gehirns. Leipzig, Germany: Georg Thieme; 1936.
2. Berry RG, Alpers BJ, White JC: The site, structure and frequency of intracranial aneurysms, angiomas and arteriovenous abnormalities. In: Millikan CH, ed. *Research Publications. Association for Research in Nervous and Mental Disease.* Baltimore, Md: Williams and Wilkins; 1966;41:4–72.
3. Bertalanffy H, Gilsbach JM, Eggert H-R, et al. Microsurgery of deep-seated cavernous angiomas: report of 26 cases. *Acta Neurochir (Wien).* 1991;108:91–99.
4. Bicknell JM, Carlow TJ, Kornfeld M, et al. Familial cavernous angiomas. *Arch Neurol.* 1978;35:746–749.
5. Brühlmann Y, de Tribolet N, Berney J. Intracerebral cavernous angiomas. *Neurochirurgie (Paris).* 1985;31:271–279. English abstract.
6. Clark JV. Familial occurrence of cavernous angiomata of the brain. *J Neurol Neurosurg Psychiatry.* 1970;33:871–876.
7. Combelles G, Blond S, Biondi A, et al. Formes familiales des hémangiomes caverneux intracrâniens: à propos de 5 cas dans deux familles. *Neurochirurgie (Paris).* 1983;29:263–269. English abstract.
8. Courville CB. Morphology of small vascular malformations of the brain with particular reference to the mechanism of their drainage. *J Neuropathol Exp Neurol.* 1963;22:274–284.

9. Curling OD Jr, Kelly DL Jr, Elster AD, et al. An analysis of the natural history of cavernous angiomas. *J Neurosurg*. 1991;75:702–708.

10. Dandy WE. Venous abnormalities and angiomas of the brain. *Arch Surg*. 1928;17:715–793.

11. Dobyns WB, Michels VV, Groover RV, et al. Familial cavernous malformations of the central nervous system and retina. *Ann Neurol*. 1987;21:578–583.

12. Fahlbusch R, Strauss C, Huk W, et al. Surgical removal of pontomesencephalic cavernous hemangiomas. *Neurosurgery*. 1990;26:449–457.

13. Fortuna A, Ferrante L, Mastronardi L, et al. Cerebral cavernous angioma in children. *Childs Nerv Syst*. 1989;5:201–207.

14. Frima-Verhoeven PAW, Op De Coul AAW, Tijssen CC, et al. Intracranial cavernous angiomas: diagnosis and therapy. *Eur Neurol*. 1989;29:56–60.

15. Gangemi M, Longatti P, Maiuri F, et al. Cerebral cavernous angiomas in the first year of life. *Neurosurgery*. 1989;25:465–469.

16. Gass TDM. Cavernous hemangioma of the retina, a neuro-oculo-cutaneous syndrome. *Am J Opthalmol*. 1971;71:799.

17. Giombini S, Morello G. Cavernous angiomas of the brain: account of fourteen personal cases and review of the literature. *Acta Neurochir (Wien)*. 1978;40:61–82.

18. Hayman LA, Evans RA, Ferrell RE, et al. Familial cavernous angiomas: natural history and genetic study over a 5-year period. *Am J Med Genet*. 1982;11:147–160.

19. Hubert P, Choux M, Houtteville JP. Cavernomes cérébraux de l'enfant et du nourrisson. *Neurochirurgie (Paris)*. 1989;35:104–105.

20. Jonutis AI, Sondheimer FK, Klein HZ, et al. Intracerebral cavernous hemangioma with angiographically demonstrated pathologic vasculature. *Neuroradiology*. 1971;3:57–63.

21. Kidd MA, Cumings JN. Cerebral angiomata in an Icelandic family. *Lancet*.1947;1:747–748.

22. Krayenbuhl H, Yasargil MG. *Der vaskularen erkrankungen im gebiet der arteria vertebralis und arteria basilaris*. Stuttgart, Germany: Thieme Verlag; 1957.

23. Kufs H. Uber heredofamiliare angiomatose des Gehirns und der Retina, ihre Beziehungen zueinander und zur angiomatose der haut. *Z Neurol Psychiatri*. 1928;113:651–686.

24. Mazza C, Scienza R, Dalla Bernardin B, et al. Cerebral cavernous malformations (cavernomas) in children. *Neurochirurgie (Paris)*. 1989;35:106–108.

25. McCormick WF. The pathology of vascular ("arteriovenous") malformations. *J Neurosurg*. 1966;24:807–816.

26. Michael JC, Levin PM. Multiple telangiectases of the brain: a discussion of hereditary factors in their development. *Arch Neurol Psychiatr (Chic)*. 1936;36:514–529.

27. Michelsen WJ. Natural history and pathophysiology of arteriovenous malformations. *Clin Neurosurg*. 1979;26:307–313.

28. Orenstein D, Kiesman M, Dietemann JL, et al. Angiographically occult vascular malformations suggestive of cavernomas: clinical study of 18 cases. *Neurochirurgie (Paris)*. 1989;35:95–97.

29. Otten P, Pizzolato GP, Rilliet B, et al. A propos de 131 cas d'angiomes caverneux (cavernomes) du S.N.C., repérés par l'analyse rétrospective de 24 535 autopsies. *Neurochirurgie (Paris)*. 1989;35:82–83.

30. Pool JL, Potts DG. *Aneurysms and Arteriovenous Anomalies of the Brain. Diagnosis and Treatment*. New York, NY: Harper and Row; 1965: 463.

31. Rigamonti D, Drayer BP, Johnson PC. The MRI appearance of cavernous malformations (angiomas). *J Neurosurg*. 1987;67:518–524.

32. Rigamonti D, Drayer BP, Johnson PC, et al. Familial cerebral cavernous malformations. *New Engl J Med*. 1988;319:343–347.

33. Rigamonti D, Johnson PC, Spetzler RF, et al. Cavernous malformations and capillary telangiectasia: a spectrum within a single pathological entity. *Neurosurgery*. 1991;28:60–64.

34. Rigamonti D, Rekate H, Pittmann H, et al. Cavernous malformations (angiomas) in children. *J Pediatr Neurosc*. 1988;4:55–59.

35. Rigamonti D, Spetzler RF, Drayer BP, et al. Appearance of venous malformations on magnetic resonance imaging. *J Neurosurg*. 1988;69:535–539.

36. Robinson JR, Awad IA, Little JR. Natural history of the cavernous angioma. *J Neurosurg*. 1991;75:709–714.

37. Russell DS, Rubenstein LJ. *Pathology of Tumors of the Nervous System*. 5th ed. Baltimore, Md: Williams and Wilkins; 1989;730–736.

38. Sarwar M, McCormick WF. Intracerebral venous angioma: case report and review. *Arch Neurol*. 1978;35:323–325.

39. Scott RM, Barnes P, Kupsky W, et al. Cavernous angiomas of the central nervous system in children. *J Neurosurg*. 1992;76:38–46.

40. Simard JM, Garcia-Bengochea F, Ballinger WE Jr, et al. Cavernous angioma: a review of 126 collected and 12 new clinical cases. *Neurosurgery*. 1986;18:162–172.

41. Steiger HJ, Markwalder TM, Reulen HJ. Clinicopathological relations of cerebral cavernous angiomas: observations in eleven cases. *Neurosurgery*. 1987;21:879–884.

42. Tagle P, Huete I, Mendez J, et al. Intracranial cavernous angioma: presentation and management. *J Neurosurg*. 1986;64:720–723.

43. Vaquero J, Cabezudo JM, Leunda G. Cystic cavernous hemangiomas of the brain. *Acta Neurochir*. 1983;67:135–138.

44. Vaquero J, Salazar J, Martinez R, et al. Cavernomas of the central nervous system: clinical syndromes, CT scan diagnosis, and prognosis after surgical treatment in 25 cases. *Acta Neurochir (Wien)*. 1987;85:29–33.

45. Voigt K, Yasargil MG. Cerebral cavernous hemangiomas or cavernomas: incidence, pathology, locclization, diagnosis, clinical features and treatment. Review of the literature and report of an unusual case. *Neurochirurgia (Stuttg)*. 1976;19:59–68.

46. Weber M, Vespignani H, Bracard S, et al. Les angiomes caverneux intracérébraux. *Rev Neurol (Paris)*. 1989;145:429–436.

47. Weskamp C, Cotlier I. Angioma cerebro y dela retina con malformations cupilares de Ia piel. *Arch Ophthalmol (Buenos Aires).* 1940;15:1.

48. Yamasaki T, Handa H, Yamashita J, et al. Intracranial and orbital cavernous angiomas: a review of 30 cases. *J Neurosurg.* 1986;64:197–208.

49. Yamasaki T, Kikuchi H, Yamashita J, et al. Subependymoma of the septum pellucidum radiologically indistinguishable from cavernous angioma: case report. *Neurol Med Chir (Tokyo).* 1989;29:1020–1025.

50. Yasargil MG. *Microneurosurgery, IIIA, IIIB.* Stuttgart, Germany: Georg Thieme Verlag; 1988:419–434.

51. Zimmerman RS, Spetzler RF, Lee KS, et al. Cavernous malformations of the brain stem. *J Neurosurg.* 1991;75:32–39.

Chapter 3

Clinical Spectrum
and Natural Course

John R. Robinson, MD, and Issam A. Awad, MD, MSc, FACS

Cavernous malformations (CMs) are vascular lesions that have received a great deal of attention in recent years, largely due to improved diagnostic evaluation with magnetic resonance imaging (MRI) and heightened clinical awareness. Numerous case reports, short series, and reviews of the literature have attempted to define CMs, characterize their natural history, and present rational guidelines for clinical management.*

This chapter reviews the spectrum of clinical manifestations associated with intracranial CMs and summarizes what is known about the natural course of these lesions, including the risk of hemorrhage and factors predisposing to an aggressive neurologic course. As much as possible, our discussion is limited to the CM as defined pathologically.[27] This lesion consists of a berrylike collection of blood-filled sinusoidal channels lined by endothelium and collagen. There is no intervening brain within the core of the lesion. The sinusoidal walls are unique in that they are devoid of smooth muscle and elastin.[11,12,29]

It is important to note in reviewing the literature, that all studies have not adhered to such a stringent definition. The clinical literature on this topic is often quite imprecise, with many CMs included in the category of *cryptic arteriovenous malformations, angiographically occult vascular malformations,* or *venous angiomas.* In a recent re-evaluation of pathologic specimens from consecutive cases of angiographically occult vascular malformations, the authors found that the initial pathologic diagnosis was incorrect or imprecise in a high proportion of cases, mostly because of unclear histopathologic defining criteria at initial evaluation. Strict definitions are essential in natural history studies so as to avoid imprecisions due to mixing and confusing clinical information from distinct lesions.[5] Vascular malformations represent a pathologically heterogenous group of lesions that may or may not exhibit corresponding heterogeneity of natural course.[18]

The survey of a large mix of pathologically and radiologically defined cases provides a broader perspective of the clinical spectrum and natural course of this lesion than studies published in the pre-MRI era that were invariably based on autopsy or

---

*References 1–5,8,10,13,15,17,19,23–25,27,31,33–36, 38–46

surgical cases.** While theoretically more specific in view of pathologic confirmation, those studies were heavily biased by symptomatic and aggressive cases. Also, pathologic definitions in those series were not always sufficiently precise or accurate. [15,18,35,43] Therefore, these cases may not accurately represent CMs occurring in the general population.

Reports based on MRI appearance of CMs provide a different perspective about these lesions. They allow an examination of the incidence, epidemiologic associations, and clinical manifestations of CMs, including asymptomatic cases. [3,4,9,17,23,27,32] While there is a theoretical lack of specificity of the MRI appearance suggestive of CM, this does not appear to impact significantly on large series of cases. [27] As has been shown in a recent series of 13,000 consecutively performed MRIs, the incidence of CMs diagnosed by MRI is identical to that recorded by two major autopsy series. [11,20,27,30] This indicates that series of consecutive MRI cases do not vastly overestimate nor underestimate the actual prevalence of this lesion, and may reflect its true representation in the general population. The recent radiologic literature has documented several characteristic MRI features that distinguish CMs from other vascular malformations.*** Furthermore, most studies of angiographically occult vascular malformations cite CMs as the most frequent subtype of such lesions. [15,39,43] Lastly, there is no firm evidence of heterogeneity of natural history among the various pathologic subtypes of angiographically occult vascular malformations. [15,34,43] Thus, at the present time MRI-based studies offer the only relatively specific noninvasive method of following the natural history of unoperated lesions. Information from such studies should be analyzed in comparison with selected and typically more aggressive cases reported in surgical or autopsy series.

**References 1,2,13,16,20,31,33,35,38–43,45,46
***References 9,10,17–19,23,25,27,32,43,45,46

This review is based on the authors' experiences with over 100 CMs, as well as an additional review of the international literature of more than 200 published cases. [1-46] These include operated and nonoperated cases, symptomatic and asymptomatic lesions that have been defined pathologically and/or radiographically.

Clinical Presentation

CMs may be associated with a variety of clinical syndromes. These have been frequently divided into the broad categories of seizures, focal neurologic deficits, and headaches. Numerous studies have noted a frequent association with seizures, described in 40% to 70% of reported CM cases. [10,27,33,35,38,41] The second most frequent presentation is that of focal neurologic deficits including diplopia, ataxia, sensory disturbances, and hemiparesis. These complaints are closely related to lesion location and size and are considered by some authors as a "pseudotumoral" form of presentation. They account for the presenting complaint in 35% to 50% of reported cases. [10,27,33,35,38,41] Headaches accompany a CM in many patients and may have prompted diagnostic evaluation uncovering the lesion. While this is a controversial presenting complaint due to its nonspecific and nonlocalizing nature, it represents a major symptom in 25% to 30% of reported CM cases. [10,27,33,35,38,41]

The published literature on CMs is dominated by pathologically defined cases, few of which are asymptomatic. Two major series based on the detection of CMs among consecutive patients undergoing MRIs have found asymptomatic lesions in 14% to 19% of the patients. [3,27] The prevalence of asymptomatic lesions in the general population would be expected to be somewhat higher, since patients generally undergo MRIs because of related or unrelated neurologic complaints.

The hemorrhagic form of CM presentation has been well characterized in the surgical literature. Table 1 summarizes the

Table 1. Prevalence of Hemorrhage in Large Published Series of Cavernous Malformations*

Series	Year	Study type	Number of cases	Percent of patients with hemorrhage
Robinson et al[27]	1991	MR	66	9.0%
Houtteville[10]	1989	MR	18	6.0%
Vaquero et al[42]	1987	Pathology	24	8.0%
Steiger et al[36]	1987	Pathology	11	18.0%
Tagle et al[39]	1986	Pathology	13	30.8%
Simard et al[34]	1986	Pathology	12	16.7%
Weighted Average (by number of cases)			144	11.6%

*Patient selection and definitions of hemorrhage are different in the various series.

prevalence of hemorrhage in large published series. This has ranged between 6% and 30% of cases.[10,27,33,35,38,41] A weighted average of 11.6% (adjusted according to number of cases in each series) of reported CMs are associated with hemorrhage, although this figure is somewhat clouded by differences in patient selection and the definition of hemorrhage among the series.

Volume Distribution

Major studies over the past few years have underscored the preponderance of supratentorial lesions. The MRI series by Houtteville and the pathologic series by Vaquero et al found 92% and 94% of the lesions, respectively, to be supratentorial.[10,40,41] Studies of lesions by Curling et al and by Robinson et al documented by MRI included 78% and 86% supratentorial lesions, respectively.[4,27] Analysis of published reports with information about lesion location reveals a lobar distribution favoring the frontal and temporal regions in the supratentorial compartment, and the cerebellum and pons in the infratentorial compartment.[8,27,39] In a recent study there was evidence of a true volume of distribution effect, with lesion prevalence in direct proportion to the volume of the respective brain region (Figure 1).[27] This is in agreement with the hypothesis of congenital origin of the lesions as opposed to theories about acquired etiologies which would be less likely to reflect a volume of distribution. Also, this distribution does not directly support the pure concept of capillary telangiectases (predominantly seen in the pons) evolving into CMs.

Sex and Age Distribution

There has been some controversy in the literature about the prevalence of CMs between sexes. Recent studies, however, have failed to demonstrate a clear gender predominance.[4,27,33] The review by Simard et al of 138 cases revealed a slight female predominance (53%),[33] while the report by Robinson et al showed a slight male predominance (55%).[27] Other reports have also failed to demonstrate a consistent gender association.*

One trend apparent in the authors' series indicates that males tend to present earlier than females (Figure 2).[27,28] Sixty percent of males came to medical attention prior to age 30, while 70% of females presented after age 30. The significance of this trend is unknown, although it is consistent with possible hormonal influences on the clinical presentation of CMs.

In most large series of CMs there are rare lesions discovered in children and neonates. The authors have personally cared for several children with these lesions, including a 4-week-old patient who was symptomatic from a CM almost from birth. These observations are further consistent with a congenital origin of this le-

*References 10,15,23,27,34,40,42–44

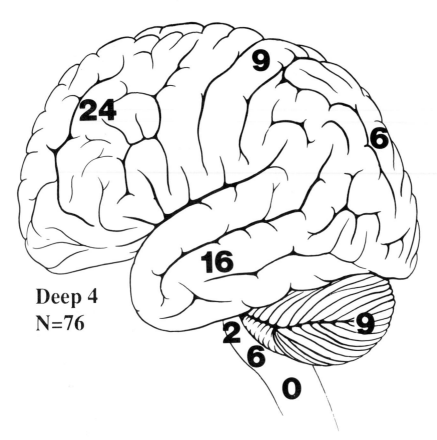

Figure 1. Distribution of 76 CMs in various brain regions. There appears to be a volume distribution with regional lesion prevalence in relation to the volume of the respective brain region. From Robinson et al.[27]

sion in at least some cases. On the other hand, the clinical presentation of most lesions later in life and the variability of clinical behavior between the sexes underscore additional factors which probably influence the biologic behavior of this lesion. A survey of several large published studies demonstrates age at clinical presentation ranging between 24 and 39 years, with a median of 34 years.[10,27,33,35,41]

Multiplicity and Inheritance

The presence of multiple lesions in the same patient has been noted by several authors. The highest prevalence of multiplicity was reported in the series of Rigamonti et al, with 5 of their 10 patients

harboring multiple lesions.[23] Simard et al reported multiplicity in 11 of 136 cases (8%),[33] while Tagle et al reported multiplicity in 1 of 13 cases (8%).[38] These two studies, which relied upon computed tomography (CT) for the diagnosis of CMs, may have underestimated the prevalence of multiplicity. More recent large studies based on more sensitive MR diagnosis have demonstrated lesion multiplicity in 11% to 19% of cases.[4,27]

Selection factors and biases may certainly account for these differences in the prevalence of CM multiplicity. Yet, some have speculated a geographic clustering of multiple lesion cases in southwestern United States and among Hispanic patients.[24] Cases with multiple CMs have a consistent familial association reflecting an

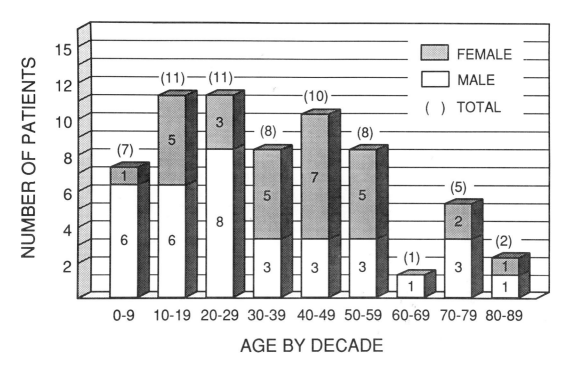

Figure 2. Age at initial diagnosis (clinical presentation) of 63 patients with CMs. Note the mismatched age at initial diagnosis in males and females. (Three patients without complete data sets not included.) From Robinson et al.[27]

autosomal dominant inheritance with variable penetrance.[24] There does not appear to be a convincing hereditary link in cases with single lesions.

Factors Affecting Clinical Behavior

There is little information in the published literature about factors that may affect the clinical behavior of CMs. The authors' series demonstrated that supratentorial lesions were more likely to present with seizures, while infratentorial lesions were more likely to present with focal neurologic deficits.[27] An additional trend indicated that 73% of patients under age 40 presented with seizures, while 69% of patients over age 40 initially complained of focal neurologic deficits.[28] The mechanisms underlying these differences remain unclear at this time.

Despite the lack of an overwhelming gender predominance in the prevalence of CMs, we have found that males are more likely to present with seizures (62% of males had seizures), and females were more likely to present with focal deficits (66% of women had focal deficits).[28] Women were also more likely to present with overt hemorrhage.[27] This may reflect hormonal influences as will be discussed later in this chapter. Lesion multiplicity did not affect clinical presentation. An equal proportion of patients presented with seizures and focal neurologic deficits regardless of having single or multiple lesions.[27] This is consistent with the notion that the lesions do not seem to influence one another and may be considered independent entities.[28] There also does not appear to be a clear relationship between lesion size and clinical presentation.[27,28]

Hemorrhage and the Hemosiderin Ring

Many published reports have attempted to identify the prevalence of hemorrhage in CMs.* After careful scrutiny of these reports, one discovers a variable and often imprecise definition for the term "hemorrhage." In some studies this has consisted of a clinical definition based on the sudden onset of new symptoms or exacerbation of old ones.[13,15,23,38-41] Most reports, but not all, have supplemented the clinical diagnosis of hemorrhage with some additional supportive diagnostic information including an imaging study or a spinal tap.[15,39,40] Other authors have supported their definition of hemorrhage with ex post facto analysis using pathologic criteria.[33,35,39] These criteria have often included microscopic evidence of hemorrhage of any age including the presence of hemosiderin staining in surrounding parenchyma.

The controversy regarding this issue arises with the presumption that the hemosiderin ring represents an index of gross hemorrhage. We and others feel that the hemosiderin ring is not necessarily representative of a gross overt hemorrhage, but may instead represent the diapedesis of red blood cells through the very thin-walled caverns that comprise these lesions.[5,17,23] This perilesional "slow ooze" is accompanied by a chronic breakdown of red blood cells and release of hemoglobin, which is subsequently converted to hematoidin and hemosiderin, accounting for the characteristic ring on both pathology specimens and MRIs. This concept inherently calls into question those studies which cite high hemorrhage rates for this lesion based on the presence of adjacent hemosiderin.

We must be careful, however, not to imply that hemosiderin has absolutely nothing to do with hemorrhage. Indeed, the rim of hemosiderin and gliotic brain may significantly encapsulate the lesion so

*References 1,2,4,13,15,19,22-24,27,31,33,35,38-41,43

as to make the path of least resistance to bleeding within the lesion itself. This may account for the intralesional collections of blood of various ages demonstrated on MRI and in pathology specimens. These are thought to represent intralesional (encapsulated) hemorrhages. As a result of this encapsulating effect, the consequences of hemorrhage would be generally limited to changes in the size and turgor of the lesion as opposed to overt bleeding into surrounding brain with disruption of functional neural tissue. In addition, factors affecting the process of red cell translocation into brain parenchyma may also influence hemorrhagic tendencies.

Another often misused definition of hemorrhage relies upon the CT or MRI appearance of blood within the CM. In fact blood flow through various parts of the CM is often quite sluggish,[14] with frequent evidence of frank thrombosis, including various stages of thrombus organization and/or calcification. Such factors combine to produce various imaging artifacts based on the appearance of thrombi and calcifications, and on the summation involved with each voxel in the tomographic imaging processes of CT and MRI.

With these factors in mind, we have proposed to differentiate "overt hemorrhages" from more subtle indications of hemorrhage, which may actually be present in all CMs (Table 2).[27] While most lesions exhibit a hemosiderin ring, thrombosis, and calcification, only 11% of cases in our series were associated with "overt hemorrhage."

Risk of Hemorrhage

The true risk of hemorrhage from a CM can be estimated by examining the prevalence of hemorrhagic lesions among all cases, and also by calculating an annualized risk of hemorrhage in lesions followed over time. Information from both figures is complementary, but not always congruous. As was discussed previously, almost all of the studies on this topic have presented the

---

Table 2. Criteria for Overt (Gross) Hemorrhage in Cavernous Malformations of the Brain*

- MR signal of acute of subacute blood *outside* the "hemosiderin ring" of the lesion.
- Evidence of hemorrhage on lumbar puncture.
- Evidence of fresh clot outside the confines of the lesion at the time of surgery or autopsy.

*From Robinson et al.[27]

---

number of patients which have, according to varying definitions, suffered a hemorrhage. All but a few of these studies are surgical series and provide little useful information regarding the natural risk of hemorrhage in unoperated lesions over time.

With the advent of noninvasive imaging, several institutions are collecting large series of unoperated patients who are being followed prospectively.[4,23,27] Our series now includes over 100 patients, the majority of whom are being followed conservatively. We have published our followup of these cases for a mean of 26 months, and have observed a single instance of subsequent hemorrhage in 143 lesions per year, leading to an estimated annualized bleeding risk of 0.7%.[27] This excludes hemorrhages that were the cause of the initial presentation, since the inclusion of these cases would introduce a selection bias. This 0.7% figure implies a significant lifelong risk of hemorrhage. A newborn with a lesion presumed present at birth would be subject to a 50% risk of overt hemorrhage over an average 73-year life span. We are awaiting the update of this figure with longer followup of patients in our registry and for the results from followup data of patients from other institutions to corroborate these initial findings.

Other workers have calculated hemorrhage risk based on an assumption of uniform risk from birth to the age at diagnosis of a hemorrhage. Curling et al used this method to estimate a risk of hemorrhage of 0.25% per lesion per year based on 3 hemorrhages in 3 lesions over 1,195 lesion-years.[4] The application of this method to our series reveals a similar hemorrhage risk of 0.27% per lesion per year based on 7

hemorrhages in 2,618 lesion-years, assuming the lesions were present from birth.

However, it may not be accurate to assume a uniform annual hemorrhage risk from birth. There is evidence to suggest that the risk of hemorrhage after a known diagnosis of CM is maximal in young adults, which may imply a variability in the risk of hemorrhage throughout life.[27] Also, the authors and others have shown a greater tendency toward hemorrhage in females.[27,39] The lesion, even if present from birth, may mature over time with various factors affecting its risk of hemorrhage. Lesions associated with overt hemorrhage may be more likely to rebleed. Although the number of unoperated lesions with overt hemorrhage is small in our series and in others, nearly 25% of unoperated cases presenting with gross hemorrhages have rebled within 1 year.[27]

It appears, therefore, that the risk of first overt hemorrhage from a CM is quite small, in the range of 0.25% to 0.7% per lesion per year, with the higher figure reflecting the risk of subsequent hemorrhage after a known diagnosis. This risk is significantly smaller than the risk of first hemorrhage from an arteriovenous malformation (AVM).[6,7,21,36,37] However, there are factors that significantly impact on hemorrhagic risk including age, sex, and previous hemorrhage. These factors may magnify substantially this baseline annualized risk.

The occurrence of overt hemorrhage does not appear to be related to the size or location of the CM. Overt hemorrhage was observed in 8.3% of cases less than 1 cm in size, and in 9.6% of cases larger than 1 cm. It occurred in 8.4% of supratentorial lesions and in 11.8% of infratentorial lesions. The proportion of patients with overt hemorrhages above and below the age of 40 were not significantly different. However, the risk of hemorrhage appears greatest in the fourth decade of life, indicating a possible complex relationship to age.[27]

There appears to be a clear association between gender and the risk of hemorrhage. In the authors' series, 86% of overt hemorrhages occurred in females despite an equal lesion prevalence in both sexes.[27] Other studies have also noted this trend. The study of Tung et al documented 71% of hemorrhages in females.[39] These findings provide at least circumstantial evidence that hormonal alterations may exert some influence over the lesion, perhaps through alterations in the vascular endothelium.

A hormonal influence is also supported by our observation that a third of the females in our study who experienced an overt hemorrhage were pregnant.[27] All of these women were in the first trimester of their pregnancy. An influence of gestation on hemorrhage risk has also been suggested in the AVM and aneurysm literature.[26]

Hormonal factors may influence the CM directly, or may exert general vascular effects that may be more overtly manifested in CMs in view of their unique morphology. Such a hormonal influence, if confirmed, may provide unique opportunities for therapeutic intervention and altering of the natural course of CMs. It also might predict an alteration of the rate of hemorrhage in those patients taking oral contraceptives or replacement estrogens. Much work must yet be performed on this topic and on defining the relationship suggested by this preliminary data.

Clinical Consequences of Hemorrhage

Our own experience and the literature indicate that catastrophic consequences of a first hemorrhage are rare in CMs, in contrast to a first hemorrhage from an aneurysm or an AVM.[6,7,21,36,37] We have identified a single case of a patient, who expired from a massive lobar hemorrhage attributed to a CM pathologically confirmed in the evacuated clot, and are aware of another patient with documented multiple CMs, who died suddenly from presumed cerebral hemorrhage. However, these anecdotal cases are a notable exception to the general experience and the published literature, where patients generally had good outcomes from a first hemorrhage. In our recently published series, 5 of 6 patients presenting with initial overt hemorrhage had good outcomes.[27] However, the remote possibility of fatal first hemorrhage should not be totally excluded.

The high prevalence of good outcome despite overt hemorrhage appears largely related to the self-limited nature of most hemorrhages associated with CMs. The one case in our initial series with hemorrhage, which had a poor outcome, did so after several documented recurrent hemorrhages. The study of Tung et al examined the issue of recurrent hemorrhage in a surgical series of angiographically occult vascular malformations consisting of 7 patients with pathologically documented CMs.[39] Several cases had as many as 4 separate episodes of clinical exacerbation attributed to hemorrhage. Nonetheless, this study by Tung et al relied on the acceptance of macrophages, fibrosis, and the presence of hemosiderin as the sine qua non of an old hemorrhage.[39] It is possible that this report overstated the risk of recurrent hemorrhage by equating a clinical change in symptom profile and the presence of the above pathologic features with the occurrence of a hemorrhage. Clinical exacerbation may be due to intralesional hemorrhage or thrombosis with sudden changes in lesion size or turgor without overt exsanguination into the parenchyma.

Another study that examined the issue of recurrent hemorrhage is the updated series from the Barrow Neurological Institute, reporting 27 patients.[22] Rigamonti described initial hemorrhagic presentation in

8 patients, 3 of whom suffered recurrent hemorrhage. Our own experience includes 4 cases of unoperated CMs with overt hemorrhage, and documents 1 rebleed during a followup of less than a year. While the risk of rebleed from a CM is unknown at this time, it appears to be significantly higher than the annualized risk of a first bleed. *Whatever factors predispose a lesion to bleed, appear to make it more likely to rebleed.* This is another significant difference between hemorrhagic tendencies of CMs and AVMs.[45]

The morbidity and mortality associated with recurrent hemorrhage are also poorly defined at this time. The one case we have documented and several cases reported by Tung et al have all resulted in debilitating consequences from recurrent hemorrhages. Tung et al concluded that there was a relationship between the number of hemorrhagic episodes and lasting neurologic deficits.[39] They also documented the influence of lesion location on the morbidity and mortality associated with a hemorrhage, with a higher proportion of persistent neurologic deficits in infratentorial hemorrhagic lesions.

The factors underlying the relatively low morbidity and mortality with overt hemorrhage from CMs and the very low incidence of catastrophic first hemorrhage in these lesions bear further discussion. One of the factors that we feel is significant in reducing the morbidity and mortality associated with hemorrhage is the low-pressure, low-flow circulation within the CM, and dampened pressure fluctuations within the lesion as demonstrated by intraoperative measurements.[14] Several authors have also proposed that the gliosis in surrounding brain may exert a limiting membranelike effect on a potential hemorrhage. In addition, many "hemorrhages" are confined within the cavernous walls of the lesion (pseudoencapsulated), and are more accurately described as intralesional hemorrhages without frank extravasation (Figure 3).

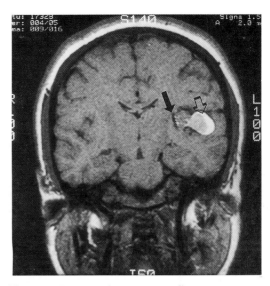

Figure 3. T1-weighted MR scan of a deep hemispheric CM presenting with acute headaches and hemiparesis in a young female during the first month of pregnancy (gestation diagnosed at same time as the CM). Note the hemosiderin ring indicating remote oozing of blood into surrounding brain (closed arrow), and acute hemorrhage within a compartment of the CM, which has expelled itself beyond the hemosiderin ring into adjacent brain (open arrow).

Natural Course of Nonhemorrhagic Lesions

It is also important to discuss the natural history and clinical course of lesions without gross hemorrhage. In the authors' experience, the outcome of patients with CMs and no gross hemorrhage is fair or poor in 16% of cases.[27]

We have examined factors that may predispose to an aggressive course in nonhemorrhagic lesions. The initial clinical presentation appears directly related to eventual outcome upon clinical followup. Patients who present with focal neurologic deficits are the group most likely to have an aggressive course with disabling symptom progression. Lesion size and multiplicity do not appear to exert a significant influence on the course of nonhemorrhagic lesions. The location of the CM in the in-

Pathophysiologic Phenomena Associated with Cavernous Angiomas

"Slow Ooze" and the Hemosiderin Ring

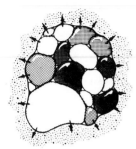

"Intralesional Hemorrhage" and Lesion Expansion

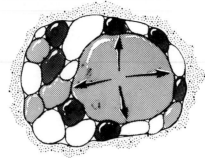

"Gross Hemorrhage" Beyond the Lesion

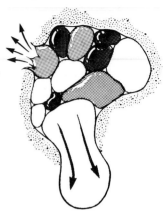

Brain Irritation

Seizures
Focal neurologic
    deficits (?)

Lesion Expansion, Increased Focal Turgor

Focal neurologic
    deficits
Headaches (?)
Seizures (?)

Contained or Non-contained Hemorrhage into Surrounding Brain

Focal neurologic
    deficits
Hemorrhagic stroke
    (apoplexy)
Headaches (acute)
Seizures (?)

Figure 4. Pathophysiologic phenomena accompanying the clinical manifestations of CMs.

fratentorial compartment is significantly correlated with an aggressive natural course. Patients presenting with focal neurologic deficits rarely become asymptomatic, and are likely to have exacerbations of the same symptoms over time, with specific symptomology directly related to lesion location.[28]

Cases presenting with seizures or headaches are also likely to remain symptomatic, with seizures becoming gradually more difficult to control over time. Fifty percent of patients who were asymptomatic at the time of initial diagnosis later developed symptoms after a mean followup of 26 months.[27]

Another observation of some interest regarding these lesions has been their possible enlargement over time. We have found this to occur in 9% of cases undergoing serial MRIs. In addition, 89% of cases with serial scans exhibited gradual darkening and increased definition of the surrounding hemosiderin ring.[27]

Summary

It appears that CMs occur in approximately 0.4% of the population and are equally prevalent in females and males. A fraction of cases harbor multiple lesions, and these are usually familial with autosomal dominant inheritance and partial penetrance. Lesions are associated with a low incidence of gross hemorrhage, estimated to be between 0.25% and 0.75% per lesion per year. Gross hemorrhage appears significantly more prevalent in females during gestation. A first hemorrhage is rarely disabling but is commonly followed by a significantly higher incidence of recurrent hemorrhages, which may become increasingly disabling or lethal. Other symptoms include seizures, focal neurologic deficits, and headaches (in order of prevalence). Supratentorial lesions are more likely associated with seizures; while infratentorial CMs and lesions in other eloquent brain regions frequently present with focal neurologic deficits. Symptoms rarely remit permanently. More often, symptomatic lesions are associated with progressive exacerbation of the same clinical signs, mostly related to the lesion location.

The pathophysiology of CMs consists of slow oozing of blood into surrounding brain with a resulting "surrounding ring" of hemosiderin and gliosis (Figure 4). In cortical regions, notably in areas adjacent to limbic structures or to central gyri, there is significant association with poorly controlled epilepsy, presumably related to chronic irritation from blood breakdown products and iron deposits. Lesions frequently exhibit sudden thrombosis of one or more caverns, with increase in size or turgor within one or more compartments, occasionally resulting in acute cavernous expansion into surrounding brain (Figure 4). Such "intralesional hemorrhage" is rarely catastrophic, but more frequently results in exacerbation of focal neurologic deficits in eloquent brain regions. "Gross hemorrhage" into surrounding brain is rare and often self-contained in view of the low-pressure, low-flow dynamics within the lesion. Factors predisposing to a gross hemorrhage appear to make lesions more likely to rebleed.

References

1. Abe M, Kjellberg RN, Adams RD. Clinical presentations of vascular malformations of the brain stem: comparison of angiographically positive and negative types. *J Neurol Neurosurg Psychiatry.* 1989;52:167–175.

2. Bell BA, Kendall BE, Symon L. Angiographically occult arteriovenous malformations of the brain. *J Neurol Neurosurg Psychiatry.* 1978;41:1057–1064.

3. Curling OD Jr, Kelly DL. The natural history of intracranial cavernous and venous malformations. *Perspect Neurol Surg.* 1990;1:19–39.

4. Curling OD Jr, Kelly DL Jr, Elster AD, et al. An analysis of the natural history of cavernous angiomas. *J Neurosurg.* 1991;75:702–708.

5. Ebeling JD, Tranmer BL, Davis KA, et al. Thrombosed arteriovenous malformations: a type of occult vascular malformations. *Neurosurgery.* 1988;23:605–610.

6. Forster D, Steiner L, Håkanson S. Arteriovenous malformations of the brain: a long-term clinical study. *J Neurosurg.* 1972;37:562–570.

7. Fults D, Kelly DL Jr. Natural history of arteriovenous malformations of the brain: a clinical study. *Neurosurgery.* 1984;15:658–662.

8. Giombini S, Morello G. Cavernous angiomas of the brain: account of fourteen personal cases and review of the literature. *Acta Neurochir (Wien).* 1978;40:61–82.

9. Gomori JM, Grossman RI, Goldberg HI, et al. Occult cerebral vascular malformations: high-field MR imaging. *Radiology.* 1986;158:707–713.

10. Houtteville J. Les cavernomes intra-craniens (Table Ronde). *Neurochirurgie (Paris).* 1989;35:73–131.

11. Jellinger K. The morphology of centrally-situated angiomas. In: Pia HW, Gleave JRW, Grote E, Zierski J, eds. *Cerebral Angiomas; Advances in Diagnosis and Therapy.* New York, NY: Springer Verlag; 1975:9–20.

12. Jellinger K. Vascular malformations of the central nervous system: a morphological overview. *Neurosurg Rev.* 1986;9:177–216.

13. Kashiwagi S, van Loveren HR, Tew JM, et al. Diagnosis and treatment of brain-stem malformations. *J Neurosurg.* 1990;72:27–34.

14. Little JR, Awad IA, Jones SC, et al. Vascular pressures and cortical blood flow in cavernous angioma of the brain. *J Neurosurg.* 1990;73:555–559.

15. Lobato RD, Perez C, Rivas JJ, et al. Clinical, radiological, and pathological spectrum of angiographically occult intracranial vascular malformations: analysis of 21 cases and review of the literature. *J Neurosurg.* 1988;68:518–531.

16. McCormick WF, Hardman JM, Boulter TR. Vascular malformations ("angiomas") of the brain, with special reference to those occurring in the posterior fossa. *J Neurosurg.* 1968;28:241–251.

17. New PFJ, Ojemann RG, Davis KR, et al. MR and CT of occult vascular malformations of the brain. *AJNR.* 1986;7:771–779.

18. Ogilvy CS, Heros RC, Lobato RD. Angiographically occult intracranial vascular malformations. *J Neurosurg.* 1988;69:960–962. Letter to the editor.

19. Ogilvy CS, Heros RC, Ojemann RG, et al. Angiographically occult arteriovenous malformations. *J Neurosurg.* 1988;69:350–355.

20. Otten P, Pizzolato GP, Rilliet B, et al. A propos de 131 cas d'angiomes caverneux (cavernomes) du S.N.C., répérés par l'analyse rétrospective de 24 535 autopsies. *Neurochirurgie (Paris)*. 1989;35:82–83.

21. Parkinson D, Bachers G. Arteriovenous malformations: summary of 100 consecutive supratentorial cases. *J Neurosurg*. 1980;53:285–299.

22. Rigamonti D. Natural history of cavernous malformations, capillary malformations (telangiectases), and venous malformations. In: Barrow DL, ed. *Intracranial Vascular Malformations*. Park Ridge, Ill: American Association of Neurological Surgeons; 1990:45–51.

23. Rigamonti D, Drayer BP, Johnson PC, et al. The MRI appearance of cavernous malformations (angiomas). *J Neurosurg*. 1987;67:518–524.

24. Rigamonti D, Hadley MN, Drayer BP, et al. Cerebral cavernous malformations: incidence and familial occurrence. *N Engl J Med*. 1988;319:343–347.

25. Rigamonti D, Spetzler RF, Johnson PC, et al. Cerebral vascular malformations. *BNI Quart*. 1987;3:18–28.

26. Robinson JL, Hall CF, Sedzimir CB. Subarachnoid hemorrhage in pregnancy. *J Neurosurg*. 1972;36:27–33.

27. Robinson JR Jr, Awad IA, Little JR. Natural history of the cavernous angioma. *J Neurosurg*. 1991;75:709–714.

28. Robinson JR Jr, Awad IA, Magdenic M. Factors predisposing to clinical disability in cavernous malformations of the brain. *Neurosurgery*. In press.

29. Russell DS, Rubenstein LJ. *Pathology of Tumours of the Nervous System*. 4th ed. Baltimore, Md: Williams & Wilkins; 1977:116–145.

30. Sarwar M, McCormick WF. Intracerebral venous angiomas: case report and review. *Arch Neurol*. 1978;35:323–325.

31. Savoiardo M, Strada J, Passerini A. Intracranial cavernous hemangiomas: neuroradiologic review of 36 operated cases. *AJNR*. 1983;4:945–950.

32. Schörner W, Bradac GB, Treisch J, et al. Magnetic resonance imaging (MRI) in the diagnosis of cerebral arteriovenous angiomas. *Neuroradiol*. 1986;28:313–318.

33. Simard JM, Garcia-Bengochea F, Ballinger WE Jr, et al. Cavernous angioma: a review of 126 collected and 12 new clinical cases. *Neurosurgery*. 1986;18:162–172.

34. Spetzler RF, Lobato RC. Angiographically occult intracranial vascular malformations. *J Neurosurg*. 1988;69:642–644. Letter to the editor and reply.

35. Steiger HJ, Markwalder TM, Reulen HJ. Clinicopathological relations of cerebral cavernous angiomas: observations in eleven cases. *Neurosurgery*. 1987;21:879–884.

36. Stein BM, Wolpert SM. Arteriovenous malformations of the brain: I. Current concepts and treatment. *Arch Neurol*. 1980;37:1–5.

37. Stein BM, Wolpert SM. Arteriovenous malformations of the brain: II. Current concepts and treatment. *Arch Neurol*. 1980;37:69–75.

38. Tagle P, Huete I, Mendez J, et al. Intracranial cavernous angioma: presentation and management. *J Neurosurg*. 1986;64:720–723.

39. Tung H, Giannotta SL, Chandrasoma PT, et al. Recurrent intraparenchymal hemorrhages from angiographically occult vascular malformations. *J Neurosurg*. 1990;73:174–180.

40. Vaquero J, Leunda G, Martinez R, et al. Cavernomas of the brain. *Neurosurgery*. 1983;12:208–210.

41. Vaquero J, Salsazar J, Martinez R, et al. Cavernomas of the central nervous system: clinical syndromes, CT scan diagnosis, and prognosis after surgical treatment in 25 cases. *Acta Neurochir (Wien)*. 1987;85:29–33.

42. Voigt K, Yasargil MG. Cerebral cavernous hemangiomas or cavernomas: incidence, pathology, localization, diagnosis, clinical features and treatment. Review of the literature and report of an unusual case. *Neurochirurgia*. 1976;19:59–68.

43. Wakai S, Ueda Y, Inoh S, et al. Angiographically occult angiomas: a report of thirteen cases with analysis of the cases documented in the literature. *Neurosurgery*. 1985;17:549–556.

44. Wilkins RH. Natural history of intracranial vascular malformations: a review. *Neurosurgery*. 1985;16:421–430.

45. Yamasaki T, Handa H, Yamashita J, et al. Intracranial and orbital cavernous angiomas: a review of 30 cases. *J Neurosurg*. 1986;64:197–208.

46. Zimmerman RS, Spetzler RF, Lee KS, et al. Cavernous malformations of the brain stem. *J Neurosurg*. 1991;75:32–39.

Chapter 4

Diagnostic Imaging of Cavernous Malformations

John Perl, MD, and Jeffrey S. Ross, MD

Introduction

Cavernous malformations (CMs) are being diagnosed antemortem in adults and children with increasing frequency as newer and more widespread use of computed tomography (CT) and magnetic resonance imaging (MRI) becomes available.[9,15,16,22,25,26,41] With the newer imaging modalities the frequency of detection of asymptomatic CMs is likely to increase.[31,39,42,47] Because of the relative lack of sensitivity and specificity of angiography and CT, the natural history of CMs was based primarily on symptomatic lesions.* MRI has provided significant improvement in the ability to image and localize angiographically occult cerebral vascular malformations, and specifically it has allowed an accurate preoperative diagnosis of cavernous malformations.[9,16,22,26,30,31,38] In addition, the newer imaging modalities have confirmed that a familial incidence can exist in some patient populations and that multiple lesions occur in a significant number of patients.[1,5,26,27,33] As a result, the natural history has become more clearly elucidated and therefore the clinical management of CMs is evolving.[25,31,39,47] CMs frequently have been included in a group of vascular malformations of different pathologic characteristics, which have been collectively called angiographically occult vascular malformations. This is a very nonspecific term whose only common feature is the absence of abnormal vascularity on angiography. Morphologically the common feature to all of these lesions is slow blood flow. They are comprised pathologically of thrombosed arteriovenous malformations, capillary telangiectases, CMs, and, occasionally, venous malformations.[19,32] More recently the CT and MRI findings have become better established, as more rigorous evaluations of angiographically occult malformations have been performed.*

There are several classifications of vascular malformations of the brain; however, the most widely accepted classification is that of McCormick and colleagues. This consists of five categories: **(1)** arteriovenous malformation, **(2)** venous malformation, **(3)** cavernous malformation, **(4)** capillary telangiectasia, and **(5)** varices.[19,35] The true incidence and prevalence of CMs are not precisely known. In Sarwar and McCor-

---

*References 4,17,30,31,37,39,42,46,47

*References 9,16,22,25,26,31,37,38,47

mick's[35] prospective autopsy study of 4,069 consecutive brains, 165 patients were found to have one or more vascular malformations of the brain. The prevalence of venous malformations comprised 105 (2.6%), capillary telangiectasia 28 (0.69%), arteriovenous malformations 24 (0.59%), CMs 16 (0.39%), and varix malformations of the brain 4 (0.1%). The fact that the highest percentage were venous malformations in this autopsy series does not correlate with surgical series as many of these venous malformations are asymptomatic. The prevalence of CMs in Sarwar and McCormick's series closely parallels that of a recent retrospective study performed by Robinson et al.[31] The reports of 14,035 MRI examinations were evaluated in a five-year period. In those 14,035 images, there were 76 lesions identified in 66 patients constituting a prevalence of 0.47%.

Location and Size

In a retrospective review by Robinson et al, MRI images of 76 lesions in 66 patients demonstrated that most intracranial CMs occur within the frontal and temporal lobes. Approximately 70% of these lesions were in the cerebral hemispheres, and approximately 5% of the lesions were considered deep lesions affecting the diencephalon and septal region. The infratentorial lesions were almost equally distributed between the cerebellar hemisphere and brain stem locations.[31] The pons is the most common site for brain stem CMs.[20] In another study of 56 CMs in 47 patients, 59% were supratentorial (the most common location being in the temporal and parietal regions) and 39% of the lesions were infratentorial (the most common locations being the pons and the cerebellum).[25] Of significant clinical and therapeutic importance is the association of venous angiomas with CMs in 5%–16% of cases.[29,31,36,47] The size of a CM can vary widely—ranging from several millimeters to 4 cm or greater.[31]

Intracranial extracerebral CMs have also been described but are considerably rarer than intracerebral lesions, most commonly involving the cavernous sinus. They have also been described arising from cranial nerves.[13,21,28,40,43]

Multiplicity of Cavernous Malformations

Pathologic studies have demonstrated that multiple lesions occur in approximately 25% of cases.[32] Rigamonti et al[26] in an MRI-based series demonstrated multiple lesions in approximately 50% of the patients. Recent studies by both Robinson et al[31] and Requena et al[25]—which are both based on the MRI diagnosis of CMs—demonstrated that approximately 11% to 13% of patients harbored multiple malformations. While many CMs appear to be sporadic, familial occurrences have been described by several authors.[1,5,27,33] Familial populations have a high incidence of multiple lesions (73%) compared to the sporadic form (10% to 15%).[32]

Pathology

CMs are hamartomatous lesions composed of enlarged sinusoidal vascular spaces with a single layer of attenuated endothelium, devoid of elastin or smooth muscle. The sinusoids are separated from each other by connective tissue with no intervening neural tissue. The brain parenchyma immediately surrounding the lesion is gliotic and may contain small, slow-flowing arteries and draining veins. In addition, a rim of gliotic parenchyma surrounding the lesion is hemosiderin stained.[12,26,32]

Imaging

In the pre-MR era, "angiographically occult malformations" were collectively grouped without using strict histologic features of lesion definition. With the more recent rigorous studies using primarily MRI with histologic confirmation, the imaging characteristics of CMs have become more firmly established. While the appearance of CMs on MRI is relatively specific, other vascular malformations and some neoplasms may demonstrate a similar morphology.[24-26,44]

Plain Films of the Skull

Russel and Rubenstein[32] have described microscopic calcifications as being a common feature of CMs. In two pathologically proven studies, 8% to 10% of patients with CMs presented abnormal fine granular or coarse calcifications on conventional skull radiographs.[26,37] Other rare skull film abnormalities may be secondary to erosions from mass effect in patients with larger CMs.[42]

Angiography

Angiography is normal in approximately 30% to 40% of patients.[18,26,30] Studies by New et al[22] and Requena et al[25] demonstrated that angiography was positive in 30% to 33%. Rarely are CMs identified directly by angiography as classically described by Liliequist. He described findings consistent of a capillary blush and early filling of veins without enlarged feeding arteries.[17] More frequently, nonspecific findings are present, such as an avascular region in the capillary phase with displacement of vessels in the absence of pathologic circulation (Figure 1).[25,26,37,39] Occasionally, venous pooling or early draining veins are seen.[17,26,37] Lobato et al summarized the hypotheses of why there is a frequent lack of angiographic identification: **(1)** compression of the CM vessel's lumen by mass effect from the adjacent hematoma; **(2)** destruction of the cavernous malformation vessels by macroscopic bleeding; **(3)** spontaneous thrombosis of the cavernous malformation; **(4)** thrombosis secondary to a gross hemorrhage; **(5)** partial thrombosis with sluggish circulation through the remaining patent vessels; **(6)** posthemorrhagic vascular vasospasm; and **(7)** dilution of the contrast media in enlarged cavernous vascular spaces of the malformation.[18]

The capillary blush and early draining vein as described by Liliequist are nonspecific findings and are also compatible with neoplastic and inflammatory conditions. Early draining veins also may be seen in other histologic types of vascular malformations.

Numaguchi et al described opacification of the capacious cavernous sinuses by prolonged slow arterial injection.[23] The value of angiography in the evaluation of CMs is primarily in recognition of coexistent vascular malformations such as a venous angioma, since they are managed by resection of the CM and preservation of the venous angioma.[24,26,29,36,47] Venous angiomas have a pathognomonic appearance consisting of a collection of dilated medullary veins radiating into an enlarged central vein, the so-called "caput-medusa."[11] The large vein either drains into the deep or superficial venous system.[7,11,29,34]

Computed Tomography

The sensitivity of CT in the detection of CM is less than that of MRI. However, CT will frequently be the first imaging study obtained in patients with acute clinical presentations. CMs on noncontrast enhanced CT appear as focal nodular heterogeneous hyperdensities relative to adjacent brain.[22,25,37,39,46] A minority of lesions are hypodense compared to brain.[22,25,37,39,46] After intravenous contrast administration there is variable but commonly faint enhancement.[22,25,37,39,46] Punctate areas of increased attenuation coefficient (probably related to calcifications) are seen in approximately 14% of cases (Figure 2A,B).[37] Transient increased attenuation is also seen with acute hemorrhage which frequently has associated mass effect.[26,39,46] Surrounding edema and mass effect have been described.[22,25,37,46] In six episodes of acute brain stem hemorrhages into pathologically proven CMs observed on CT by Zimmerman et al,[47] none

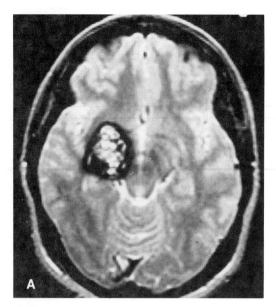

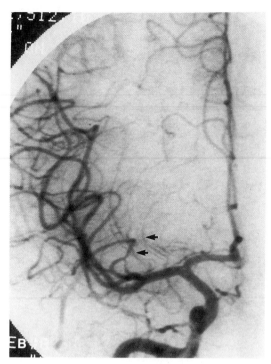

Figure 1. Cavernous malformation. **(A)** A spin-echo axial long TR/TE image demonstrates a typical appearance of a large CM, heterogeneous central signal intensity and very hypointense rim due to hemosiderin. **(B)** Anterior-posterior and **(C)** lateral digital subtraction angiogram demonstrate a subtle mass effect on the lenticulostriate vessels (arrows). No enlarged vessels are demonstrated. The venous phase was normal. Normal or nonspecific secondary signs of mass effect are the most common angiographic findings of CMs.

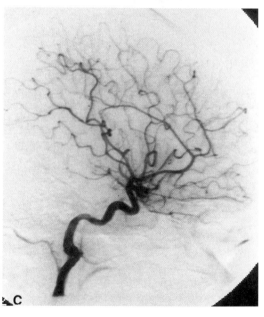

had evidence of subarachnoid or fourth ventricular hemorrhage. This is not the case for cryptic arteriovenous malformations which are thought to be the result of a lack of a capsule in the true arteriovenous malformations so that the hemorrhage follows the path of least resistance into the ventricle or subarachnoid space.[47]

Magnetic Resonance Imaging

The high sensitivity of MRI makes it the examination of choice in the evaluation of CMs.* The absence of artifact from overlying bones is particularly advantageous for the evaluation of CMs in both the high subcortical regions as well as in the posterior fossa.

*References 8,10,14–16,22,25,26,31,39,41,47

Evolution of hemorrhage, as documented by MRI, from the hyperacute to the chronic stages has been described extensively.[3,8,45] Acute hematomas (1–7 days) are isointense or slightly hypointense to gray matter and brain on short relaxation time/echo time (TR/TE) (T1-weighted) spin-echo

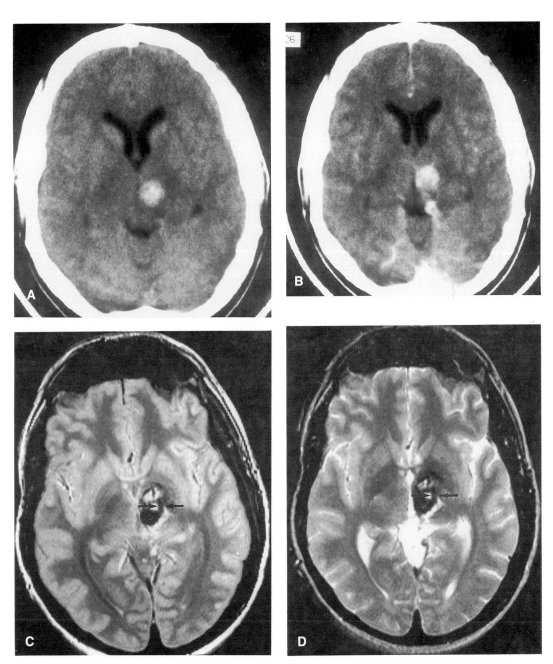

Figure 2. Cavernous malformation. **(A)** Noncontrast-enhanced CT scan reveals a well-defined, dense lesion without mass effect in the left thalamus. The density is probably related to calcifications. **(B)** There is mild contrast enhancement. **(C)** A spin-echo long TR/short TE image of a CM demonstrates heterogeneous signal intensity with a dark rim due to hemosiderin. The heterogeneous central signal intensity is also due to blood by-products. **(D)** The spin-echo long TR/TE image demonstrates thickening of the hemosiderin rim (arrows) when compared to the spin-echo long TR/short TE image due to more prominent susceptibility changes. No flow void from an enlarged vessel is seen.

Table 1. **Appearance of Intracerebral Hematomas on Spin-Echo MRI***

Time	State	T1-W	T2-W
Acute	Intracellular Deoxyhemoglobin	Isointense	Hypointense
Early subacute	Intracellular Methemoglobin	Hyperintense	Hypointense
Late subacute	Extracellular Methemoglobin	Hyperintense	Hyperintense
Chronic	Hemosiderin	Hypointense	Hyperintense with hypointense rim

*References 3,8,10,45

images and are markedly hypointense centrally on long TR/TE (T2-weighted) spin-echo images. This is a result of preferential T2-proton relaxation enhancement by deoxyhemoglobin in the intact red blood cells. Subacute hematomas (weeks to months) are hyperintense to brain on both short TR/TE and long TR/TE images as a result of the paramagnetic free intracellular methemoglobin. In subacute and chronic hematomas there is a hypointense rim on short TR/TE-weighted images which becomes markedly hypointense on long TR/TE-weighted images. This is due to hemosiderin deposition which also demonstrates preferential T2-proton relaxation enhancement.[2,3,10] The preferential T2-relaxation enhancement in acute hematomas and with hemosiderin is field dependent, and increases as the square of the magnetic field.[8-10] For this reason it is less advantageous to image patients with suspected or known CMs on lower field MR units.[9,26] This has been supported clinically in the detection of occult cerebrovascular malformations.[9,26] In addition, the susceptibility effect due to the hemosiderin is directly related to the length of the TE. Therefore, the hypointense rim thickens with longer TE-weighted images (Figure 2C,D).[8] Gradient-echo MRI can detect both acute and chronic hemorrhage not seen on conventional spin-echo techniques. This is attributed to the greater sensitivity of the gradient echo technique to magnetic field inhomogeneities susceptibility that arise

from the paramagnetic blood break-down products (Figure 3).[2,3] Thus, with patients with suspected CMs a gradient-echo sequence could be quite helpful, especially if the patient is being imaged on a low-field MRI unit. (Table 1 summarizes the MRI findings of hemorrhage.)

CMs on T1-weighted and T2-weighted images have well-defined rounded or multi-lobulated margins. A peripheral hypointense rim with a heterogeneous central signal is the typical appearance. The peripheral decreased signal intensity is due to the hemosiderin rim, and the heterogeneous central portion is a result of blood and blood by-products in various states of evolution. In addition, some of the mixed signal intensity may be due to calcifications. Occasionally small regions of high signal surrounding the hemosiderin rim may be seen due to vasogenic edema and/or brain parenchymal gliosis.[24-26] No large vessels (which would typically have a serpentine course and a decreased signal intensity due to a flow void) are typically identified, although a vessel adjacent to the CM may represent a coexistent venous angioma. Small CMs may appear as petechial areas of decreased signal intensity only.[24,25]

Since the MRI appearance of CMs is mostly related to hemorrhage in evolution, it is not surprising that its appearance is not absolutely specific. Other diagnostic considerations include a thrombosed arteriovenous malformation and hemorrhagic neoplasms.[24,25,44] Differentiation from neoplasm may be possible as most metastases

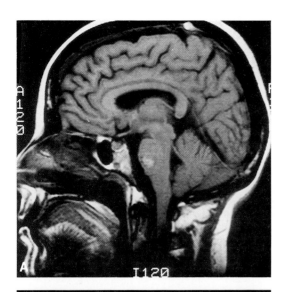

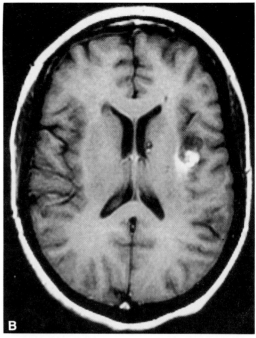

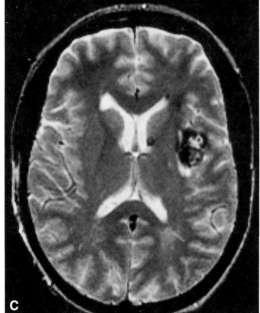

Figure 3. Multiple CMs. **(A)** Spin-echo short TR/TE sagittal image demonstrates high-signal intensity in the pons with a faint hypointense rim. **(B)** Spin-echo short TR/TE axial image demonstrates multiple lesions with heterogeneous or a high-signal intensity center with a hypointense rim identified in the insular cortex in the left caudate head. A third punctate hypointensity is identified in the frontal lobe. **(C)** Spin-echo long TR/TE image at the same level demonstrates multiple lesions with thickening of the hypointense peripheral rim. **(D)** Gradient-echo axial image reveals a fourth lesion in the left frontal lobe (arrow)

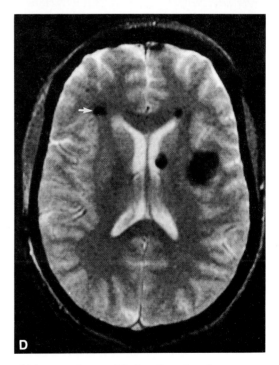

which was not appreciated on the spin-echo sequences illustrating the increased sensitivity of this sequence to hemosiderin deposition.

greater than 5mm have moderate-to-extensive vasogenic edema, while CMs have little or no vasogenic edema.[44] If the patient is being treated with steroids the amount of edema is frequently diminished. Multiplicity of lesions, especially if not all are hemorrhagic, would favor metastatic disease.[44] CT may be helpful in some situations as metastases are frequently hypodense and do not commonly contain calcifications.[24] CMs on the other hand are most often hyperintense and often contain calcifications.[37]

The MR appearance of a CM may be difficult to distinguish from other vascular malformations, especially in the presence of resolving hematoma. The presence of subarachnoid or intraventricular hemorrhage, or dilated prominent feeding or draining vessels adjacent to the lesion, suggests an arteriovenous as opposed to a cavernous malformation. Multiple lesions or lobulated extensions of the lesions strongly suggest a CM. While other types of angiographically occult vascular malformations may theoretically mimic the MR appearance of a CM, this does not appear to be a frequent occurrence clinically. In two recently published series, all lesions with typical MR features of CMs that were resected surgically, proved to be CMs on pathologic examination.[26,31]

More recently, magnetic resonance angiography (MRA) has been used in the diagnosis of CMs. The hemosiderin and other complex paramagnetic signals within such lesions have resulted in MRA visualization of the lesion, mimicking angiographically overt lesions. This artifactual visualization on the time-of-flight MRA techniques is eliminated in more sophisticated phase-contrast techniques (Figure 4).

Positron Emission Tomography (PET)

In a small series of four patients with pathologically proven CMs, positron emission

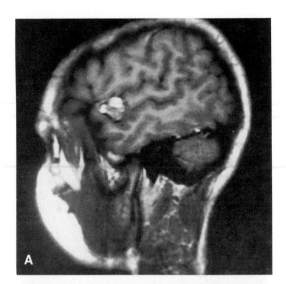

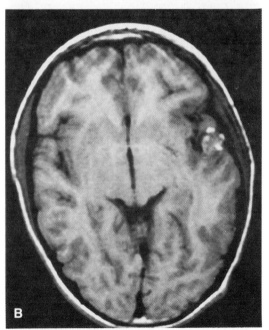

Figure 4. Cavernous malformation with a venous angioma. **(A & B)** Spin-echo short TR/TE sagittal and axial images demonstrating a heterogeneous central signal intensity with a small peripheral hypointense rim. **(C)** Spin-echo long TR/TE axial image at the same level. **(D & E)** Spin-echo short TR/TE axial images before and after the administration of contrast demonstrating moderate enhancement and a draining vein. The degree of enhancement in the draining vein are more typical of a venous angioma. **(F)** 3D time-of-flight lateral MRA demonstrates a hyperintense mass due to hemosiderin (arrow). No enlarged vessels are identified. **(G)** Phase contrast MRA of the same

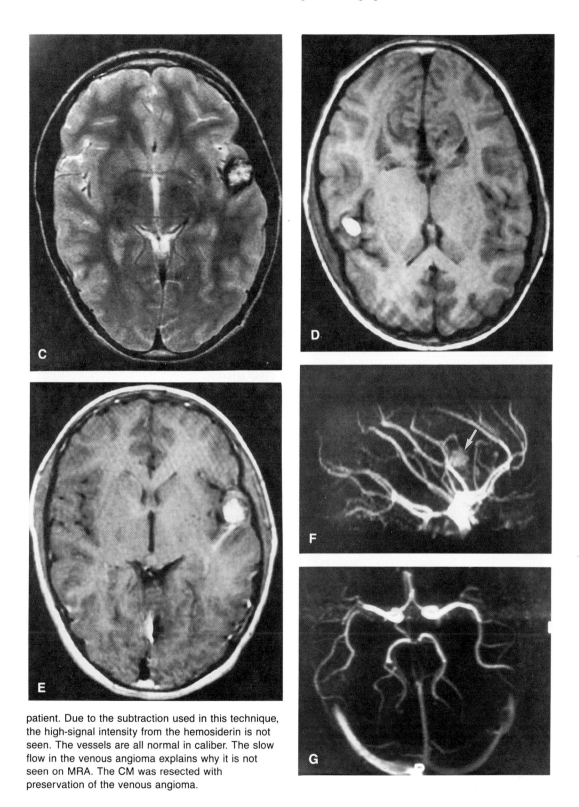

patient. Due to the subtraction used in this technique, the high-signal intensity from the hemosiderin is not seen. The vessels are all normal in caliber. The slow flow in the venous angioma explains why it is not seen on MRA. The CM was resected with preservation of the venous angioma.

tomography (PET) scanning was performed. The findings demonstrated normal or decreased uptake of ^{11}C-methionine and ^{11}C-glucose.[6] This is not the case for tumors in which the finding demonstrates markedly increased uptake of the methionine.[6] These findings in combination with a CT or MRI examination consistent with cavernous malformation may help differentiate CMs from neoplasms.

Extracerebral Cavernous Malformations

Extracerebral intracranial CMs are rare. Approximately 40 of these malformations have been reported in the literature.[21] These malformations are most commonly located in the middle cranial fossa in close association with the cavernous sinus.[21,28,40] These lesions tend to affect women much more frequently than intracerebral CMs.[21,28] The clinical presentation is usually of an acute or subacute onset of diplopia, impaired visual acuity and visual field defects. Other findings including exophthalmos and facial weakness may occur.[21,24,40,43]

The plain skull radiographs and CT demonstrate secondary changes of bony erosion of the adjacent structures: specifically the orbital fissure, middle cranial fossa floor, the dorsum sella and the posterior clinoid.[28] In addition, a discrete hyperdense mass with homogeneous enhancement is usually present after contrast administration.[21] Calcifications are not a frequent finding.[13] The amount of enhancement and the rarity of calcifications are in contrast to the intracerebral CMs. The appearance on angiography is less clear. Momoshima et al[21] and Kaard et al[13] describe CMs in the cavernous sinus as avascular or hypovascular masses. Rigamonti et al describe early staining in the cavernous sinus.[28] When early staining is demonstrated it usually arises from small branches arising from the intracavernous internal carotid artery or the middle meningeal artery.[13,21,28]

Of significant clinical importance is that although the extracerebral CMs may appear hypovascular on imaging studies, they bleed profusely at surgery causing life-threatening hemorrhages.[13,28] The appearance on MRI also does not share the same features of the intracerebral CMs. Extracerebral CMs tend to be isointense with gray matter on short TR/TE and hyperintense on the long TR/TE images.[21,23] They avidly enhance after the administration of contrast.[21] The most common differential diagnosis is that of a meningioma that is commonly isointense to brain on T1- and T2-weighted images, although some meningiomas may be hyperintense on T2-weighted images.[21] Other features which may allow differentiation between meningiomas and CMs is the frequent association of hyperostosis with meningiomas, which has not been described with *extra*cerebral CMs. In contrast to *intra*cerebral CMs, meningiomas lack the markedly hypointense rim due to the absence of the hemosiderin-laden macrophages peripherally.[13]

Summary

MRI, especially high-field, has emerged as the diagnostic study of choice in evaluating either intracerebral or extracerebral CMs. The appearance of intracerebral CMs is relatively specific on MRI, although the appearance is not pathognomonic. Often the clinical history and imaging findings should allow confident diagnosis in a majority of cases. Evaluation for coexistent venous angioma should be performed in the case of intracerebral CMs. In the evaluation of a parasellar mass, the possibility of an extracerebral intracranial cavernous malformation should be entertained.

References

1. Allard JC, Hochberg FH, Franklin PD, et al. Magnetic resonance imaging in a family with hereditary cerebral arteriovenous malformations. *Arch Neurol.* 1989;46:184–187.

2. Atlas SW, Mark AS, Fram EK, et al. Vascular intracranial lesions: applications of gradient-echo MR imaging. *Radiology.* 1988;169:455–461.

3. Atlas SW, Mark AS, Grossman RI, et al. Intracranial hemorrhage: gradient-echo MR imaging at 1.5 T: comparison with spin-echo imaging and clinical applications. *Radiology.* 1988;168:803–807.

4. Bell BA, Kendall BE, Symon L. Angiographically occult arteriovenous malformations of the brain. *J Neurol, Neurosurg and Psychiatry.* 1978;41:1057–1064.

5. Clark JV. Familial occurrence of cavernous angiomata of the brain. *J Neurol Neurosurg Psychiatry.* 1970;33:871–876.

6. Ericson K, von Holst H, Mosskin M, et al. Positron emission tomography of cavernous haemangiomas of the brain. *Acta Radiologica Diagnosis.* 1986;27:379–383.

7. Fierstein SB, Pribram HW, Hieshima G. Angiography and computed tomography in the evaluation of cerebral venous malformations. *Neuroradiology.* 1979;17:137–148.

8. Gomori JM, Grossman RI, Goldberg HI, et al. Intracranial hematomas: imaging by high-field MR. *Radiology.* 1985;157:87–93.

9. Gomori JM, Grossman RI, Goldberg HI, et al. Occult cerebral vascular malformations: high-field MR imaging. *Radiology.* 1986;158:707–713.

10. Gomori JM, Grossman RI, Hackney DB, et al. Variable appearances of subacute intracranial hematomas on high-field spin-echo MR. *AJNR.* 1987;8:1019–1026.

11. Heinz ER. Pathology involving the supratentorial veins and dural sinuses. In: Newton TH, Potts DG, eds. *Radiology of the Skull and Brain.* St. Louis, Mo: CV Mosby Co; 1974;2:1878–1902.

12. Jellinger K. Vascular malformations of the central nervous system: a morphological overview. *Neurosurg Rev.* 1986;9:177–216.

13. Kaard HP, Khangure MS, Waring P. Extraaxial parasellar cavernous hemangioma. *AJNR.* 1990;11:1259–1261.

14. Kucharczyk W, Lemme-Pleghos L, Uske A, et al. Intracranial vascular malformations: MR and CT imaging. *Radiology.* 1985;156:383–389.

15. Lee BCP, Herzberg L, Zimmerman RD, et al. MR imaging of cerebral vascular malformations. *AJNR.* 1985;6:863–870.

16. Lemme-Pleghos L, Kucharczyk W, Brant-Zawadzki M, et al. MR imaging of angiographically occult vascular malformations. *AJNR.* 1986;7:217–222.

17. Liliequist B. Angiography in intracerebral cavernous hemangioma. *Neuroradiology.* 1975;9:69–72.

18. Lobato RD, Perez C, Rivas JJ, et al. Clinical, radiological, and pathological spectrum of angiographically occult intracranial vascular malformations: an analysis of 21 cases and review of the literature. *J Neurosurg.* 1988;68:518–531.

19. McCormick WF. The pathology of vascular ("arteriovenous") malformations. *J Neurosurg.* 1966;24:807–816.

20. McCormick WF, Hardman JM, Boulter TR. Vascular malformations ("angiomas") of the brain,

with special reference to those occurring in the posterior fossa. J Nuerosurg. 1968;28:241–251.

21. Momoshima S, Shiga H, Yuasa Y, et al. MR findings in extracerebral cavernous angiomas of the middle cranial fossa: report of two cases and review of the literature. *AJNR.* 1991;12:756–760.

22. New PF, Ojemann RG, David KR, et al. MR and CT of occult vascular malformations of the brain. *AJR.* 1986;147:985–993.

23. Numaguchi Y, Kishikawa T, Fukui M, et al. Prolonged injection angiography for diagnosing intracranial cavernous hemangiomas. *Radiology.* 1979;131:137–138.

24. Rapacki TF, Brantley MJ, Furlow TW Jr, et al. Heterogeneity of cerebral cavernous hemangiomas diagnosed by MR imaging. *J Comput Assist Tomogr.* 1990;14:18–25.

25. Requena I, Arias M, Lopez-Ibor L, et al. Cavernomas of the central nervous system: clinical and neuroimaging manifestations in 47 patients. *J Neurol. Neurosurg Psychiatry.* 1991;54:590–594.

26. Rigamonti D, Drayer BP, Johnson PC, et al. The MRI appearance of cavernous malformations (angiomas). *J Neurosurg.* 1987;67:518–524.

27. Rigamonti D, Hadley MN, Drayer BP, et al. Cerebral cavernous malformations: incidence and familial occurrence. *N Engl J Med.* 1988;319:343–347.

28. Rigamonti D, Pappas CTE, Spetzler RF, et al. Extracerebral cavernous angiomas of the middle fossa. *Neurosurgery.* 1990;27:306–310.

29. Rigamonti D, Spetzler RF. The association of venous and cavernous malformations: report of four cases and discussion of the pathophysiological, diagnostic, and therapeutic implications. *Acta Neurochir (Wien).* 1988;92:100–105.

30. Rigamonti D, Spetzler RF, Johnson PC, et al. Cerebral vascular malformations. *BNI Quart.* 1987;3:18–28.

31. Robinson JR, Awad IA, Little JR. Natural history of the cavernous angioma. *J Neurosurg.* 1991;75:709–714.

32. Russel DS, Rubenstein LJ. *Pathology of the Nervous System.* 5th ed. Baltimore, Md: Williams & Wilkins; 1989.

33. Rutka JT, Brant-Zawadzki M, Wilson CB, et al. Familial cavernous malformations: diagnostic potential of magnetic resonance imaging. *Surg Neurol.* 1988;29:467–474.

34. Saito Y, Kobayashi N. Cerebral venous angiomas. *Radiology.* 1981;139:87–94.

35. Sarwar M, McCormick WF. Intracerebral venous angioma: case report and review. *Arch Neurol.* 1978;35:323–325.

36. Sasaki O, Tanaka R, Koike T, et al. Excision of cavernous angioma with preservation of coexisting venous angioma: case report. *J Neurosurg.* 1991;75:461–464.

37. Savoiardo M, Strada L, Passerini A. Intracranial cavernous hemangiomas: neuroradiologic review of 36 operated cases. *AJNR.* 1983;4:945–950.

38. Schörner W, Bradac GB, Treisch J, et al. Magnetic resonance imaging (MRI) in the

diagnosis of cerebral arteriovenous angiomas. *Neuroradiology.* 1986;28:313–318.

39. Scott RM, Barnes P, Kupsky W, et al. Cavernous angiomas of the central nervous system in children. *J Neurosurg.* 1992;76:38–46.

40. Sepehrnia A, Tatagiba M, Brandis A, et al. Cavernous angioma of the cavernous sinus: case report. *Neurosurgery.* 1990;27:151–155.

41. Sigal R, Krief O, Houtteville JP, et al. Occult cerebrovascular malformations: follow-up with MR imaging. *Radiology.* 1990;176:815–819.

42. Simard JM, Garcia-Bengochea F, Ballinger WE, et al. Cavernous angioma: a review of 126 collected and 12 new clinical cases. *Neurosurgery.* 1986;18:162–172.

43. Steinberg GK, Marks MP, Shuer LM, et al. Occult vascular malformations of the optic chiasm: magnetic resonance imaging diagnosis and surgical laser resection. *Neurosurgery.* 1990;27:466–470.

44. Sze G, Krol G, Olsen WL, et al. Hemorrhagic neoplasms: MR mimics of occult vascular malformations. *AJR.* 1987;149:1223–1230.

45. Vaquero J, Leunda G, Martinez R, et al. Cavernomas of the brain. *Neurosurgery.* 1983;12:208–210.

46. Vaquero J, Salazar J, Martinez R, et al. Cavernomas of the central nervous system: clinical syndromes, CT scan diagnosis, and prognosis after surgical treatment in 25 cases. *Acta Neurochir (Wien).* 1987;85:29–33.

47. Zimmerman RS, Spetzler RF, Lee KS, et al. Cavernous malformations of the brain stem. *J Neurosurg.* 1991;75:32–39.

Chapter 5

Cavernous Malformations and Epilepsy

Issam A. Awad, MD, and John R. Robinson, MD

Seizures and epilepsy are frequent clinical manifestations of a cavernous malformation (CM) and represent the most frequent symptomatic presentation of supratentorial lesions.* Clinicians often uncover the diagnosis of a CM following a first seizure, or in some cases after performing neuroimaging studies for chronic epilepsy previously thought to be idiopathic.[2,13,27,29,30,40,49,51,56,72] In some instances, the sole clinical significance of the lesion is related to its epileptogenicity, while in other cases there may be concern about potential hemorrhage or focal neurologic deficits from the same lesion.

In this chapter, we review current pathophysiologic concepts related to partial epilepsy associated with focal structural lesions of the brain including CMs. We present the spectrum of seizure disorders associated with this lesion, and the natural history, prognosis, and options for therapeutic intervention.

Pathophysiology of Partial Epilepsy

Convergence of Focal Pathology in the Epileptogenic Zone

Seizure disorders associated with structural lesions of the brain including CMs generally consist of partial (focal) epilepsy.[1,9,36] The clinical phenomenology of the seizures is associated with a stereotyped generation and propagation in time and space of specific regional electroencephalographic (EEG) phenomena. These are spatially related in a consistent fashion to the epileptogenic structural lesion.** The CM of the brain exerts a pathologic effect on nearby brain parenchyma, rendering this region of the brain epileptogenic (Figure 1). The vascular malformation itself cannot generate seizures. It is the impact of the lesion on surrounding brain that may render neural

---

*References *3–5,8,14,20,21,26,28,35, 45–48,50,52,53,55,59–62,65,67-69,71,73

**References 1,2,6,11,13,15,18,24,33,37, 41–44,57,66,70,73

Convergence of Focal Pathology in Focal Epilepsy

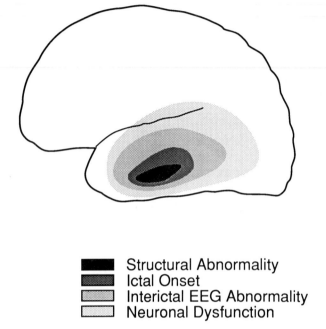

■ Structural Abnormality
▨ Ictal Onset
▧ Interictal EEG Abnormality
☐ Neuronal Dysfunction

Figure 1. Convergence of focal pathology in partial (focal) epilepsy. The zone of neuronal dysfunction is usually quite extensive. Within it is a large area of interictal EEG abnormality. A smaller area of ictal onset is generally closely associated with a well-defined structural pathologic abnormality. The convergence of multiple abnormalities assists in the definition of the epileptogenic zone.

tissue epileptogenic. The effect of the CM on surrounding brain may be mechanical (pressure, ischemia, etc.) or may be related to specific trophic factors (blood leakage and hemosiderosis).[1,2,10,25,63,64]

Just beyond the epileptogenic structural lesion lies a critical mass of neural tissue responsible for the generation of seizures. This zone of ictal onset is consistent for every stereotyped seizure attack in a given patient.[1,36] Electrophysiologists can identify such an area by recording epileptiform EEG activity from it prior to or simultaneous with clinical ictal onset.[15,44]

The ability of electrophysiologists to detect and map the zone of ictal onset is limited by the number and location of electrodes.[1,36] If electrodes are placed on the surface of the scalp, they may detect regional propagation of seizure activity as opposed to a spatially precise ictal onset. Even implanted electrodes may mislocalize the zone of ictal onset if they are placed just outside this zone. For example, partial complex seizures may originate in the cingulate gyrus with rapid propagation to the ipsilateral mesiotemporal structures, causing clinical manifestations of epilepsy indistinguishable from seizures originating

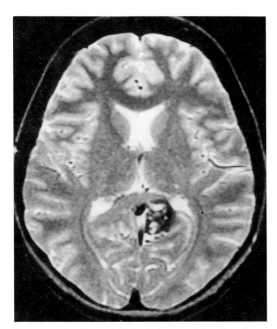

Figure 2. CM located in the isthmus of the cingulate gyrus presented with partial complex seizures, including an aura of visual oscillopsia and a feeling of *déja vu*, followed by loss of awareness, staring, and lip smacking. EEG epileptiform activity was recorded from both temporal lobes in the interictal state and during seizures. The patient has become seizurefree (on anticonvulsant medications) following lesion resection.

associated EEG abnormalities may represent **(1)** diffuse regional epileptogenicity (a large epileptogenic area) or **(2)** secondary spread of ictal phenomena from another area of the brain that was not accessible to simultaneous recording. Therefore, the ability of electrophysiologists to detect the zone of ictal onset is strongly dependent on clinical suspicion (location of the structural lesion or clinical manifestations of the seizure) and the type, location, and number of electrodes used.

Just beyond the region of epileptogenic structural pathology and seizure onset lies a more extensive zone of the brain exhibiting interictal epileptiform EEG activity (Figure 1). The intensity and frequency of the interictal activity is greatest at or near the region of ictal onset. Unlike EEG abnormalities associated with ictal onset, interictal activity is not stereotyped and is not consistent from patient to patient and from seizure to seizure. Furthermore, it is affected by the type and level of anticonvulsant medication, patient arousal and activity, and the frequency and clustering of recent seizures.

Definition of the zone of interictal abnormality is therefore strongly dependent on the conditions and duration of EEG recording. As with ictal-onset EEG activity, information can only be gathered from areas of the brain accessible to specific electrodes used for recording. Interictal EEG activity picked up by scalp electrodes usually represents synchronous interictal activity in a large region of underlying brain. Scattered focal cortical interictal epileptiform activity may not always be detectable by scalp recording, especially when it is not synchronous, does not involve a large enough region of the brain, or is limited to deep or basal cortical lesions.

Within and beyond the zone of interictal epileptiform abnormality lies a larger area of the brain that exhibits interictal neuronal dysfunction and apparent inhibition (Figure 1).

in mesiotemporal structures (Figure 2). If electrodes are placed solely within mesiotemporal structures in such patients, they will only detect propagated ictal activity, and the clinician may misinterpret seizure onset as arising in mesiotemporal structures.

Simultaneous invasive recording from the cingulate gyrus and mesiotemporal regions may be the only way to elucidate the actual pattern of ictal generation and propagation. The clinician must have an index of suspicion that seizures may actually be arising elsewhere, so as to seek specific recording from suspected areas outside the temporal lobe. The index of suspicion may be raised by the presence of a CM outside the mesiotemporal area.

As a corollary of the above observations, the detection of diffuse, regional ictal-

This zone of interictal inhibition can be detected by hypometabolism on positron emission tomography (PET), and by hypoperfusion on single-photon emission computed tomography (SPECT). It also can be manifested by modality-specific neuropsychologic testing. For example, a patient with right temporal CM and epileptogenicity may exhibit an area of hypometabolism and hypoperfusion involving the whole ipsilateral frontotemporal region, and may manifest abnormalities on visual memory testing. The zone of neuronal dysfunction and inhibition can be quite useful in lateralization and general localization of the epileptogenic zone. Because of its extent, it is of limited value in precise localization of the zone of ictal onset, unless the specific epileptogenic structural lesion or the zone of ictal onset is well localized.

Regional dysfunction and inhibition are certainly not specific to the zone of epileptogenicity. They simply indicate a zone of focal functional pathology that may contain within it focal structural pathology, which may in turn be epileptogenic. Nonepileptogenic structural lesions, including CMs, may also be surrounded by a zone of inhibition related to focal brain dysfunction. Therefore, the zone of neuronal dysfunction and inhibition are neither precisely localizing nor specific to the area of epileptogenicity.

Usefulness of Convergence

The convergence of focal structural abnormality, ictal-onset epileptiform EEG abnormality, interictal epileptiform EEG abnormality, and neuronal dysfunction and inhibition in a given region of the brain provides powerful evidence of focal epileptogenicity.[1,36] In instances where there is not such absolute convergence, the clinician should be suspicious of possible mislocalization of epileptogenicity. In an individual case, missing or imprecise information (such as poor recording of ictal onset) may be overcome if all other localizing information is convergent. More precise electrophysiologic information may help to make up for imprecise imaging or neuropsychologic testing.

From a practical standpoint, the presence of partial epilepsy in the setting of a CM of the brain may be attributed to the CM if the seizure type and one or more of the diagnostic electrophysiologic tests point to epileptogenicity in the same region. A question should be raised about the relation of a CM to a particular seizure disorder if one or more items are discordant in relation to focal epileptogenicity. For example, one should be hesitant to automatically attribute electroclinical right temporal seizures to a CM in the left parietal lobe. In this setting, further testing should be made to clarify the nature of epileptogenicity.

Limitations of Convergence

The principle of convergence of focal pathology does not hold true in all cases of focal epilepsy.* A patient may harbor several structural lesions, one or more of which may be surrounded by zones of neuronal dysfunction, but only one of which is responsible for intractable seizures. This situation is extremely common in the case of multiple CMs (Figure 3).

One or more of the CMs may be too small to be visualized clearly by neuroimaging, yet may be responsible for the seizure disorder. A visible structural lesion or the most impressive structural lesion may therefore not always be the epileptogenic lesion or the sole source of seizures in a given patient. Other lesions may cause epileptiform abnormalities in regions (notably limbic structures) remote from the lesions.

Spectrum of Seizure Disorders

Focal epilepsy implies the presence of an epileptogenic structural lesion and a host

---

*References 1,2,6,11,15,18,24,33,37,41–44,57,66,70,73

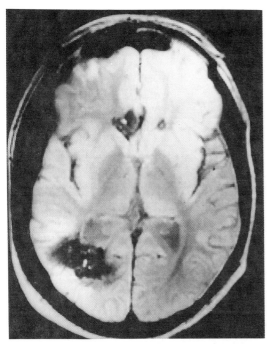

Figure 3. Patient presenting with intractable partial complex seizures without clear clinical localizing or lateralizing features. Interictal and ictal EEG information was also nonlocalizing. Any one of the multiple CMs may be responsible for this seizure disorder.

brain susceptible to epileptogenicity.[10,17] A similar lesion does not predictably cause the same seizure disorder in every patient. Yet, lesion location is critical to the type of seizure disorder and also to vulnerability to epilepsy.

Mesiotemporal structures are particularly vulnerable to epileptogenicity from a variety of structural lesions including CMs.[12,17,24,33,41] Lesions adjacent to mesiotemporal structures often result in secondary epileptogenicity in these structures.[13,16,33] Lesions located near limbic structures may also present with epileptic spells originating near the lesion and rapidly spreading to the limbic system, with clinical and EEG ictal manifestations indistinguishable from mesiotemporal epilepsy. Such is the case with partial complex seizures secondary to lesions in medial or basal frontal areas, in the cingulate gyrus, or in calcarine or occipitotemporal regions—all possibly manifesting as partial complex epilepsy similar to epilepsy of temporal lobe origin (Figure 4).

The location of the structural lesion, associated EEG activity, and/or clinical manifestations of the seizures (auras and postictal symptomatology) may all assist in the localization of the primary zone of epileptogenicity and in seizure propagation phenomenology. CMs in cortical supratentorial locations are most likely associated with epilepsy (Table 1). Recent clinical behavior of the lesion, including overt hemorrhage or enlargement, may also result in exacerbation of seizures.

The threshold of epileptogenicity of a given structural lesion is also related to the host brain. There appears to be genetic predisposition to epilepsy as well as environmental factors that trigger the onset of focal epilepsy. We documented many cases of mesiotemporal epilepsy related to a CM that became clinically manifest following trauma or other neurologic insult (Figure 5). There are also patients who harbor multiple cortical CMs and yet remain seizure-free all of their lives; while other patients have intractable epilepsy from a single CM.

There is a wide spectrum of vulnerability to epilepsy, with multiple interacting factors influencing seizure symptoms (Table 2). Epilepsy associated with CMs is not an all-or-nothing phenomenon. As indicated above, patients may be seizurefree until a lesion bleeds or enlarges, or until an environmental or other triggering factor results in clinically manifest epilepsy. Patients may exhibit a single seizure and remain seizure-free the rest of their lives with or without medications. Other patients may only exhibit seizure activity when their anticonvulsant medications are tapered down or withdrawn. Another group of patients may exhibit frequent disabling seizures despite compliance with near-toxic doses of multiple antiepileptic medications.

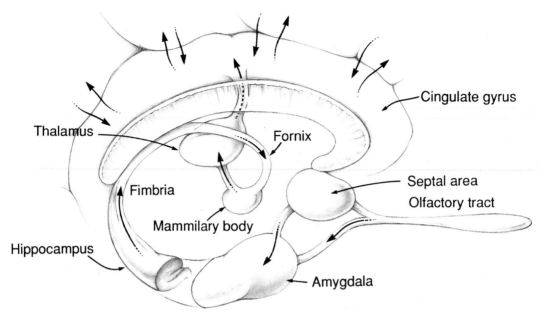

Figure 4. Schematic diagram of limbic structures comprising the circuit of Papez. The amygdala and hippocampus are particularly vulnerable to epileptogenicity from intrinsic lesions or from adjacent regions with intimate connections to the limbic system.

Table 1. Prevalence of Seizure Disorder Among 84 Patients Harboring 100 Intracranial Cavernous Malformations*

Lesion location	No seizures	Well-controlled seizures	Intractable seizures
Frontal (n = 26)	9	12	5
Temporal (n = 22)	6	8	8
Parieto-occipital (n = 21)	6	9	6
Deep supratentorial (n = 9)	7	1	1
Infratentorial (n = 22)	20	1	1
Total			
Lesions (n = 100)	48	31	21
Patients (n = 84)	41	26	17

*Registry of CMs prospectively followed at the Cleveland Clinic Foundation. This registry does not include other cases referred directly for evaluation and treatment of intractable epilepsy.

Epilepsy and Cavernous Malformations

The spectrum of seizure disorders associated with the CM is highly variable, relating in part to variability of lesion size, multiplicity, and location in different patients, and to variability of vulnerability to seizures and triggering events in the host. In relative terms, the CM is a highly epilep-togenic lesion (Table 1). In a review of all published clinical series, seizure disorder was by far the most frequent clinical manifestation of a CM.[53] It is often the only clinical manifestation of cortical supratentorial lesions. Seizures occur in 50% to 70% of patients with CMs, as compared to 20% to 40% of those with AVMs, and 10% to 30% of those with gliomas. This higher frequency of seizures cannot be accounted for

Table 2. **Factors Influencing Epileptogenicity of Cavernous Malformations**

1. Lesion location (cortical supratentorial, proximity to limbic structures)
2. Lesion behavior (hemorrhage, enlargement)
3. Genetic predisposition (to epilepsy)
4. Environmental factors (trauma, other neurologic insult)

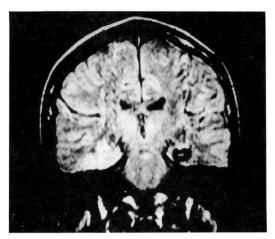

Figure 5. This 29-year-old male presented with partial complex seizures of 10 years duration. Seizures began following a serious motor vehicle accident causing prolonged loss of consciousness and multisystem trauma including documented left carotid dissection (with near-complete left carotid occlusion). There was left temporal lobe dysfunction as documented by neuropsychologic studies, Wada testing, and positron emission tomography (PET) scans. Interictal and ictal onset epileptiform activity was localized to the left anteromesial temporal lobe region. The magnetic resonance image (MRI) (shown) demonstrates a small CM in the left anterior hippocampus. An anteromesial temporal lobectomy including the CM rendered the patient seizurefree.

The pathophysiology of epilepsy in the setting of CMs may be different than epileptogenicity of other structural lesions. Vascular steal and ischemia in neighboring brain are not likely important factors associated with CMs.[19,34,49,51] In addition to mechanical causes of mass effect, a CM is characterized by the slow oozing of blood and blood products into the surrounding brain, and a characteristic gliotic reaction to hemosiderin and other blood products in adjacent brain. Such trophic factors have been shown to be highly epileptogenic in the experimental setting and may explain the vulnerability to seizures and the intractability of epilepsy in the setting of CMs.

Cleveland Clinic Experience with Intractable Epilepsy and Cavernous Malformations

We analyzed in detail 27 cases of truly intractable epilepsy as the sole clinical manifestation of a brain vascular malformation. All patients had frequent seizures disabling enough to interfere seriously with psychosocial or neurologic function despite maximal, competent, and compliant medical therapy. Twenty-four of these patients manifested complex partial seizures, while 3 patients manifested simple partial seizures (visual, motor, or sensory). The partial seizures were associated with secondary generalization, in at least some instances, in 20 of the patients. The lesion consisted of a CM in 21 cases (of which there was 1 with concurrent venous malformation, 1 familial, and 3 cases with multiple lesions), a venous malformation in 3 cases (1 with concurrent CM), and an AVM in 4 cases. Since AVMs are slightly more prevalent than CMs in the general population, pre-

by lesion location alone, since the three clinical entities occur in a similar volume distribution.[53]

A seizure disorder is more likely intractable in the setting of a CM. Among 387 consecutive cases evaluated for intractable epilepsy at the Cleveland Clinic Foundation in 1987–1989, there were 13 vascular malformations (3.3% prevalence), all but one of which were CMs. Seven vascular malformations were among 77 consecutive resective procedures for intractable epilepsy (9% prevalence) performed during that same period, and all but one were CMs.

Table 3. Vascular Malformations and Intractable Epilepsy*

| Sex, Age at Seizure Onset and Diagnostic Evaluation | | |
	M/F	Mean age seizure onset	Mean age at time of evaluation
Arteriovenous malformation	4/0	17.7 years	32.0 years
Venous malformation	2/1	13.7 years	23.7 years
Cavernous malformation	1.6/1	14.9 years	25.5 years

*Cases evaluated for *intractable epilepsy* at the Cleveland Clinic Foundation, 1982–1990.

Table 4. Vascular Malformations and Intractable Epilepsy*

| | Lesion Location | | |
	Temporal	Frontal	Parieto-occipital
Arteriovenous malformation	2	2	
Venous malformation	2		1
Cavernous malformation	13	5	5

*Cases evaluated for *intractable epilepsy* at the Cleveland Clinic Foundation, 1982–1990.

Table 5. Vascular Malformations and Intractable Epilepsy*

| Electroencephalographic Findings | | |
	Localize to lesion	Lateralize to lesion	Remote, undeterminate, or normal
Arteriovenous malformation	3		1
Venous malformation		1	2
Cavernous malformation	5	4	12

*Cases evaluated for *intractable epilepsy* at the Cleveland Clinic Foundation, 1982–1990.

ponderance of CMs in this series emphasizes once again the vulnerability to intractable epilepsy associated with this lesion.

Table 3 summarizes the sex distribution, mean age at seizure onset, and mean age at diagnostic evaluation of patients with various vascular malformations. In general, regardless of lesion type, intractable epilepsy arose in the mid-teens and presented to our epilepsy center following 10 or more years of seizures. Table 4 summarizes the location of various vascular malformations associated with intractable epilepsy. CMs in the temporal lobe are particularly likely to cause intractable epilepsy.

Table 5 summarizes the EEG findings in these patients. In many instances, and notably with CMs and intractable epilepsy, the EEG was totally normal or revealed remote or indeterminate localizing features difficult to attribute directly to the vascular malformation.

All patients with intractable epilepsy and vascular malformations at the Cleveland Clinic underwent prolonged video-EEG monitoring with the aim (1) of registering interictal activity during a lengthy period of recording, and (2) attempting to characterize the clinical features and EEG manifestations of the patients' usual seizures. Results of this evaluation are summarized in Table 6. In more than half the patients, focal or regional epileptogenicity was demonstrated that corresponded to the specific location or the general region of the vascular malformation. In 5 patients with a CM, there was evidence of bitemporal epileptiform abnormality despite the presence of a sin-

Table 6. **Vascular Malformations and Intractable Epilepsy***

	Prolonged Video-EEG Evaluation			
	Focal in area of lesion	Regional at and beyond lesion	Bitemporal single lesion	Multifocal/ undeterminate
Arteriovenous malformation	2	1		
Venous malformation		2		1
Cavernous malformation	3	7	5	5+

*Cases evaluated for *intractable epilepsy* at the Cleveland Clinic Foundation, 1982–1990.
+Includes 1 case of pseudoseizures and 3 cases of multiple vascular malformations.

gle lesion. In another 5 CM cases there was multifocal or undeterminate localization of the epilepsy; these included 1 case with psychogenic seizures and 3 cases with multiple CMs where the offending epileptogenic lesion(s) could not be determined with certainty.

The above experience illustrates the greater likelihood of intractable epilepsy from CMs of the brain in comparison with other intracranial vascular malformations. It also illustrates the frequent difficulty in attributing the seizure disorder to a particular vascular malformation. This is in part due to the problem of multiple lesions. In other patients, the epilepsy may be idiopathic and the visible CM may be incidental and unrelated to the seizure disorder.

Natural History and Prognosis

The natural history of seizures associated with CMs is not well understood. Much information about epilepsy and vascular malformations does not accurately differentiate among various lesion types,[39,51,54,58] which may exhibit varying degrees and mechanisms of epileptogenicity, or does not define precisely the seizure disorder. The CM is obviously highly epileptogenic when involving cortical supratentorial areas. This tendency toward epileptogenicity and also toward intractability of seizures is more pronounced than with other vascular malformations of the brain or with gliomas. Lesions in temporal lobe locations appear to be most likely to result in intractable epilepsy, although this trend is more obvious among

patients evaluated for intractable epilepsy (see Table 3) than among prospectively followed patients with CMs (see Table 1). There is little or no additional information in the published literature to supplement these broad observations.

Anecdotally, clinical experience suggests a wide spectrum of epilepsy associated with lesions of all sizes and locations. Patients may harbor multiple lesions and yet remain seizurefree. Others may experience a single seizure or rare spells, while some patients will have truly intractable epilepsy despite optimal medical therapy. In some patients, epilepsy is truly disabling and may represent the sole clinical significance of a CM.

We recently analyzed data in the Cleveland Clinic registry of cavernous malformations regarding the prognosis of patients with seizures (see Table 1). Of 43 patients with seizure disorder who were followed prospectively for 1 to 8 years through the registry, epilepsy remained under excellent control in 26 (60%) cases, and was truly intractable in the remaining 17 (40%). No prospective information reliably predicts either the likelihood of intractability in an individual case, or factors predisposing to such intractability.

Therapeutic Intervention and Outcome

The primary line of therapy for seizures associated with CMs is medical treatment with anticonvulsants. The choice of anticonvulsant therapy should be dictated by seizure type, as in other patients with epilepsy. Since the majority of cases are associated with partial complex seizures, carbamazepine therapy appears to be the most optimal drug in the majority of patients unless there is specific allergy or contraindication. The dose of anticonvulsant medications should be gradually titrated in the individual case so as to achieve complete seizure control (elimination of symptomatic spells of seizure activity) or documented clinical toxicity.

Monotherapy should be pursued until one of these endpoints is achieved prior to the addition of a second drug. Rarely would the combination of more than two anticonvulsant medications be necessary or effective. Compliance and competent use of medical therapy should achieve seizure control without undue side effects in a substantial portion of symptomatic patients. We are following numerous patients whose epilepsy is under excellent control with medical therapy despite multiple lesions, large lesions, and lesions in a variety of locations.

Other patients do not fare so well with medical therapy. Some may continue to have limited spells, which do not interfere whatsoever with their lives. Other patients have occasional "breakthrough" seizure activity related to decreased compliance with medications or environmental factors. The remaining patients continue to have frequent seizure activity interfering to varying degrees with their lives despite the most optimal medical therapy. Each patient is a bit different in this regard, and the influence of epilepsy on a patient's psychosocial milieu is highly variable. While there are strict criteria of intractability (disabling seizure activity despite optimal medical therapy), there are also degrees of intractability.

Surgical Intervention for Seizure Control

Consideration must sometimes be given to surgical intervention to achieve seizure control. The literature is confusing on this topic, and is rarely specific about the type

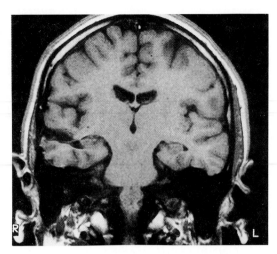

Figure 6. This 34-year-old male presented with partial complex seizures, which were moderately difficult to control. Seizures have persisted despite excellent resection of a single CM within the right temporal lobe. It is possible that the seizure disorder was not related to the CM, or that additional resection of temporal lobe parenchyma would have rendered this patient seizurefree.

of surgical intervention and/or the spectrum of seizure disorders prior to surgical intervention. In general, it is agreed that surgical excision of the lesion improves seizure control in the majority of patients.* Yet, the outcome of specific surgical interventions for cases with truly intractable epilepsy continues to be debated. The surgical outcome of lesion excision for patients with a single seizure or rare seizures cannot be used to justify the same surgical intervention as for patients with truly intractable epilepsy.

Several studies have shown that lesion excision is necessary for seizure control in the majority of patients where the lesion is shown to be responsible for the seizure disorder.[2] It also is well documented that lesion excision alone is not always sufficient for seizure control, especially in patients with truly intractable epilepsy (Figure 6). The natural history of the seizure disorder following excision of the lesion is not well documented, and there are cases of "gradual rundown" of seizures over several months and years following

---

*References 2,10,13,16,18,22,29,31,33,53,60–62,73

lesion excision.[15] Outcome of surgical intervention is complex, and may change over time. It is strongly influenced by the specific type and degree of preoperative seizure disorder and the exact type of surgical intervention.

Lesion Surgery Versus Epilepsy Surgery

Lesion excision alone is likely to result in excellent postoperative control of seizure activity in many patients. The likelihood of postoperative seizure control following simple lesion excision is greater in patients with less intractable preoperative epilepsy, and also in patients with extratemporal lesions.[7] It is not known if duration of seizures prior to surgery influences the effectiveness of lesion excision.

Many cases with persistent intractable seizures following lesion excision have involved lesions in the temporal lobe (see Figure 6).[7] Some of these patients were rendered seizurefree by additional resection of epileptogenic brain in the same region. It is presumed that in these cases the brain around the CM was irreversibly kindled so as to remain epileptogenic despite lesion resection.* The likelihood of this phenomenon appears to be greater in patients with temporal lobe lesions.[7,12,13,33,64] Resection at first operation of epileptogenic brain in addition to the lesion may accomplish seizure control, sparing the patient a second surgical intervention.

There are other limitations to simple lesion excision for epilepsy associated with CMs. As indicated in our own experience and from numerous published cases, a possibility exists that the visualized lesion is not responsible for the seizure disorder. In many instances of multiple lesions it is not possible to "guess" which lesion is in fact epileptogenic (see Figure 3). Patients with CMs may also harbor microscopic telangiectasia elsewhere in the brain, which may not be visualized on imaging studies

*References 7,11,12,13,15,16,18,22,24,25, 33,41,42,43,63,70,73

but may be epileptogenic. These are not theoretic considerations, but could result in unsatisfactory and possibly dangerous clinical outcomes if the wrong operation was performed. Patients with CM and possible epileptogenicity in the contralateral temporal lobe may have disastrous neurocognitive outcomes if the "wrong lobe or lesion" is resected.

For these reasons, we review patients with CMs according to the severity of their seizure disorder. Patients with well-controlled seizures are not considered for lesion excision unless there is indication for lesion excision other than for seizure control. We do not believe that the risk of surgical intervention for any lesion is warranted in the setting of well-controlled epilepsy unless there exists another indication for lesion excision.

Patients with epilepsy that is difficult to control, but not truly intractable or disabling, fall into a "gray zone." An abbreviated electrophysiologic workup is often performed so as to define the epileptogenic lesion. If the epileptogenic CM is identified with certainty and is easily accessible to resection with minimal risk, the patient may be offered the option of lesion excision with the aim of improved seizure control. The majority of patients operated on for this indication benefit from improved seizure outcome following seizure excision.

Patients with truly intractable epilepsy deserve a different consideration. In these patients, the objective of surgery is solely or primarily to realize seizure control. In our opinion, all such patients should undergo sufficient preoperative electrophysiologic evaluation so as to ensure that the intractable seizure disorder is related primarily to one or more CMs. If the CM is located within a general noneloquent brain region, excision of the lesion and surrounding brain would be recommended. In the temporal lobe, a modified temporal lobectomy would generally be undertaken so as to include the lesion and the mesiotemporal structures (unless there is neuropsychologic contraindication against such resection). For example, a patient with highly functional verbal memory would not undergo resection of extensive left temporal lobe structures beyond the structural lesion if that temporal lobe was responsible for his verbal memory function. We would be more likely to consider resection of mesiotemporal structures if the patient's temporal lobe was dysfunctional. Because of these considerations, we recommend extensive preoperative evaluation as with other patients undergoing epilepsy surgery.*

In these same situations, it may be acceptable to offer the patient resection of the lesion and surrounding gliotic brain tissue without additional resection of brain parenchyma at the first procedure.[7] However, the patient must be informed of the possibility of persistent seizures following this operation, and that further brain resection could minimize this risk or could be required as a staged operation. The patient would often have a strong choice in this regard, taking into consideration the risk and cost of a staged procedure versus the equally small risk of additional primary resection of epileptogenic brain parenchyma.

In patients where there is any question whatsoever about the relationship of a CM to the intractable seizure disorder, the patient should not undergo empiric lesion resection with the remote hope that intractable epilepsy might resolve. While there is a possibility that this outcome might be achieved with empiric lesion resection, there may be frequent clinical disappointments as well as occasional significant morbidity related to resection of the wrong lesion or a wrong region of the brain.

Several major epilepsy centers have followed the above strategy, especially with regard to mapping and resection of epileptogenic tissue associated with CMs.[2,7,13,15,22,29–31,33,73] Published results from these centers confirm a greater than 90% likelihood of a seizurefree outcome with this surgical strategy.

---

*References 1,2,6,13,15,22–24,32,33,37,38,44,56,73

Our results at the Cleveland Clinic Foundation are in agreement with these reports. Of 15 cases of CMs operated on strictly for intractable epilepsy, 11 had complete lesion resection and excision of the epileptogenic zone; 8 of these patients are totally seizure-free and 3 have significantly improved seizure frequency (greater than 90%) for more than 1 year after surgery. Of 4 cases with incomplete resection of the epileptogenic zone, only 1 patient is seizurefree, 2 have significantly improved (greater than 90%) seizures, and 1 patient has unchanged seizures.

Summary

The spectrum of seizure disorders associated with CMs of the brain is highly variable. This is in part due to the great variability in lesion location, size, clinical behavior, and multiplicity. It is also due in part to host-related predisposition and to environmental factors influencing susceptibility to epilepsy. A seizure disorder may range from single, rare, or well-controlled seizures to medically intractable and disabling epilepsy.

Seizures are most likely partial or focal in type, with secondary propagation into limbic structures (clinical manifestation as partial complex seizures) and/or secondary generalization. Electroclinical scenarios are highly variable, often involving a variety of seizure propagation pathways, and often difficult to define by scalp recording alone. The relationship of the seizure disorder to an individual CM is not always evident or clear-cut, especially in situations of apparent multifocal epileptogenicity or multiple lesions.

While medical therapy can be highly effective at controlling seizures in many cases, other patients will gradually develop intractability to maximal medical therapy or will develop unacceptable side effects of anticonvulsant therapy. Lesion excision can greatly improve seizure control, and may be more effective if it includes the gliotic hemosiderin-stained brain surrounding the lesion. In patients with truly intractable epilepsy, and notably in patients with temporal lobe lesions, lesion excision alone may not be sufficient for seizure control. Mapping and resection of additional epileptogenic brain results in excellent postoperative seizure control in all but rare cases. Resection of additional epileptogenic brain may be carried out as a primary procedure (in conjunction with lesion resection) or as a second operation (following failure of simple lesion excision).

References

1. Awad IA, Nayel M. Epilepsy surgery: introduction and overview. *Clin Neurosurg.* 1992;38:493–513.

2. Awad IA, Rosenfeld J, Ahl J, et al. Intractable epilepsy and structural lesions of the brain: mapping, resection strategies, and seizure outcome. *Epilepsia.* 1991;32:179–186.

3. Becker DH, Townsend JJ, Kramer RA, et al. Occult cerebrovascular malformations: a series of 18 histologically verified cases with negative angiography. *Brain.* 1979;102:249–287.

4. Bell BA, Kendall BE, Symon L. Angiographically occult arteriovenous malformations of the brain. *J Neurol Neurosurg Psychiatry.* 1978;41:1057–1064.

5. Bicknell JM, Carlow TJ, Kornfeld M, et al. Familial cavernous angiomas. *Arch Neurol.* 1978;35:746–749.

6. Black PMcL, Ronner SF. Cortical mapping for defining the limits of tumor resection. *Neurosurgery.* 1987;20:914–919.

7. Cascino GD, Kelly PJ, Sharbrough FW, et al. Long-term efficacy of stereotactic lesionectomy in intractable partial epilepsy. *Epilepsia.* 1991;32 (suppl 3):87. Abstract.

8. Cohen HC, Tucker WS, Humphreys RP, et al. Angiographically cryptic histologically verified cerebrovascular malformations. *Neurosurgery.* 1982;10:704–714.

9. Commission on Classification and Terminology of the International League Against Epilepsy. Proposal for revised classification of epilepsies and epileptic syndromes. *Epilepsia.* 1989;30:389–399.

10. Crawford PM, West CR, Shaw MDM, et al. Cerebral arteriovenous malformations and epilepsy: factors in the development of epilepsy. *Epilepsia.* 1986;27:270–275.

11. Crowell RM. Distant effects of a focal epileptogenic process. *Brain Res.* 1970;18:137–154.

12. Dam AM. Epilepsy and neuron loss in the hippocampus. *Epilepsia.* 1980;21:617–629.

13. Drake Jr, Hoffman HJ, Kobayashi J, et al. Surgical management of children with temporal lobe epilepsy and mass lesions. *Neurosurgery.* 1987;21:792–797.

14. El-Gohary EM, Tomita T, Guiterrez FA. Angiographically occult vascular malformations in childhood. *Neurosurgery.* 1978;20:759–766.

15. Engel J Jr, Driver MV, Falconer MA. Electrophysiological correlates of pathology and surgical results in temporal lobe epilepsy. *Brain.* 1975;98:129–156.

16. Estes ML, Morris HH III, Lüders H, et al. Surgery for intractable epilepsy: clinicopathologic correlates in 60 cases. *Cleve Clin J Med.* 1988;55:441–447.

17. Falconer MA. Genetic and related etiological factors in temporal lobe epilepsy: a review. *Epilepsia.* 1971;12:13–31.

18. Falconer MA, Kennedy WA. Epilepsy due to small focal temporal lesions with bilateral independent spike-discharging foci: a study of seven cases relieved by operation. *J Neurol Neurosurg Psychiatry.* 1961;24:205–212.

19. Feindel W. The influence of cerebral steal: demonstration of fluorescent angiography and focal cerebral blood flow measurement. In: Pia HW, Gleaves EG, Zierski J, eds. *Cerebral Angiomas. Advances in Diagnosis and Therapy.* New York, NY: Springer-Verlag; 1975:87–99.

20. Giombini S, Morello G. Cavernous angiomas of the brain: account of fourteen personal cases and review of the literature. *Acta Neurochir (Wien).* 1978;40:61–82.

21. Golden JB, Kramer RA. The angiographically occult cerebrovascular malformation: report of three cases. *J Neurosurg.* 1978;48:292–296.

22. Goldring S, Gregorie EM. Surgical management of epilepsy using epidural recordings to localize the seizure focus: review of 100 cases. *J Neurosurg.* 1984;60:457–466.

23. Gotman J, Gloor P, Schaul N. Comparison of traditional reading of the EEG and automatic recognition of interictal epileptic activity. *Electroencephalogr Clin Neurophysiol.* 1978;44:48–60.

24. Gupta PC, Dharampaul, Pathak SN, et al. Secondary epileptogenic EEG focus in temporal lobe epilepsy. *Epilepsia.* 1973;14:423–426.

25. Hanna GR. Morphological changes in primary and secondary epileptic foci. In: Mayersdorf A, Schmidt RP, eds. *Secondary Epileptogenesis.* New York, NY: Raven Press; 1982:115–130.

26. Hashim ASM, Asakura T, Koichi U, et al. Angiographically occult arteriovenous malformations. *Surg Neurol.* 1985;23:431–439.

27. Heinz ER, Heinz TR, Radtke R, et al. Efficacy of MR vs. CT in epilepsy. *AJR.* 1989;152:347–352.

28. Houtteville JP, ed. Les cavernomas intra-crâniens: table ronde. *Neurochirurgie.* 1989;35:73–131.

29. Jabbari B, Huott AD, Di Chiro G, et al. Surgically correctable lesions detected by CT in 143 patients with chronic epilepsy. *Surg Neurol.* 1978;10:319–322.

30. Jabbari B, Huott AD, Di Chiro G, et al. Surgically correctable lesions solely detected by CT scan in adult-onset chronic epilepsy. *Ann Neurol.* 1980;7:344–347.

31. Leblanc R, Feindel W, Ethier R. Epilepsy from cerebral arteriovenous malformations. *Can J Neurol Sci*. 1983;10:91–95.

32. Lesser RP, Lüders H, Dinner DS, et al. The location of speech and writing functions in the frontal language area: results of extraoperative cortical stimulation. *Brain*. 1984;107:275–291.

33. Lévesque MF, Nakasato N, Vinters HV, et al. Surgical treatment of limbic epilepsy associated with extrahippocampal lesions: the problem of dual pathology. *J Neurosurg*. 1991;75:364–370.

34. Little JR, Awad IA, Jones SC, et al. Vascular pressures and cortical blood flow in cavernous angioma of the brain. *J Neurosurg*. 1990;73:555–559.

35. Lobato RD, Perez C, Rivas JJ, et al. Clinical, radiological, and pathological spectrum of angiographically occult intracranial vascular malformations: analysis of 21 cases and review of the literature. *J Neurosurg*. 1988;68:518–531.

36. Lüders H, Awad IA. Conceptual considerations. In: Lüders H, ed. *Epilepsy Surgery*. New York, NY: Raven Press; 1992:51–62.

37. Lüders H, Lesser RP, Dinner DS, et al. Commentary: chronic intracranial recording and stimulation with subdural electrodes. In: Engel JP Jr, ed. *Surgical Management of the Epilepsies*. New York, NY: Raven Press; 1987:297–321.

38. Lüders H, Lesser RP, Hahn JF, et al. Cortical somatosensory evoked potentials in response to hand stimulation. *J Neurosurg*. 1983;58:885–894.

39. McCormick WF. The pathology of vascular "arteriovenous" malformations. *J Neurosurg*. 1966;24:807–816.

40. McGahan JP, Dublin AB, Hill RP. The evaluation of seizure disorders by computerized tomography. *J Neurosurg*. 1979;50:328–332.

41. McNamara JO. Kindling model of epilepsy. In: Delgado-Escueta AV, Ward AA Jr, Woodbury DM, et al, eds. *Basic Mechanisms of the Epilepsies. Molecular and Cellular Approaches. Advances in Neurology. Vol. 44.* New York, NY: Raven Press; 1986:303–318.

42. Morrell F. Secondary epileptogenesis in man. *Arch Neurol*. 1985;42:318–335.

43. Morrell F, Whisler WW. Secondary epileptogenic lesions in man: prediction of the results of surgical excision of the primary focus. In: Canger R, Angeleri F, Penry JK, eds. *Advances in Epileptology: XIth Epilepsy International Symposium*. New York, NY: Raven Press; 1980:123–128.

44. Morris HH III, Lüders H, Hahn JF, et al. Neurophysiological techniques as an aid to surgical treatment of primary brain tumors. *Ann Neurol*. 1986;19:559–567.

45. Ogilvy CS, Heros RC, Ojemann RJ, et al. Angiographically occult arteriovenous malformations. *J Neurosurg*. 1988;69:350–355.

46. Ogilvy CS, Heros RC. Angiographically occult intracranial vascular malformations. *J Neurosurg*. 1988;69:960–962. Letters to the editor.

47. Otten P, Pizzolato GP, Rilliet B, et al. A propos de 131 cas d'angiomes caverneux (cavernomes) du S.N.C., repérés par l'analyse rétrospective de 24,535 autopsies. *Neurochirurgie*. 1989;35:82–83.

48. Pozzati E, Padovani R, Morrone B, et al. Cerebral cavernous angiomas in children. *J Neurosurg*. 1980;53:826–832.

49. Rigamonti D, Drayer BP, Johnson PC, et al. The MRI appearance of CMs (angiomas). *J Neurosurg*. 1987;67:518–524.

50. Rigamonti D, Hadley MN, Drayer BP, et al. Cerebral cavernous malformations: incidence and familial occurrence. *N Engl J Med*. 1988;319:343–347.

51. Rigamonti D, Johnson PC, Spetzler RF, et al. Vascular malformations and MRI. *Ann Neurol*. 1988;23:208–209. Letter.

52. Rigamonti D, Spetzler RF. The association of venous and CMs: report of four cases and discussion of the pathophysiological, diagnostic, and therapeutic implications. *Acta Neurochir (Wien)*. 1988;92:100–105.

53. Robinson JR, Awad IA, Little JR. Natural history of the cavernous angioma. *J Neurosurg*. 1991;75:709–714.

54. Russel DS, Rubinstein LJ, Lumsden CE. Tumors and hamartomas of the blood vessels. In: Russel DS, Rubenstein LJ, Lumsden CE, eds. *Pathology of Tumours of the Nervous System*. London: Edward Arnold Publishers; 1959:72–92.

55. Simard JM, Garcia-Bengochea F, Ballinger WE Jr, et al. Cavernous angioma: a review of 126 collected and 12 new clinical cases. *Neurosurgery*. 1986;18:162–172.

56. Spencer DD, Spencer SS, Mattson RH, et al. Intracerebral masses in patients with intractable partial epilepsy. *Neurology*. 1984;34:432–436.

57. Sperling MR, Cahan LD, Brown WJ. Relief of seizures from a predominantly posterior temporal tumor with anterior temporal lobectomy. *Epilepsia*. 1989;30:559–563.

58. Spetzler RF. Cavernous angiomas and AVMs. *J Neurosurg*. 1989;70:500. Letters to the editor.

59. Steiger HJ, Markwalder TM, Reulen HJ. Clinicopathological relations of cerebral cavernous angiomas: observations in eleven cases. *Neurosurgery*. 1987;21:879–884.

60. Steiger HJ, Tew JM Jr. Hemorrhage and epilepsy in cryptic cerebrovascular malformations. *Arch Neurol*. 1984;41:722–724.

61. Stein BM, Wolpert SM. Arteriovenous malformations of the brain, I: current concepts and treatment. *Arch Neurol*. 1980;37:1–5.

62. Stein BM, Wolpert SM. Arteriovenous malformations of the brain, II: current concepts and treatment. *Arch Neurol*. 1980;37:69–75.

63. Spielmeyer W. The anatomic substratum of the convulsive state. *Arch Neurol Psychiatry*. 1930;23:869–875.

64. Sutula T, Cascino G, Cavazos J, et al. Mossy fiber synaptic reorganization in the epileptic human temporal lobe. *Ann Neurol*. 1989;26:321–330.

65. Tagle P, Huete I, Méndez J, et al. Intracranial cavernous angioma: presentation and management. *J Neurosurg*. 1986;64:720–723.

66. Torres F, Jacome D. Secondary epileptogenesis in the human. In: Mayersdorf A, Schmidt RP, eds. *Secondary Epileptogenesis.* New York, NY: Raven Press; 1982:15–26.

67. Vasquero J, Leunda G, Martínez R, et al. Cavernomas of the brain. *Neurosurgery.* 1983;12:208–210.

68. Vasquero J, Salazar J, Martínez P, et al. Cavernomas of the central nervous system: clinical syndromes, CT scan diagnosis, and prognosis after surgical treatment in 25 cases. *Acta Neurochir (Wien).* 1987;85:29–33.

69. Waltimo O. The relationship of size, density, and localization of intracranial arteriovenous malformations to the type of initial symptom. *J Neurol Sci.* 1973;19:13–19.

70. Westmoreland BF, Hanna GR, Bass NH. Cortical alterations in zones of secondary epileptogenesis: a neurophysiologic, morphologic and microchemical correlation study in the albino rat. *Brain Res.* 1972;43:485–499.

71. Wharen RE Jr, Scheithauer BW, Laws ER Jr. Thrombosed arteriovenous malformations of the brain. *J Neurosurg.* 1982;57:520–526.

72. Wilkins RH. Natural history of intracranial vascular malformations: a review. *Neurosurgery.* 1985;16:421–430.

73. Wyllie E, Lüders H, Morris HH III, et al. Clinical outcome after complete or partial cortical resection for intractable epilepsy. *Neurology.* 1987;37:1634–1641.

Chapter 6

Cavernous Malformations and Hemorrhage

Daniel L. Barrow, MD, and Ali Krisht, MD

Improvements in neuroimaging techniques have enhanced our recognition of a variety of central nervous system (CNS) disorders. These technological innovations have had a particular impact on our understanding and management of intracranial lesions presenting with hemorrhage.

At the turn of the century, a variety of congenital vascular malformations were recognized as the cause of spontaneous intracranial hemorrhage. The etiology of hemorrhage was confirmed through autopsy studies and later by examination of surgical specimens. The introduction of cerebral angiography into clinical practice provided a means of diagnosing intracranial vascular malformations prior to surgical exploration. There remained, however, a subgroup of vascular malformations that could not be demonstrated by cerebral angiography and were therefore categorized as "cryptic" or "angiographically occult."[1,2,5,10,16,18,29,38] Included in this subset were small or partially thrombosed arteriovenous malformations (AVMs), venous malformations, cavernous malformations (CMs), and capillary malformations. As discussed in Chapter 4, the majority of CMs are not readily apparent on angiography. Clearly, the appellation of "angio-graphically occult vascular malformations" to all lesions that share only the characteristic of angiographic invisibility is a misnomer for such a diverse group.

The development of computed tomography (CT) provided a means of imaging an intracerebral hemorrhage and its relationship to the surrounding brain. CT permitted some of the small, angiographically occult AVMs to be identified as enhancing lesions related to the hemorrhage; and some CMs were directly apparent on CT as well. However, it was not until the introduction of magnetic resonance imaging (MRI) in clinical practice that CMs were readily imaged (Figure 1). This elegant imaging technique provides exquisite images of CMs that are quite characteristic and nearly pathognomonic. Since the advent of MRI, many more CMs are being identified than previously, which has shaped considerably our understanding of the natural history and pathophysiology of these lesions. As a result of the widespread use of MRI and its accuracy in identifying CMs, our ability to detect these lesions has, for the present, surpassed our understanding of their natural history.

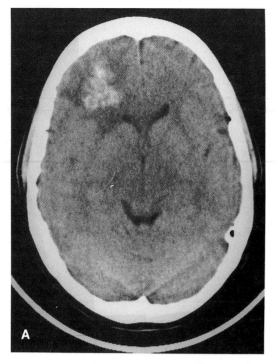

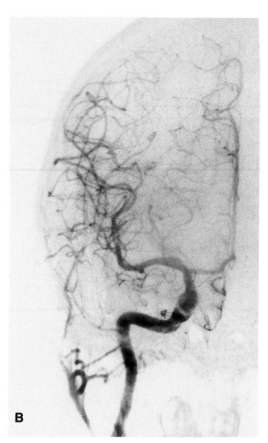

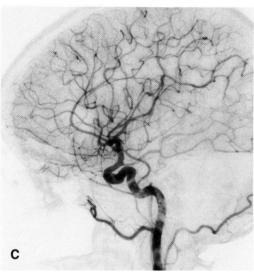

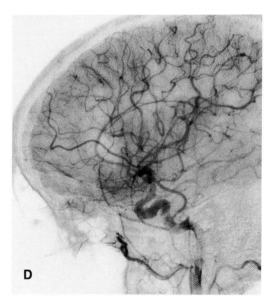

Figure 1. **(A)** Axial nonenhanced CT demonstrates an intraparenchymal hematoma in the right frontal lobe. **(B)** Anteroposterior, **(C)** early, and **(D)** late arterial phase of right carotid angiogram. There is no clear abnormality in the angiogram to suggest the cause of hemorrhage. **(E)** Axial T2-weighted MRI. **(F)** Coronal and **(G)** sagittal T1-weighted MRI of lesion demonstrating the typical appearance of a CM.

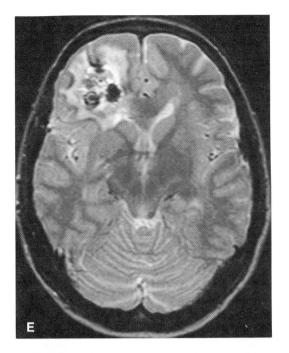

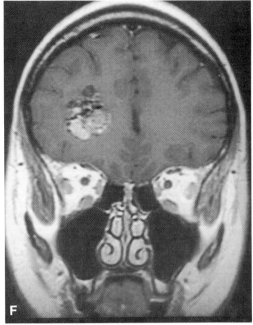

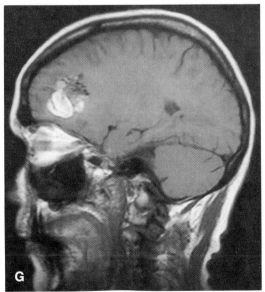

Incidence

Hemorrhage is the most serious conse-quence of a CM. Thus, prevention of hem-orrhage, initial or recurrent, is a common indication for surgical treatment. The clini-cian's knowledge of the incidence of hem-orrhage from a CM is critical when coun-seling an individual patient.

Older literature from the pre-MRI era may overestimate the incidence of clinically significant hemorrhage from CMs, as those patients would most likely come to clinical attention and undergo surgical removal of the hematoma and malformation. CT and angiography are much less sensitive in detecting CMs; and patients presenting with seizures or headaches would not be readily identified.

The reported incidence of hemorrhage from CMs has declined, probably due to a number of factors. Earlier reports included CMs in the group of "angiographically occult" vascular malformations. This group included small AVMs, which may have a much higher incidence of bleeding.[1,2,5,10,18,38] For example, the review by Wakai et al re-ported the incidence of hemorrhage from angiographically occult vascular malforma-tions as high as 65%.[38]

In more recent reports on studies treat-ing CMs as a separate group, the highest incidence of hemorrhage at the initial pre-sentation was 36.6%[40] (varying between 0.7% and 36.6%). The advent of MRI brought many more asymptomatic and

Table 1. **Incidence of Hemorrhage from Cavernous Malformations**

Source	Year	Total Number of Patients	Patients with Hemorrhage (%)
Yamasaki et al[40]	1986	30	11 (36.6%)
Tagle et al[34]	1986	13	4 (30.8%)
Simard et al[30]	1986	138	40 (29.0%)
Steiger et al[31]	1987	11	2 (18.0%)
Farmer et al[8]	1988	31	3 (9.7%)
Weber et al[39]	1989	34	3 (11.3%)
Curling and Kelly[7]	1990	32	3 (9.5%)*
Robinson et al[27]	1991	57	7 (12.3%)**

*An estimated 3% per year risk of bleeding was calculated assuming lesions are congenital with a uniform annual risk of bleeding during life.
**Data allows calculation of a 3% per year risk of bleeding based on the assumptions of Curling and Kelly. Among lesions followed prospectively following diagnosis, there was a 0.7% per year risk of new overt hemorrhage.

relatively asymptomatic lesions to clinical attention. In the past, these lesions were infrequently diagnosed unless they were the source of a clinically significant hemorrhage. Table 1 shows the declining incidence of hemorrhage from CMs reported during the last few years.

When discussing hemorrhage from CMs, one must distinguish between chronic, subclinical microhemorrhages, or diapedesis of blood from the lesion, and acute, clinically significant hemorrhages. MRI is so sensitive in imaging blood and its breakdown products that the presence of some blood constituents is virtually universal on the MRIs of CMs (Figure 2).

The significance of this microhemorrhage is uncertain. Several studies recorded the incidence of old hemorrhage associated with CMs.* These hemorrhages are usually microscopic and subclinical. Histologic evidence of old hemorrhage was found in almost all patients studied and appears to occur very early in life. Pozzati et al reported 5 cases of CMs in children, the youngest being 10 years old.[23] Hemosiderin discoloration of the surrounding brain, consistent with an old hemorrhage, was noted in 3 of the patients. In another report, Tung et al studied 13 patients with

*References 3–5,10,14,16,18,21,23,30,31,35,37,38,40

recurrent hemorrhage from "occult vascular malformations"[35]; 7 of the 9 surgical specimens were CMs, and evidence of old hemorrhage was present in all the specimens.

MRI findings in patients with asymptomatic CMS confirm that subclinical microhemorrhages occur in almost all patients.[8,14,21,22,25] Rigamonti et al reported on the MRI findings of 27 CMs and found decreased signal intensity on the T2-weighted images in 100% of the cases.[25] This signal abnormality was consistent with hemosiderin deposition in the surrounding brain, secondary to the old microhemorrhages.

Earlier reports of CMs included other angiographically occult vascular malformations[1,2,5,10,16,29,38]; as a result, the incidence of hemorrhage in CMs alone was not well studied. Wakai et al reviewed 159 cases of angiographically occult vascular lesions.[38] Hemorrhage occurred in 65% of the cases. CMs constituted 37% of the cases, but the exact incidence of hemorrhage in the group of CMs was not given. In another study, Lobato et al reviewed 254 cases of angiographically occult vascular malformations.[16] CT scans were obtained in 189 patients; and hematoma was found in 48% of the scanned patients. CMs constituted 38% (81 cases) of the total number of cases, but the incidence of hemorrhage due to these lesions was not given.

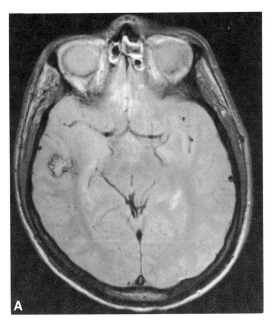
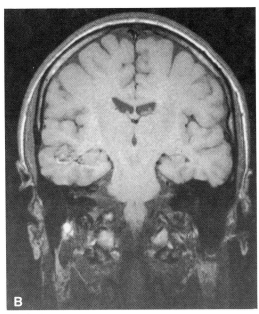

Figure 2. **(A)** Axial and **(B)** coronal MRI demonstrating a surgically proven CM in a patient who presented with a seizure disorder. Despite the low intensity signal surrounding the lesion, suggesting the presence of hemosiderin, this patient had no clinical evidence of a prior hemorrhage.

Farmer et al studied 31 patients with histologically verified intracerebral CMs.[8] Intracranial hemorrhage occurred in 3 patients (9.7%). In another reported series, Curling and Kelly found a 9.5% (3 patients) rate of hemorrhage in 32 patients with CMs.[7] In a review of 138 cases of CMs in the literature, Simard et al reported clinical evidence of hemorrhage in 29% (40 patients) of the cases.[30] Yamasaki et al studied 30 patients with intracerebral and orbital CMs and reported hemorrhage in 36.6% (11 of the 38 cases).[40] Robinson et al[27] retrospectively reviewed 14,035 MRI studies and identified 76 lesions that had the typical appearance of a CM in 66 patients. Follow-up studies in 86% of the cases over a mean period of 26 months provided 143 lesion-years of clinical survey. There was a clinically significant hemorrhage in 7 of the 57 symptomatic patients and only 1 overt hemorrhage during the follow-up interval for an annualized bleeding rate of 0.7% per lesion per year. Table 1 summarizes the incidence of hemorrhage in the various reported series. It must be noted that these various series included vastly different patient selection criteria and varying definitions of "hemorrhage."

Rebleeding from a CM may occur at any time from days to years following the initial bleed.[9,23,24,32,35] In Giombini and Morello's series, a rebleed occurred in one-third of the cases initially presenting with hemorrhage (4 out of 12).[9] Tung et al reported a rebleed in 13 patients with angiographically occult vascular malformations[35]; 7 of the 9 operated cases were confirmed to be CMs. Pozzati reported a child with several rebleeds from a surgically confirmed CM.[23]

The hemorrhages that occur with CMs are usually parenchymal. CMs may present with a subarachnoid hemorrhage,[35,36,40] although this is not usual. Ueda et al reported a patient with a CM of the cauda equina[36] who presented with a sudden headache and low-back pain and was found to have a subarachnoid hemorrhage. Zentner et al[41] reported a patient with a

CM of the optic tract who presented with an intracerebral and subarachnoid hemorrhage.

Pathophysiology

The pathophysiologic factors that lead to hemorrhage from CMs are not well understood. Available radiologic and pathologic data suggest that microscopic and clinically undetected hemorrhage occurs in the majority of cases. This may lead to local changes in the surrounding brain, which may, in some cases, act as a seizure focus.[16,23] The mechanisms by which microhemorrhages occur, and the reason why they are usually self-limited are not fully understood. Little et al studied the hemodynamic aspects of CMs in 5 adult patients.[15] The mean pressure in the lesion was 38.2 ± 0.5 mm Hg in patients operated in the supine position and 7 mm Hg in the 1 patient who was operated in the sitting position. These authors concluded that CMs are low-pressure lesions with a slow circulation. This "low driving pressure" may explain the self-limited bleeds that remain, in the majority of cases, at a microscopic level.

Clinically significant hemorrhages are the more sizable bleeds that present with acute symptoms. CMs may enlarge over time[20,22,30]; and as the lesion increases in size, surrounding mass effect may make the adjacent brain less tolerant of a hemorrhage and clinically more significant. The precise factors that trigger the bleed are unknown as is the reason why some CMs enlarge without a clinically significant hemorrhage.[22]

Pozzati et al described CMs as dynamic and aggressive lesions.[22] Steiger et al report that the lesions appear to develop internal hemorrhages, which leads to the formation of an internal hematoma capsule.[31] This newly formed membrane reinforces the malformation capsule, as it organizes and develops a neocapillary network. By osmotically attracting water, it may then behave in a similar fashion to the membrane of a chronic subdural hematoma, leading to enlargement of the malformation. Steiger et al suggest that the degree of encapsulation may protect against rupture and intracranial hemorrhage.[31] Likewise, a defect in the capsule would behave as a weak-point and a potential site for bleeding.

In addition to the properties of the malformation capsule, hemodynamic changes may contribute to hemorrhage. In the study by Little et al,[15] an increase in pressure within the CM occurred after jugular vein compression—an indication that hemodynamic changes result in immediate and direct changes in the pressures recorded in the malformation. It seems plausible that a weakened capsule, if associated with the proper hemodynamic changes, could result in a hemorrhage. Although these pathophysiologic suggestions are valid, the exact mechanism by which hemorrhage from a CM occurs remains an enigma.

It may be useful in the analysis of reported cases and in subsequent clinical reports on CMs to differentiate among types of hemorrhage. The "slow ooze" is essentially a characteristic feature of all CMs including asymptomatic and quiescent lesions. Other lesions undergo intralesional expansion by thrombosis or contained hemorrhages. Gross hemorrhage beyond the confines of the lesion is quite rare, but may represent an important clinical phenomenon with overt clinical symptomology and with possible propensity to rebleed.[27]

Clinical Presentation

Symptoms from CMs, including hemorrhage, occur with the highest incidence between the second and third decades of life. Males and females are equally affected.[40] The clinical effects of a hemorrhage from a CM depend on a variety of factors, including the location and size of the bleed. Old microhemorrhages are often clinically silent and are usually detected incidentally on MRI.[14,21] These smaller hemorrhages may result in a seizure disorder or, if repetitive, may result in a progressive neurologic deficit. A discussion of the subgroup of patients presenting with seizure disorders is well covered in Chapter 5. The clinical presentation varies with the location of the bleed. CMs may occur anywhere in the CNS, including the spinal cord. They may be located above and below the tentorium in proportion to the volume of the brain above and below the tentorium.[9] In the supratentorial region, they are usually located in the white matter and occasionally surface to the cortex (Figure 3). Hemorrhage from supratentorial lesions are usually intraparenchymal and only occasionally dissect into the ventricles or the subarachnoid space,[24] depending on the depth of the malformation.[24,37,38] The next most common location of supratentorial hemorrhage from these lesions is in the region of the basal ganglia and the thalamus.

The clinical presentation is acute but usually not as dramatic as the hemorrhages occurring from intracranial aneurysms or even AVMs. They usually present with a sudden onset of headache that may be followed by a focal neurologic deficit. In the review of angiographically occult vascular malformations by Wakai et al, a sudden headache or a focal deficit with or without a change in the level of consciousness occurred in 70 of 101 patients.[38] Depending on the size and location of the hematoma, there may be associated changes in the level of consciousness.[9,30,31,38-40] Not infrequently, supratentorial hemorrhage from a CM may mimic the clinical presentation of a brain tumor (Figure 4). Murakami et al reported a patient with a large frontal lesion and no focal neurologic deficit.[20] The patient was later found to have an encapsulated hematoma associated with a CM. Pozzati et al reported 3 similar cases in which the CM enlarged on a follow-up CT scan.[22]

A rare subgroup of supratentorial CMs is located within the optic nerve or chiasm and may be appreciated on MRI. Fewer than 10 histologically confirmed CMs have been reported in this location. The hemorrhage can extend to the subarachnoid space or produce an intracerebral clot. Even small hemorrhages in this region will often result in sudden or progressive visual loss and/or a chiasmal syndrome, depending on the exact location of the lesion.[3,11,12,33,41]

Infratentorial CMs may be located in the cerebellum or the brain stem (Figures 5 and 6).[2,5,6,8,13,28,30,35] Although it has been suggested that posterior fossa CMs have a greater tendency to bleed, the literature does not support this assumption. Curling and Kelly found that CMs appear to have the same likelihood of hemorrhage, irrespective of location.[7] Smaller hemorrhages in critical areas such as the brain stem may be more likely to produce neurologic symptoms than a similar-sized bleed in a more silent area of the brain. Ishikawa et al reviewed nine cerebellar hemorrhages secondary to CMs.[13] Headache, vomiting, ataxia, and nystagmus occurred in all the cases.

Brain stem hemorrhages from CMs are usually located in the pons but may occur in the midbrain or medulla.[5,8,38] They present with vertigo, diplopia, hemiparesis, associated sensory deficits, and changes in the level of consciousness. Occasionally, they produce signs of increased intracranial pressure due to obstructive hydrocephalus, more commonly with lesions located on the surface of the brain stem or the fourth ventricle.[24] CMs in the brain stem frequently present with repeated small hemorrhages that result in acute neurologic deficits, which resolve, often completely. These patients may be misdiagnosed with a demyelinating disorder because of exacerbation and remission of symptoms.

The association of CMs and adjacent but separate venous malformations was recently appreciated.[42] This association has been noted predominantly in the cerebellum, often following a hemorrhage. Angiography will demonstrate the venous malformation but high-resolution MRI is required to image the CM (Figure 7). When a hemorrhage occurs in this situation, it is the CM, not the venous malformation, that is the source of bleeding. Therefore, surgical treatment should include

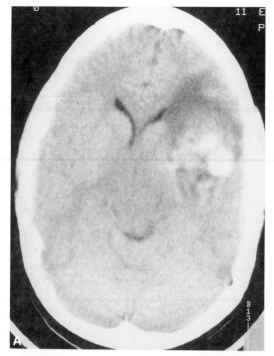

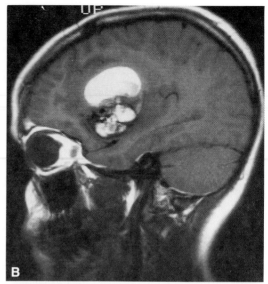

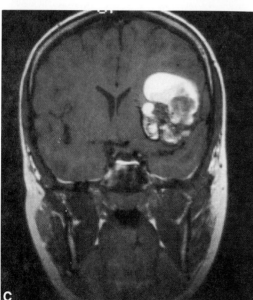

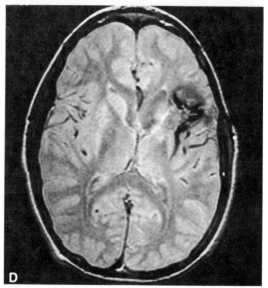

Figure 3. (A) Axial nonenhanced CT demonstrates acute hemorrhage in left sylvian fissure with surrounding edema and mass effect. **(B)** Sagittal and **(C)** coronal T1-weighted MRIs show CM within the left sylvian fissure with associated acute hemorrhage. **(D)** Axial, **(E)** sagittal, and **(F)** coronal T1-weighted postoperative MRIs following removal of CM and associated hematoma; despite postoperative changes, there is no evidence of any residual CM.

complete removal of the hematoma and the CM, but the venous malformation should be left alone. The venous malformation functions as a normal draining vein, and resection will result in catastrophic consequences of venous infarction.

CMs also occur in the spinal cord.[6,28] Spinal cord CMs generally present with an acute or subacute myelopathy.[6] Four of the 5 patients with spinal cord CMs reported by Cosgrove et al[6] presented with acute, lower extremity sensory disturbances very similar

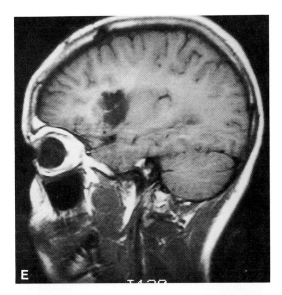

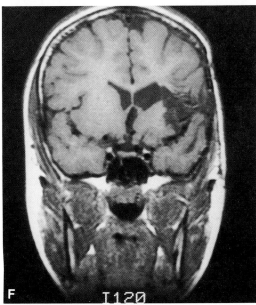

to those seen in acute transverse myelitis. As with brain stem lesions, however, they may also present with a slowly progressive neurologic deficit or an episode of neurologic worsening separated by periods of improvement, suggestive of a demyelinating disorder. These lesions are discussed more completely in Chapter 12.

A recurrent hemorrhage may occur after the initial bleed from a CM.[9,21,24,35,38] These patients present in much the same manner as

patients with a first hemorrhage, and the resulting neurologic deficit may resolve completely. Tung et al found a correlation between the number of recurrent bleeds and the extent of the residual permanent deficit, implying progressive damage to neural tissue with recurrent bleeds.[35]

Outcome

The natural history of CMs has been the subject of several reports.[6,26,27] These authors concur that CMs behave in a more benign manner than previously thought. This is supported by data showing that they have a very low risk of hemorrhage. In their series, Curling and Kelly[7] found the risk of hemorrhage from a CM to be as low as 0.1% per person per year for each lesion. In their study on the natural history, Robinson et al[27] estimated the annual bleeding rate to be 0.7% per year for each lesion.

As noted earlier, some reports grouped CMs with small AVMs under the term "angiographically occult vascular malformations." In general, the outcome of these lesions varied with the location of the lesion. Lobato et al[16] studied the outcome in 195 patients undergoing surgery for angiographically occult vascular malformations. Lesions located in the brain stem carried a 26% mortality, while those located in the cortical region carried a 5% mortality. In the series of Wakai et al,[38] 7 of the 172 patients with angiographically occult vascular malformations died. In 4 of these 7 patients, the lesion was located in the pons.

In reports that studied CMs as a separate group, the outcome after hemorrhage is better. Tung et al[35] found zero mortality from initial and recurrent hemorrhages in 13 patients with CMs. Robinson et al[27] also reported no mortality in 57 cases of symptomatic CMs. Of the 7 patients presenting with evidence of overt bleeding, 6 had good outcomes and only 1 had a poor outcome.

Some evidence in the reported literature suggests that CMs become more aggressive

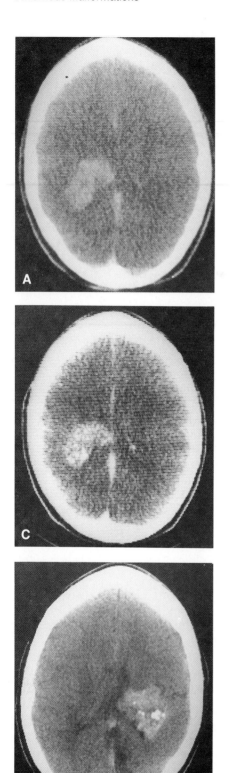

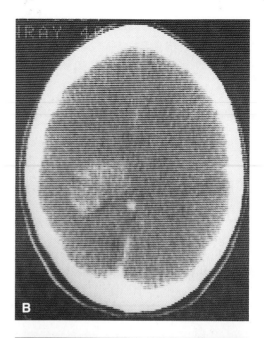

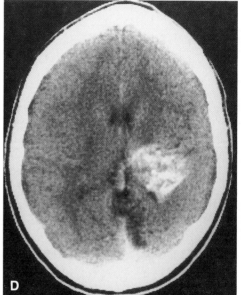

Figure 4. Progressive enlargement of CM over 15-year period. Axial contrast-enhanced CT scans demonstrate left parietal enhancing mass with calcification in **(A)** 1976, **(B)** 1977, **(C)** 1978, **(D)** 1980, **(E)** 1985, and **(F)** 1991. T1-weighted **(G)** axial, **(H)** coronal, and **(I)** sagittal MRIs illustrate this huge CM located in the deep parietal region adjacent to the region of the atrium of the lateral ventricle. At the time of surgery, there were multiple pockets of variably aged hemorrhages that likely were responsible for the progressive enlargement of the lesion. Postoperative **(J)** axial and **(K)** sagittal MRIs document complete removal of the lesion.

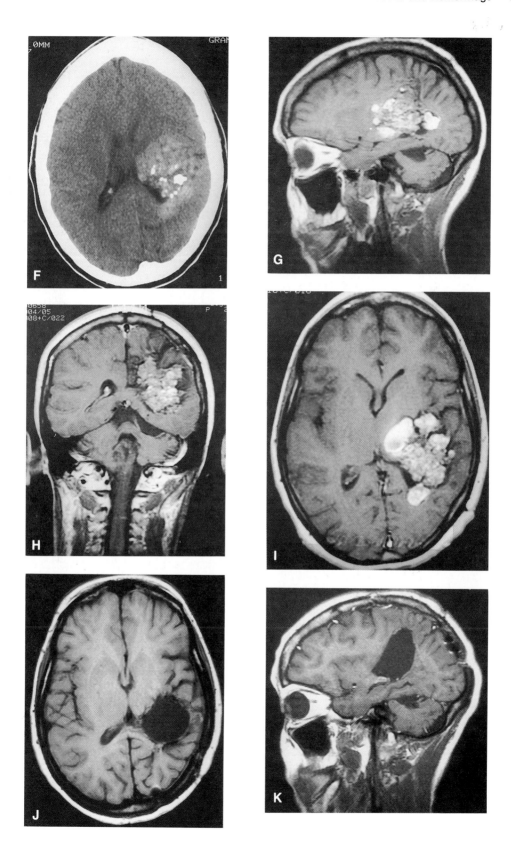

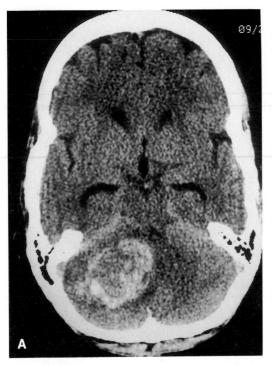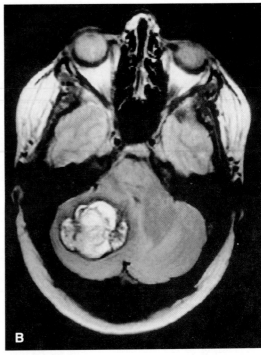

Figure 5. (A) Axial nonenhanced CT demonstrating a large right cerebellar hematoma with compression of the fourth ventricle and associated hydrocephalus. **(B)** Axial MRI reveals lesion with multiple intensities compatible with CM, proven to be such at surgery.

after they bleed. In the study by Giombini and Morello,[9] immediate mortality occurred in 3 of the 12 patients presenting with hemorrhage. A rebleed occurred in 5 patients and was fatal in 2 patients. Tung et al[35] followed 13 patients with a recurrent hemorrhage from CMs. Two-thirds of the patients had more than 1 rebleed; and in 1 patient it was as early as 1 week after the previous bleed. They also found that the extent of the residual permanent deficit correlated with the number of recurrent hemorrhages.

Zimmerman et al reviewed 24 patients with brain stem CMs, 10 of whom had experienced a recent or old hemorrhage.[42] The authors concluded that once symptomatic, CMs of the brain stem tend to cause progressive morbidity from recurrent hemorrhages. They recommend surgical excision when feasible.

Summary

Hemorrhage is the most worrisome consequence of a CM. Our past inability to image these lesions dependably, and their inappropriate classification as angiographically occult vascular malformations, made it difficult to accurately determine the incidence of hemorrhage. Although virtually all CMs are associated with MRI or histologic evidence of microscopic hemorrhage, recent studies suggest that **(1)** the incidence of clinically significant hemorrhage is low, and **(2)** hemorrhages, when they do occur, are associated with a relatively low morbidity and mortality. This morbidity is more significant if the hemorrhage occurs in an eloquent or functionally important region of the CNS, such as the optic pathways or brain stem.

Although the mechanism and the incidence of hemorrhage from CMs are incompletely understood, we believe that a

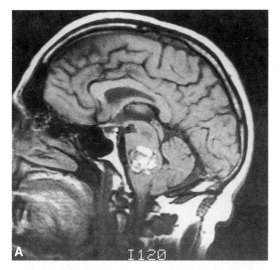

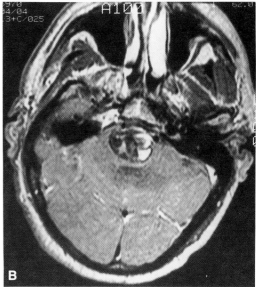

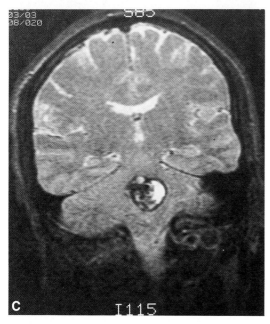

Figure 6. **(A)** Sagittal, **(B)** axial, and **(C)** coronal MRIs demonstrate large pontine CM with varying aged hemorrhage.

References

1. Becker DH, Townsend JJ, Kramer RA, et al. Occult cerebrovascular malformations: a series of 18 histologically verified cases with negative angiography. *Brain.* 1979;102:249–287.

2. Bitoh S, Hasegawa H, Fujiwara M, et al. Angiographically occult vascular malformations causing intracranial hemorrhage. *Surg Neurol.* 1982;17:35–42.

3. Castel JP, Delorges-Kerdiles C, Rivel J. Angiome caverneux du chiasma optique. *Neurochirurgie (Paris).* 1989;35:252–256.

4. Chin D, Harper C. Angiographically occult cerebral vascular malformations with abnormal computed tomography. *Surg Neurol.* 1983;20:138–142.

5. Cohen HCM, Tucker WS, Humphreys RP, et al. Angiographically cryptic histologically verified cerebrovascular malformations. *Neurosurgery.* 1982;10:704–714.

6. Cosgrove GR, Bertrand G, Fontaine S, et al. Cavernous angiomas of the spinal cord. *J Neurosurg.* 1988;68:31–36.

7. Curling OD Jr, Kelly DL Jr. The natural history of intracranial cavernous and venous malformations. *Perspect Neurol Surg.* 1990;1:19–39.

8. Farmer J-P, Cosgrove GR, Villemure J-G, et al. Intracerebral cavernous angiomas. *Neurology.* 1988;38:1699–1704.

9. Giombini S, Morello G. Cavernous angiomas of the brain: account of fourteen personal cases and review of the literature. *Acta Neurochir (Wien).* 1978;40:61–82.

clinically significant hemorrhage or multiple hemorrhages are associated with a poorer prognosis, and surgical excision of a CM that has caused an overt hemorrhage should be strongly considered. If an associated venous malformation is discovered, it is likely that the CM is the source of bleeding; and surgery should be considered for the excision of the CM, but the venous malformation should be left alone.

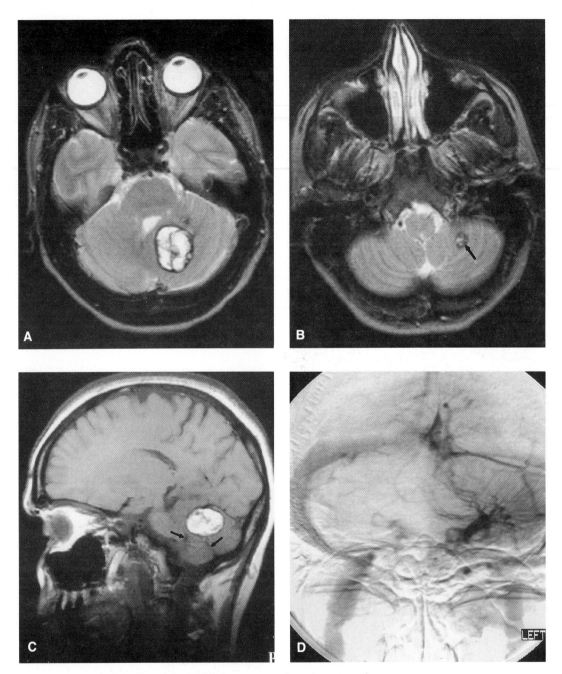

Figure 7A–D. (A) Axial T2-weighted MRI demonstrates large hematoma in
left cerebellar hemisphere, with multiple intensities apparent in the lesion. **(B)**
A second and separate lesion, seen anterior and inferior to hematoma, has
an appearance compatible with a CM (arrow). **(C)** Sagittal T1-weighted MRI
shows hematoma and flow void anterior and inferior to hematoma (arrows).
(D) Anteroposterior and lateral venous phase angiographs (in E) demonstrate
a venous malformation in left cerebellar hemisphere.

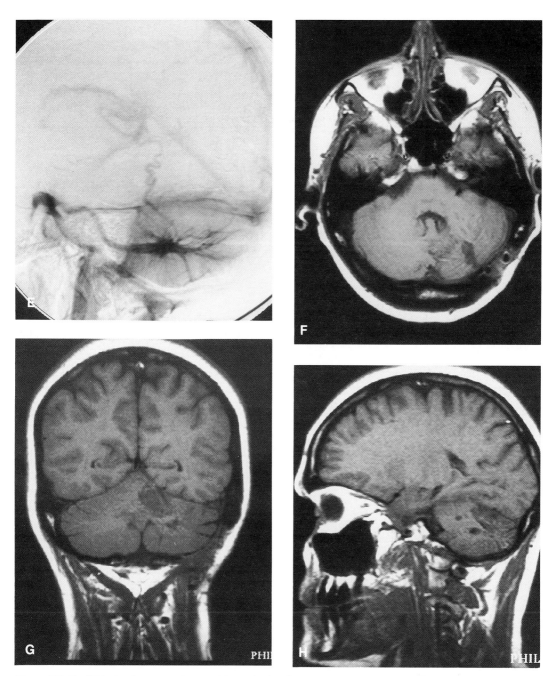

Figure 7E–H. **(E)** Lateral venous phase angiograph showing venous malformation in left cerebellar hemisphere. **(F)** Postoperative axial, **(G)** coronal, and **(H)** sagittal T1-weighted MRIs document complete removal of the two CMs—the larger being the source of the hemorrhage. The venous malformation was left intact at the time of surgery.

10. Hashim ASM, Asakura T, Koichi U, et al. Angiographically occult arteriovenous malformations. *Surg Neurol.* 1985;23:431–439.

11. Hassler W, Zentner J, Petersen D. Cavernous angioma of the optic nerve: case report. *Surg Neurol.* 1989;31:444–447.

12. Hassler W, Zentner J, Wilhelm H. Cavernous angiomas of the anterior visual pathways. *J Clin Neurol Ophthalmol.* 1989;9:160–164.

13. Ishikawa S, Kuwabara S, Fukuma A, et al. Cavernous angioma of the cerebellum: case report. *Neurol Med Chir (Tokyo).* 1989;29:35–39.

14. Kurchaczyk W, Lemme-Pleghos L, Uske A, et al. Intracranial vascular malformations: MR and CT imaging. *Radiology.* 1985; 156:383–389.

15. Little JR, Awad IA, Jones SC, et al. Vascular pressures and cortical blood flow in cavernous angioma of the brain. *J Neurosurg.* 1990;73:555–559.

16. Lobato RD, Perez C, Rivas JJ, et al. Clinical, radiological, and pathological spectrum of angiographically occult intracranial vascular malformations: analysis of 21 cases and review of the literature. *J Neurosurg.* 1988;68:518–531.

17. McCormick PC, Michelsen WJ. Management of intracranial cavernous and venous malformations. In: Barrow DL, ed. *Intracranial Vascular Malformations.* Park Ridge, Ill: American Association of Neurological Surgeons; 1990:197–217.

18. McCormick WF, Nofzinger JD. "Cryptic" vascular malformations of the central nervous system. *J Neurosurg.* 1966;24:865–875.

19. Monma S, Ohno K, Hata H, et al. Cavernous angioma with encapsulated intracerebral hematoma: report of two cases. *Surg Neurol.* 1990;34:245–249.

20. Murakami S, Sotsu M, Morooka S, et al. Chronic encapsulated intracerebral hematoma associated with cavernous angioma: a case report. *Neurosurgery.* 1990;26:700–702.

21. New PFJ, Ojemann RG, Davis KR, et al. MR and CT of occult vascular malformations of the brain. *AJNR.* 1986;7:771–779.

22. Pozzati E, Giuliani G, Nuzzo G, et al. The growth of cerebral cavernous angiomas. *Neurosurgery.* 1989;25:92–97.

23. Pozzati E, Padovani R, Morrone B, et al. Cerebral cavernous angiomas in children. *J Neurosurg.* 1980;53:826–832.

24. Rigamonti D. Natural history of cavernous malformations, capillary malformations (telangiectases), and venous malformations. In: Barrow DL, ed. *Intracranial Vascular Malformations.* Park Ridge, Ill: American Association of Neurological Surgeons; 1990:45–51.

25. Rigamonti D, Drayer BP, Johnson PC, et al. The MRI appearance of cavernous malformations (angiomas). *J Neurosurg.* 1987;67:518–524.

26. Rigamonti D, Hadley MN, Drayer BP, et al. Cerebral caverous malformations: incidence and familial occurrence. *N Engl J Med.* 1988;319:343–347.

27. Robinson JR, Awad IA, Little JR. Natural history of the cavernous angioma. *J Neurosurg.* 1991;75:709–714.

28. Saito N, Yamakawa K, Sasaki T, et al. Intramedullary cavernous angioma with trigeminal neuralgia: a case report and review of the literature. *Neurosurgery.* 1989;25:97–101.

29. Shuey HM Jr, Day AL, Quisling RG, et al. Angiographically cryptic cerebrovascular malformations. *Neurosurgery.* 1979;5:476–479.

30. Simard JM, Garcia-Bengochea F, Ballinger WE Jr, et al. Cavernous angioma: a review of 126 collected and 12 new clinical cases. *Neurosurgery.* 1986;18:162–172.

31. Steiger HJ, Markwalder TM, Ruelen H-J. Clinicopathological relations of cerebral cavernous angioma: observations in eleven cases. *Neurosurgery.* 1987;21:879–884.

32. Steiger HJ, Markwalder TM, Ruelen H-J. Das zerebrale Kavernom als Ursache von rezidivierenden Hirnbltungen und epileptischen Anfällen. *Schweiz Med Wochenschr.* 1988;118:471–477.

33. Steinberg GK, Marks MP, Shuer LM, et al. Occult vascular malformations of the optic chiasm: magnetic resonance imaging diagnosis and surgical laser resection. *Neurosurgery.* 1990;27:466–470.

34. Tagle P, Huete I, Mendez J, et al. Intracranial cavernous angioma: presentation and management. *J Neurosurg.* 1986;64:720–723.

35. Tung H, Giannotta SL, Chandrasoma PT, et al. Recurrent intraparenchymal hemorrhages from angiographically occult vascular malformations. *J Neurosurg.* 1990;73:174–180.

36. Ueda S, Saito A, Inomori S, et al. Cavernous angiomas of the cauda equina producing subarachnoid hemorrhage: case report. *J Neurosurg.* 1987;66:134–136.

37. Voigt K, Yasargil MG. Cerebral cavernous hemangiomas or cavernomas: incidence, pathology, localization, diagnosis, clinical features and treatment: review of the literature and report of an unusual case. *Neurochirurgia.* 1976;19:59–68.

38. Wakai S, Ueda Y, Inoh S, et al. Angiographically occult angiomas: a report of thirteen cases with analysis of the cases documented in the literature. *Neurosurgery.* 1985;17:549–556.

39. Weber M, Vespignani H, Bracard S, et al. Les angiomes caverneux intracérébraux. *Rev Neurol (Paris).* 1989;145:429–436.

40. Yamasaki T, Handa H, Yamashita J, et al. Intracranial and orbital cavernous angiomas: a review of 30 cases. *J Neurosurg.* 1986;64:197–208.

41. Zentner J, Grodd W, Hassler W. Cavernous angioma of the optic tract. *J Neurol.* 1989;236:117–119.

42. Zimmerman RS, Spetzler RF, Lee KS, et al. Cavernous malformations of the brain stem. *J Neurosurg.* 1991;75:32–39.

Chapter 7

Conservative Management

W. Jost Michelson, MD

General Considerations

Cavernous malformations (CMs) of the central nervous system may be associated with seizures or a small or large parenchymal hemorrhage, may enlarge like a neoplasm, or be associated with all the aforementioned phenomena. CMs may occur as a single malformation or multiple lesions in the brain or spinal cord or both, in a single individual or in several members of a family.

Hemorrhage due to a CM may cause death; although we have little idea as to the frequency of this complication, as natural history studies are small and incomplete.[1,8,10] CMs may recur, even if "complete" removal is accomplished, and a new malformation may appear where one has been removed.[9] If, as Rigamonti et al[7] have suggested, this lesion is a part of a phakamatosis-type disorder, the appearance of new lesions should not be surprising. It should not be forgotten that histologically similar CMs occur in other organ systems, i.e. liver, gastrointestinal tract, bone, and lungs.

Rational treatment of any disorder, including CMs, requires a complete understanding of the disease. A careful perusal of the literature on CMs results in great confusion.

Patients with CMs may be categorized into one of a variety of subsets. One subset of patients can be identified under the term "cryptic" vascular malformations or "angiographically occult" vascular malformations.[5,9] CMs remain angiographically occult, but because of high-resolution computed tomography (CT) and magnetic resonance imaging (MRI), they are no longer *cryptic* as noted by Wilson.[9] The pathology in these reported cases includes (1) arteriovenous malformation (AVM), (2) cavernous malformations (CMs), (3) venous malformations (angiomas), and (4) capillary malformations (telangiectasia). It is my personal opinion that these pathologic reports are highly unreliable and that most of these lesions are CMs.

A second subset of reported patients includes those in whom an intracranial or intraspinal neurologic event has occurred and in whom one or more CMs are identified on MRI.

A third group of patients includes those with multiple malformations and a family history. A fourth group includes patients who have undergone an MRI for perhaps an unrelated problem and are analyzed retrospectively. A fifth group includes patients with CMs that are extra-axial, associated with cranial nerves, attached to the dura, or in the region of the pineal gland. These lesions are histologically identical to those found in the brain but have rarely been reported to hemorrhage. A further distinct group includes lesions which are intraparenchymal and have been documented to enlarge over time.

The only common feature of all the clinical subsets of CMs mentioned above is the pathology: large cavernous spaces filled with blood, a virtually acellular mass with no brain parenchyma between the sinusoids of "blood vessels."

It has been noted by Zimmerman et al[11] and others that subarachnoid hemorrhage is virtually never a clinical feature of bleeding associated with a CM in the posterior fossa. This observation is also true in the author's experience, although these lesions often "bulge or protrude" well into the fourth ventricle and are easily identified by the hemosiderin discoloration of the distended floor. Why does subarachnoid hemorrhage not occur? As noted earlier, subarachnoid hemorrhage does not occur in the extramedullary lesions either. Wilson[9] has excluded the extramedullary lesions from his discussion of cryptic vascular malformations. However, for purposes of rational deductions regarding treatment we must include them here, as pathologically they are identical to those lesions located within the substance of the central nervous system. Their behavior and natural history will become crucial when we discuss conservative therapy.

Zimmerman et al[11] reported a series of 24 patients with CMs in the brain stem. Surgery was performed in 16 patients. More than one neurologic event or "hemorrhage" had occurred in 75% of the patients undergoing surgery. Eight patients were followed and only 1 patient in this group had a second "hemorrhage." Somewhat more than 50% of these 24 patients had more than one hemorrhage or neurologic event. How can

we reconcile these data with the very careful studies of Curling et al[1] and Robinson et al[8] where the presumed rate of bleeding ranged from 0.25% to 0.70% per patient per year? It appears that these lesions "bleed" only when located within brain parenchyma, although location within the brain (i.e. brain stem) might also predispose to "hemorrhage."

Lobato et al[5] reviewed 260 reported cases of angiographically occult intracranial malformations and added 21 cases of their own. All of their patients with posterior fossa lesions had repeated hemorrhage. CMs are found throughout the brain in equal proportion to the brain tissue; therefore a minority are in the posterior fossa. Yet, they are drawn to our attention by their seemingly increased propensity to hemorrhage; a fact that is not substantiated by other series.[1,8]

It is abundantly clear that major catastrophic hemorrhage from a CM is rare. The decision to perform brain surgery on an individual harboring a CM must be based on more than emotion; it must be based on fact. If, as is sometimes the case, the CM is enlarging in an eloquent region of the brain, there is no conservative therapy other than operative excision of the mass. We are then left with two broad categories of patients with CMs: **(1)** those that present with a seizure; **(2)** those that present with a hemorrhage, albeit a small one. (In fact, every CM within the substance of the brain or spinal cord exhibits some radiographic (MRI) evidence of previous hemorrhage.)

Patients with supratentorial CMs will more likely present with seizures, whereas lesions in the brain stem, cerebellum, and spinal cord are more likely associated with "hemorrhage" or neurologic event. These phenomena have been discussed extensively by Wilson,[9] who suggests that a small hemorrhage is part of the formation of the CM, and that later hemorrhages occur in a similar fashion to those seen from a subdural hematoma membrane, causing enlargement of the lesion and increasing neurologic deficit. There are several difficulties with this hypothesis for the enlargement of CMs. First, and most important, there are no recognizable arteriovenous shunts or other hemodynamic factors in a CM which might predispose to hemorrhage. There are no vessels with a recognizable normal structure within CMs. Secondly, there is virtually never a membrane surrounding these lesions but rather an area of hemosiderin-stained white matter. Further, this hypothesis does not explain why some patients have major brain hemorrhages. The author suspects that other mechanisms must be invoked to explain the behavior of this lesion.

Most supratentorial CMs are located in the gray-white junction or in the white matter where a 1 cc hemorrhage causes little or no disturbance. The same size hemorrhage in the thalamus, midbrain, or internal capsule will cause a deficit as will a bleed of this size in the brain stem, or spinal cord. It would therefore be attractive to propose that all CMs hemorrhage to a small degree and symptoms occur when the lesion is in a critical location (e.g. brain stem). This hypothesis is attractive, but does not account for a major hemorrhage, nor does it explain in a satisfactory fashion why CMs abutting the floor of the fourth ventricle rarely, if ever, cause a subarachnoid hemorrhage.

I would like to propose a general hypothesis regarding CMs and hemorrhages from the lesion. I suggest that a CM never hemorrhages but rather somehow causes nearby blood vessels in brain parenchyma (either capillaries or small arterioles) to break, perhaps through a toxic effect, resulting in small or large hemorrhages. The malformation itself, in spite of the studies by Little et al,[4] does not bleed profusely when broken, torn, cut into, or otherwise assaulted by a surgeon. This is supported by the large number of lesions stereotaxically biopsied without incident. Furthermore, the lesion has never been implicated

in a hemorrhage when found in an extra-axial location.

Thus, having redefined the role of a CM in causing hemorrhage due to its presence in the tissue of the central nervous system, I am prepared to approach the role of conservative therapy for the various manifestations of this disease.

Brain Cavernous Malformations

Seizure is the most common presenting symptom of brain CMs. Epilepsy is a disorder associated with a 20-year reduction in average lifespan.[2] If we could be assured of curing seizures by removal of the CM, the most conservative approach to a single malformation in a patient presenting with a seizure history would be excision. Robinson et al[8] in their study of the natural history of CMs, reported 32 patients with a severe seizure disorder. The 18 patients treated with medication only continued to have seizures. Fourteen patients with seizures (10 with intractable epilepsy) and a CM, underwent surgical resection and 7 patients continued to have seizures postoperatively. McCormick and this author reported a similar percentage.[6] Thus, a recommendation for surgery in this group of patients will have to await further data on seizure control, and for the present time, operation does not appear to be indicated for control of seizures unless the seizure disorder is intractable and warrants "epilepsy surgery." If, however, a patient has a seizure and is found on MRI to have a large hemorrhage associated with a CM, the most conservative approach is to allow the hemorrhage to resorb, if the patient is stable, and then to excise the malformation. Here I make an assumption that the malformation again may "erode" adjacent vessels.

A somewhat more difficult situation to resolve is the approach to a patient with a single malformation in the brain stem that has caused symptoms. Our review of the available data suggests an increased risk of multiple hemorrhages from these lesions.[1,5,8,10,11] The neurosurgeon has two choices when confronted with a patient with a symptomatic brain stem CM. The first choice is to follow the patient clinically, which would be the more conservative course. If the patient experiences a second neurologic event and the lesion is surgically accessible, operative excision would appear to be the more "conservative" approach. Recently, a third approach to CMs of the thalamus, midbrain, and brain stem has been utilized, namely stereotaxic radiosurgery. The largest reported series to date includes 24 patients.[3] Only 12 of these patients have been followed for more than 1 year. Almost 90 patients with CMs have been treated with proton-beam radiosurgery by the group at Massachussetts General Hospital but have not been reported on (Adams RD, personal communication, 1990). If the lesion is truly an angiographically occult AVM, as evidenced by subarachnoid hemorrhage or biopsy, then radiosurgery may have a role to play. This does not appear to justify this form of treatment for a CM, either on radiobiologic or pathologic grounds.

A patient with multiple CMs and a symptomatic lesion should be treated as if the symptomatic lesion was the only one. All other lesions should be followed expectantly. No justification exists for treating such patients in any other fashion.

A family with multiple members harboring one or more CMs discovered on screening MRI scans presents a psychological challenge for the physician and the family. Suppose that one family member undoubtedly has symptoms that lead to the diagnosis of CM and that an enterprising and well-meaning physician has decided to test the rest of the family, having recently learned of the genetic predisposition for this lesion. Our scientific curiosity has created a psychosocial dilemma for the medi-

cal care system and the involved family. What is our next step? We could inform the family members with great confidence that we do not know what should be done. Certainly, a serious hemorrhage with associated neurologic deficit or seizure could occur. However, we can reduce the patients' anxiety by performing a series of small brain operations, removing all of the patients' malformations. Indeed, some new lesions may grow but we can always reoperate. Ridiculous? Yes, but think of the poor family as they trudge out of the doctor's office having been informed that they have "several time bombs" in their brains and that they are going to pass these on to their children ad infinitum. Where does good science stop and good medicine begin? This author would make a strong argument against screening for CMs in asymptomatic relatives.

Spinal Cord Cavernous Malformations

There is not a great deal of information available on CMs within the spinal cord.[9] I have treated three patients surgically, all of whom had more than one neurologic event. One patient had three intracranial lesions, interpreted on a CT scan in 1978 as calcified granulomas. The spinal lesions in these patients were clearly symptomatic and were relatively easy to remove, and thus the conservative approach would seem to be surgery.

The potential for neurologic devastation from bleeding seems very high in the spinal cord. This could be invoked as a rationale for prophylactic surgery on all spinal lesions. However, this could very well be an emotional predisposition that will not stand up to the scrutiny of a careful study.

On the other hand, I know of no case where a lesion has recurred in the spinal cord, where multiple lesions occurred, or where a new lesion has grown; therefore, we may be justified in suggesting surgery as the conservative approach.

Summary

CM is a poorly understood lesion found in the brain and spinal cord. It is associated with mostly small but occasionally large parenchymal hemorrhage. The frequency of this occurrence is unclear. CMs may be single or multiple in one patient and may occur in the brain or spinal cord. Multiple family members may have one or more CMs, and in these families, the disorder is an autosomal dominant one.

The natural history of this disorder is not known. Recent studies suggest that major morbidity is rare without prior exacerbating symptoms. Older pathologic studies suggest that although the lesion is common, associated disability and death are rare. There is a suggestion that the occurrence of this disorder in the general population is increasing but we have no accurate information about its frequency in the pre-CT and pre-MRI eras. It is more likely that lesions are better detected with widespread use of MR imaging.

Nonoperative therapy would seem the best course of action in most incidentally discovered lesions. In lesions with previous focal neurologic deficit, intractable seizures, and in cases with brain stem CMs, surgical resection of the lesion may be the most "conservative treatment" in light of what is known about the natural history of these lesions. It is the author's belief that patients with a lesion in the spinal cord also should undergo surgical excision of the lesion. At the present time, there is no additional published data to guide conservative therapy, including indications for repeat imaging studies and prophylactic anticonvulsants. The clinician must individualize these considerations for each patient and lesion.

References

1. Curling OD Jr, Kelly DL Jr, Elster AD, et al. An analysis of the natural history of cavernous angiomas. *J Neurosurg.* 1991;75:702–708.

2. Jay GW, Leestma JE. Sudden death in epilepsy. *Acta Neurol Scand Suppl.* 1981;63(suppl 81):14.

3. Kondziolka D, Lunsford LD, Coffey RJ, et al. Stereotactic radiosurgery and angiographically occult vascular malformations: indications and preliminary experience. *Neurosurgery.* 1990;27:892–900.

4. Little JR, Awad IA, Jones SC, et al. Vascular pressures and cortical blood flow in cavernous angioma of the brain. *J Neurosurg.* 1990;73:555–559.

5. Lobato RD, Perez C, Rivas JJ, et al. Clinical, radiological, and pathological spectrum of angiographically occult intracranial vascular malformations. *J Neurosurg.* 1988;68:518–531.

6. McCormick PC, Michelsen WJ. Management of intracranial cavernous and venous malformations. In: Barrow D, ed. *Intracranial Vascular Malformations.* Park Ridge, Ill: American Association of Neurological Surgeons; 1990:197–217.

7. Rigamonti D, Johnson PC, Spetzler RF, et al. Cavernous malformations and capillary telangiectasia: a spectrum within a single pathological entity. *Neurosurgery.* 1991;28:60–64.

8. Robinson JR, Awad IA, Little JR. Natural history of the cavernous angioma. *J Neurosurg.* 1991;709–714.

9. Wilson CB. Cryptic vascular malformations. *Clin Neurosurg.* 1992;38:49–94.

10. Zeller RS, Chutorian AM. Vascular malformations of the pons in children. *Neurology.* 1975;25:776–780.

11. Zimmerman RS, Spetzler RF, Lee KS, et al. Cavernous malformations of the brain stem. *J Neurosurg.* 1991;75:32–39.

Chapter **8**

Indications for Surgical Intervention

Stephen L. Huhn, MD, Daniele Rigamonti, MD, and Frank Hsu, BS

Vascular malformations of the central nervous system (CNS) have been classified into four types: capillary telangiectases, cavernous malformations (CMs), venous malformations, and arteriovenous malformations (AVMs).[18,32] CMs comprise approximately 5% to 13% of all vascular malformations in most clinical series and have traditionally been considered rare CNS lesions.[36] The CM is thought to be a congenital lesion consisting of a hamartomatous collection of dilated vessels coalescing into sinusoids without intervening neural tissue. Although most common in the cerebral hemispheres, these lesions may occur throughout the CNS. Clinical presentation usually consists of seizures, hemorrhage, and/or neurologic deficits related to mass effect. With the advent of computed tomography (CT) and more recently, magnetic resonance imaging (MRI), the diagnosis and surgical management of these lesions have been facilitated. In addition to advances in neuroimaging, microsurgical techniques and approaches to vascular malformations have been refined, rendering CMs more amenable to operative therapy. As knowledge of the natural history of CMs increases, and the results of surgical series are analyzed, the issues involving

management and operative indications may now be more clearly addressed.

Historic Perspective

One of the earliest reports of successful surgical excision of a cerebral cavernous hemangioma was described by Englehart in 1904.[9] In 1928, Dandy reported a series of 44 cases (including five of his own) collected from the literature, of which seven were surgically extirpated.[7] However, a review by Bergstrand et al of the histopathology in these cases revealed that some did not meet the histologic criteria for a CM.[2] One of the first major reviews of the subject was by Voigt and Yasargil in 1976, in which a total of 164 cases of cerebral CMs were collected from the literature.[40] At that time, they found 21 cases, in addition to one of their own patients, who had undergone successful surgical resection of the lesion. In that review, the authors concluded that if "technically feasible," CMs should be resected in order to prevent intracranial hemorrhage, and that lesions located in the mesencephalon precluded safe surgical excision. Since that time, however, improved neuroimaging has significantly influenced the treatment of these lesions. There have been many subsequent reports describing successful resection of symptomatic CMs throughout the neuroaxis.

Surgical Anatomy

CMs may be located throughout the CNS, including the basal ganglia, lateral ventricles, brain stem, cerebellum, spinal cord, orbit, and floor of the middle fossa. CMs are characterized by a well-circumscribed collection of vascular channels or sinusoids with walls lined by a single layer of endothelial cells.[19,32] Smooth muscle fibers generally are absent, but disorganized elastic fibers may be found occasionally in the periphery of the CM. Usually there is no neural tissue located within the collection of vessels, and the diameter is less than 3 cm for most lesions. In general, CMs are mulberrylike lesions, delineated from surrounding tissue by a plane of gliosis. Areas of microcalcification, thrombosis, and hemosiderin deposition may be found within the lesion, and most cases show evidence of prior microhemorrhage. CMs also may become cystic and demonstrate a capability for growth.[25] The adjacent brain is often gliotic and does not contain abnormal arteries and/or veins. In cases of hemorrhage and/or cyst formation, there may also be a component of transient edema in the surrounding brain parenchyma. Associated vascular anomalies include venous malformations, which because of proximity may influence surgical planning.[28]

Preoperative Evaluation

Beyond a thorough history (including a family history) and physical examination, appropriate neuroimaging studies are crucial in the preoperative evaluation of CMs. CT is very useful; however, MRI is more sensitive. MRI improves preoperative localization and may diagnose multiple lesions not recognized on CT.[27] This is particularly helpful for those lesions located in the brain stem. With MRI, CMs appear as a reticulated core of mixed-signal intensity with a hypointense ring surrounding the lesion. Cerebral angiography is not necessary when the MRI pattern is distinctive. Angiography is, however, very useful when an associated venous malformation is suspected or when other vascular anomalies need to be excluded (particularly with regard to patients presenting with spontaneous intracerebral hemorrhage). For those patients with seizure disorders, electroencephalography (EEG) is necessary to confirm that the epileptic focus is related anatomically to the location of the CM. More extensive seizure monitoring may be wise if any discrepancy exists between the suspected seizure focus and the location of the CM, or in cases with multiple CMs and epilepsy.

Operative Technique

Standard microsurgical techniques are employed for resection of CMs. The use of microscopic visualization has significantly advanced the surgical treatment of CMs, particularly lesions located deep within the cerebral hemispheres or brain stem. Microsurgical instrumentation and dissection is usually sufficient, and occasionally may be supplemented by the use of the CO_2 laser as described by both Ondra and Seifert.[24,34] The laser has been advocated for delicate opening of the brain stem surface or nontraumatic vaporization of the lesion from adjacent critical structures; but in general, the CO_2 laser does not appear necessary for extirpation of CMs.[34] Davis et al described a series of 26 occult vascular malformations resected by stereotaxic technique, but only two cases of CMs were included (without reference to location or surgical result).[8] This technique may be used to enhance accuracy of flap planning and intraoperative localization of deep-seated lesions.

In fact, with the exception of extracerebral CMs, significant intraoperative hemorrhage is not encountered. The cerebral blood flow (CBF) in the region of the CM has been found to be normal (60.5 $\pm$ 8.3 ml/100 gm/min) and the CO_2 reactivity of adjacent cortex retained.[17] Little et al found that vascular pressures within the CM (38.2 $\pm$ 0.5 mm Hg) were lower than the mean arterial blood pressure (99.6 $\pm$ 15.1 mm Hg) but substantially higher than central venous pressure (CVP) (5.0 $\pm$ 1.0 mm Hg).[17] Moreover, the pressures would vary with head position and CVP, indicating that maximal strain on the vascular channels might occur with head-dependent positions. These vascular dynamics help to explain why many hemorrhagic episodes are fairly restricted, secondary to the relative absence of arterial driving pressure within the CM.

Operative Series

Since Voigt and Yasargil's review in 1976, many authors have reported surgical series of CMs involving various and diverse locations within the CNS. A review of these individual series helps to underscore the evolution and direction of the surgical therapy for CMs.

Prior to CT, Giombini and Morello reviewed a series of 51 patients with CMs, 37 of whom were selected from the literature with the prerequisite of complete clinical and histopathologic data to allow analysis.[13] Of this group, 33 patients were known to have undergone "radical resection," with results known in 30. All but three cases (one each in the pons, cerebellum, and suprasellar cistern) had lesions located in the cerebrum. A total of three deaths were noted in this series and these patients were those with CMs located in the pons, suprasellar cistern, and frontoparietal region. Of the remaining patients, all were considered either to have improved or remained with stable deficits after an average of several years followup. Patients with seizures either significantly improved or were cured by surgical resection. Two reasons were cited for the surgical successes: (1) the presence of a clear boundary for dissection

from adjacent brain tissue, and (2) the poor vascular supply of the CM. Of 6 patients who received "palliative" therapy, such as exploration, evacuation of the hematoma, or a cerebrospinal fluid (CSF) shunt, four patients later died secondary to recurrent hemorrhage. On the basis of suspected neoplasm, 2 patients had received radiotherapy. The authors considered this form of treatment to be ineffective and concurred with the results of other reports at that time on the use of radiation on vascular malformations. This series, prior to CT and largely inclusive only of CMs restricted to the supratentorial compartment, demonstrated that surgical excision of these lesions was both safe and effective when restricted to the cerebral hemisphere.

One of the first surgical series concerning CMs reported after the advent of CT was by Tagle et al.[37] Thirteen patients treated from 1979–1985 were described. The series included four lesions located in the posterior fossa (including one in the pons) while the remaining nine cases were all located in the cerebrum. The patient with the pontine lesion was not subjected to surgery because of unacceptable operative risk and remained asymptomatic after a 4-year followup. The remaining patients all underwent surgery with a good outcome in each case. This series also helped to illustrate that surgery done for the treatment of uncontrolled seizures is effective. In fact, of 7 patients presenting with seizures, all but 1 were described as being asymptomatic 1–5 years postoperatively. The authors recommended surgical excision for accessible lesions in order to avoid neurologic complications related to possible hemorrhage, as well as to exclude a neoplastic process (even though no neoplasms were uncovered in their series).

Another series of CMs diagnosed by CT was reported by Vaquero et al.[38] Twenty-five patients with CM were successfully treated from 1977–1987. Nineteen CMs were located in the cerebral hemisphere, 1 in the thalamus, 2 in the pineal region, 1 in the cerebellum, and 1 in the spinal cord. Patients presented with seizures (70%), symptoms from mass effect (40%), or hemorrhage (10%). Of the 19 patients with lesions located in the cerebral hemisphere and presenting with seizures, 17 had excellent results (no seizures without medication), and 2 were classified as good outcomes (occasional seizure with medication). Those patients with poor outcomes had lesions located in the thalamus, pineal region, and/or in the spinal cord. The authors concluded that the location of the CM as assessed by CT was "the most significant factor in determining prognosis." One death in the series occurred in the case of a thalamic lesion in a patient who had undergone surgery because of progressive neurologic deterioration.

Yamasaki et al reported their series of patients with CMs in 1986.[43] Of 30 patients, 22 underwent definitive surgical removal of the CM with one operative mortality. Total removal was accomplished in 17 and partial removal in 5 cases. Though the majority of lesions were located in the cerebral hemisphere, the operative series included 1 lesion in the basal ganglia, 3 in the middle fossa, 1 in the lateral ventricle, 3 in the third ventricle, 1 in the fourth ventricle, and 1 in the cerebellar tentorium. The one operative death occurred in a female with a CM in the middle fossa who suffered an intraoperative hemorrhage. Of the patients undergoing surgery, most improved, showing either increased seizure control or resolution of neurologic deficit. In patients undergoing total removal, 60% had complete improvement and 40% had mild-to-moderate improvement. Those patients with partial resection also did well. The authors chose not to operate on the lesions which involved the midbrain, pons, caudate, or paraventricular region. Four patients received radiation therapy (2 pontine, 1 midbrain, and 1 middle fossa); 3 showed some improvement after a mean followup of 5.4 years. The patient with a midbrain lesion remained vegetative until death 2 years later. The authors concluded that the treatment of choice for CMs was "radical surgical extirpation as is feasible." They suggested that, with regard to incidental or asymptomatic lesions, management should consist of periodic clinical and radiologic evaluation. It should be noted that 4 of the 5 patients with brain stem CMs without radiotherapy or surgical intervention remained unchanged after a 5-year followup.

In addition to a thorough review of the literature, Villani et al in 1989 described 14 cases of CMs.[39] Eleven were located in the cerebral hemispheres, 1 in the pons, and 3 in the spinal cord. With the exception of a CM located in the pons, all of the supratentorial cases underwent total resection. Good outcomes were noted in all the cases involving the cerebrum. Most of the patients presented with seizures and the result, although characterized as positive, did not specifically quantify the effect on seizure frequency. The three spinal cord CMs had only partial removal, with a good outcome in one, and clinical improvement of the paraparesis in the other two. In analysis of the other spinal cord CMs collected from the literature, Villani et al found that total removal of the lesion was possible, but was often accompanied by temporary or permanent deterioration of pre-existing neurologic deficits. Overall, Villani et al concurred with conservative management of deep-seated, asymptomatic CMs. Surgical resection was indicated in symptomatic cases involving cortical and subcortical lesions. In the review, lesions located in the thalamus, basal ganglia, pineal region, brain stem, and spinal cord, or cases in which only a partial resection was done, were associated with worse surgical outcomes. Preoperative radiotherapy was indicated for extracerebral lesions such as in the middle fossa in order to reduce intraoperative hemorrhage. The role of stereotaxic irradiation for deep lesions was considered limited by Villani et al because of the possibility of incomplete exclusion and the inherent risk of the "latency period" prior to vascular exclusion.

In contrast to the above studies, comprised mostly of lesions within the cerebral hemispheres, other recent reports have focused on the operative experience with CMs in less surgically accessible locations such as the thalamus and brain stem. In patients with CMs located in these areas, the indications for surgery become more complex as the risk of surgical complications must be weighed against the incomplete knowledge of the natural history of these vascular anomalies and the neurologic condition of the patient.

Bertalanffy et al recently completed a thorough review of the surgical outcome related to deep-seated CMs.[3] Twenty-six patients underwent microsurgical removal of symptomatic CMs located either in the brain stem, insula, basal ganglia, or thalamus. The main indication for surgical intervention was the development of progressive neurologic deficits, which developed in 18 patients. Fifteen patients had symptoms related to a hemorrhagic episode. Eleven of the patients had successful total resection without additional neurologic dysfunction. Seven patients suffered transient neurologic deterioration and/or new deficits in the immediate postoperative period. Roughly one-third or 28% (8 patients) had severe complications, according to the authors. The complications were characterized by distinct "pathogenetic mechanisms" and included: **(1)** recurrent hemorrhage from residual angioma, **(2)** damage to the internal capsule by manipulation, **(3)** injury to the lenticulostriate arteries, **(4)** damage to venous drainage, and **(5)** air embolism and resultant cortical infarction.[3] These complications seem to be related more to lesions located deep within the cerebral hemisphere than to those within the brain stem. Of the 8 patients with poor outcomes, 5 had lesions located either in the basal ganglia, thalamus, or insula. It is not clear from the report which of these patients suffered from hemorrhage and perhaps would have benefitted from a trial of observation prior to surgery. Nonetheless, given the proximity of critical white-matter fasci-

culi and/or vascular structures, the risk of microsurgical intervention in these areas is not insignificant. In this series, the operative risk was high for lesions involving the basal ganglia, thalamus, and insula. Conservative therapy in a neurologically stable patient may be an alternative to surgery, as illustrated by these cases. Bertalanffy et al noted that the surgical results improved with experience, but questioned whether the indication for surgical resection of deep-seated CMs should be limited, based upon the unsatisfactory results in this series.[3]

Thalamic CMs are rare. In Simard and colleagues' 1986 review of 138 cases with proper histologic diagnosis, only 1 patient with a thalamic CM was identified.[36] This patient underwent surgery with increased deficit postoperatively.[1] Vaquero et al also documented the case of a single patient with a thalamic CM who eventually died from respiratory complications 4 years following a radical resection without neurologic improvement.[38] Roda et al in 1990 published a report of a patient with a left thalamic CM. Following a transcallosal interhemispheric approach, this patient had worsening of preoperative neurologic function. From this experience, Roda et al advised conservative or nonsurgical therapy in patients with "benign" clinical presentation and definitive MR diagnosis of CM.[31] In response to and in support of this position, Cappabianca and coworkers' discussion of 2 conservatively managed cases of thalamic CMs also agreed with conservative therapy for patients with stable neurologic function "unless very favorable surgical features exist."[4] The poorer surgical results in cases of thalamic CM as described by Bertalanffy and Villani also support conservative therapy for deep cerebral lesions.[3,39] Although the definitive risk is not known, it appears that thalamic CMs have a significant surgical complication rate, and nonoperative approaches should be strongly considered in the stable patient. Conservative therapy, of course, always should be augmented by routine clinical and radiologic examinations to assess potential growth of the CM, which may prompt surgical intervention.

CMs located within the brain stem present a great surgical challenge and only recently have more successful results been reported. To a large extent MRI has significantly facilitated surgical planning regarding brain stem locations, by allowing precise localization of CMs.

In 1986, Yoshimoto et al reported good surgical outcomes in 3 patients. One case involved a CM located in the third ventricle and 2 cases involved the dorsal pons/floor of the fourth ventricle.[44] The remaining patient in the series, a 2-year-old male, did not undergo surgery and subsequently died as a result of recurrent hemorrhage. At autopsy he was found to have had an extensive brain stem malformation. Prevention of recurrent hemorrhage formed the basis for operative therapy in this series. The authors noted that with regard to surgical technique, the plane of adjacent gliotic tissue provided a safe boundary for excision.

Le Doux et al, in a review of 16 surgical cases of CMs involving the brain stem, reported overall good results.[16] Surgical outcome was poor in 3 patients (including 2 deaths) and unimproved in 1 patient. The remaining patients all had outcomes that were classified as either "good" or "excellent"; the 2 deaths occurred prior to the introduction of CT. The authors also presented 2 personal cases involving a pontomesencephalic CM resected successfully through splitting the cerebellar vermis and incising the floor of the fourth ventricle and a cerebellar-pontine lesion approached in an identical manner. Both patients significantly improved after surgery. Le Doux et al concluded that surgical resection of brain stem CMs could lead to neurologic improvement and that symptomatic patients were candidates for surgery.[16]

Fahlbusch et al, in 1990, described a series of 12 patients with CMs restricted to the brain stem, 6 of whom underwent successful surgical resection after presenting with recurrent hemorrhage.[10] The lesions involving the pontomesencephalic junction or the pontomedullary junction, were approached by either subtemporal, supracerebellar infratentorial, or suboccipital vermian techniques. Morbidity was low overall. Some patients suffered transient internuclear ophthalmoplegia and one-and-a-half syndromes postoperatively; and 1 patient with a pontine CM suffered an asymptomatic posterior cerebral artery infarct. Although Fahlbusch et al pointed out that reactive gliosis seemed to form a plane for dissection, they suggested that surgery should occur soon after recurrent hemorrhage once the patient was neurologically stable (thereby taking advantage of dissection through an incomplete and less-organized hematoma). Four patients who presented with a single hemorrhagic episode did not undergo surgery, and all had complete neurologic resolution within 6 weeks of the ictus. Two other patients with incidental CMs remained asymptomatic after 1 year. The authors recommended that brain stem CMs with recurrent hemorrhage and negative angiography associated with progressive deficits should undergo resection. They found no rationale for surgical removal of CMs associated with a complete recovery from a single hemorrhagic episode.

The largest series to date on brain stem CMs was reported by Zimmerman et al in 1991.[45] Twenty-four patients with symptomatic brain stem CMs were described; 16 underwent surgical resection. All 8 nonsurgical patients recovered from acute symptoms with minimal or no residual neurologic deficits; and surgery was not advised in view of their clinical improvement (of this group, 1 patient died from recurrent hemorrhage 1 year after evaluation; the remaining patients were all doing well at the time of followup). Of those patients undergoing surgery, an average of 2 hemorrhages with significant associated symptoms were documented. The outcome was the same or improved in 12; and 4 patients suffered new, but transient deficits after surgery. The only mortality occurred 6 months after surgery secondary to a shunt infection. The authors stressed the importance of determining a safe "surgical corridor" for approaching the lesion by combining clinical and MRI examination data. They also observed, in contrast to other reports, that separation from the glial surface of the brain stem was sometimes more difficult than expected. Moreover, associated venous malformations must be diagnosed and incorporated into the surgical planning so as to avoid interruption of the venous drainage. Overall, Zimmerman et al recommended surgical excision for symptomatic brain stem CMs because of the poor ability of the brain stem to withstand mass expansion either from hemorrhage or growth of the CM. A possible exception to conservative therapy in a stable patient might occur if the malformation was located superficially rather than deep within the brain stem. With surface presentation, both intraoperative localization and exposure of the CM becomes simpler, and better surgical outcomes therefore may be expected. In this series, there was a tendency for the neurologic status to progressively worsen once the lesion became symptomatic, thus forming the basis for surgical intervention. As further information regarding the natural history of CMs becomes available, particularly those associated with the brain stem, questions regarding surgical versus nonsurgical therapy and appropriate timing of intervention will be answered.

Although major, single-institution series are best suited for developing a perspective regarding the operative management and outcomes, numerous other case reports have detailed the surgical experience with CMs found in more rare locations within the CNS. Ogawa et al reported successful excision of CMs in the anterior third ventricle using bifrontal craniotomy and interhemispheric translamina terminalis approaches.[23] In addition to 3 personal cases,

Chadduck and colleagues reviewed a total of 16 intraventricular cases from the literature up to 1985.[5] A total of 15 patients underwent surgery with good results reported for all patients having total resection after 1980. CMs may also be associated with the optic nerve, chiasm, or optic track, and successful surgical treatment in these locations has been reported by Hassler and coworkers.[14]

Surgery for Pediatric Cavernous Malformations

CMs manifest themselves in any age group. A CM has even been diagnosed in utero by ultrasonography with subsequent extirpation from the tentorium.[21] CMs affecting children pose special problems regarding surgical indications and possible misdiagnosis with neoplastic processes. In addition to the usual symptoms of seizures, focal neurologic deficits, and hemorrhage, children (particularly in the first year of life) may also present with macrocephaly.[12] Pozzati et al discussed 5 patients with supratentorial CMs (age range 4–14 years) who underwent surgery. Postoperatively 3 improved, 1 was unchanged, and 1 had increased hemiparesis.[26] In addition to 2 personal cases, Gangemi et al reviewed 11 patients from the literature who presented during the first year of life.[12] Nine patients had gross total removal. Excellent outcomes were obtained in 6, with some improvement noted in the remaining 3 cases. As an additional surgical consideration, Gangemi et al stressed the importance of obtaining diagnostic tissue in order to differentiate between teratomas and mixed tumors that occur more commonly in children, but which may have a similar radiographic appearance to that of the CM.[12]

Fortuna et al reviewed 50 CM patients from the literature who presented in the first 16 years of life and added 6 cases of their own.[11] The presentation consisted of epilepsy in 45.4%, hemorrhage in 27.3%, intracranial hypertension in 16.4%, and focal deficits in 10.9%. The most common locations involved either the parietal lobe, ventricular system, frontal or temporal lobes. Total surgical removal was accomplished in 87.2% of cases, and perioperative mortality was 4.6%. After an average followup of 2.4 years, 72.1% of the patients had complete resolution of neurologic symptoms, 18.6% had some improvement, and in 4.6% deficits remained stable or worsened. Of particular interest, 65% of patients presenting with epilepsy were seizure-free off medication; the remaining 35% had reduced frequency in combination with anticonvulsant therapy.

Scott et al discussed the surgical results of 19 children ranging in age from 7 months to 17 years.[33] Ten CMs were located in the cerebral hemispheres, 4 in the brain stem, 2 in the cerebellum, 2 in the basal ganglia, and 1 in the spinal cord. Most patients presented with acute or subacute onset of focal neurologic deficit. Significant morbidity occurred in 3 patients. One case involved residual facial paresis and hemiparesis following 3 separate resections of an extensive diencephalic lesion presenting with recurrent hemorrhage. The 2 other complications involved increased hemiparesis—in one, following surgery for a hemorrhagic midbrain CM, and in the other, following a resection near the precentral gyrus. The remaining 16 patients in the series had favorable outcomes. Of the 5 patients who received subtotal resection, 2 had recurrent hemorrhage and only 1 required repeat surgery for stabilization. The remaining patients remained asymptomatic after followup ranging from 9 months to 9 years. The authors recognized that, especially in eloquent areas of the brain, partial resection could occur inadvertently by failing to identify residual malformation within the gliotic tissue adjacent to the CM. Similar to Fortuna et al, Scott and colleagues[33] concluded that in the pediatric age group, surgical intervention is indicated for symptoms related to mass effect, hem-

orrhage, and/or seizures, if the CM is safely accessible. For lesions located in the eloquent areas of the brain or brain stem, the risks of surgery should be cautiously weighed even in cases of recurrent hemorrhage. In the pediatric age group, it was not felt that small-field stereotaxic irradiation could be an alternative, given the increased risk of inducing deficits secondary to radiation necrosis and the uncertain long-term effects on the developing brain. Thus, the management of CMs in children should be biased more in favor of surgery, given the increased hemorrhagic risks and epileptic potential faced by a child.

Extracerebral Cavernous Malformations

The majority of CMs are intraparenchymal. Extracerebral CMs, although similar in histopathology to their intracerebral counterparts, have significantly distinctive surgical implications and deserve special operative consideration. Intracranial extracerebral dural CMs have been described in the frontal fossa, the middle fossa, tentorium, cavernous sinuses, and dural convexity.[15,20,22,29] These lesions occur predominantly in females. Presentation usually involves extraocular palsies, exophthalmus, and/or decreased visual acuity for those cases involving the middle fossa. Angiography usually shows a vascular blush similar to that of meningiomas, and the MR appearance may differ significantly from that of intraparenchymal CMs. These malformations are known to be more vascular and less delineated from adjacent tissue, and as such pose more of a surgical challenge. Of 29 patients reported in the literature and analyzed by Rigamonti et al, 8 patients died secondary to intraoperative hemorrhage. In order to reduce the vascularity of extracerebral CMs, the use of preoperative irradiation has been suggested.[29,35] The recommended management for extracerebral CMs would then involve initial biopsy followed by a course of external irradiation prior to surgical extirpation.

Pregnancy and Cavernous Malformations

The effect of pregnancy on vascular anomalies remains a source of speculation. Most reviews examining the effects of pregnancy on CNS vascular lesions have dealt with AVMs or aneurysms. Extrapolation of similar concepts to CMs should at best be made cautiously. Nonetheless, it has been suggested that growth and/or hemorrhage of CMs during pregnancy may be related to the endocrine changes required for vascular proliferation of the endometrium.[30,42] Although a statistically significant association between hemorrhage and pregnancy has yet to be established, Robinson et al described a series of patients in which females accounted for 86% of the hemorrhagic cases; two of the six females were in the first trimester of pregnancy. Yamasaki et al reported a case of a rapidly expanding middle fossa CM in a pregnant female who underwent a subtotal resection in the eighth month of pregnancy.[43] Ondra et al reported successful excision of a hemorrhagic rostral brain stem CM in a 23-year-old in her first trimester of pregnancy.[24] Villani et al proposed that growth of CMs during pregnancy and the subsequent decrease after parturition would be due to estrogenic sensitivity of the CM.[39]

The optimal management of CMs with regard to pregnancy should be based upon the neurologic condition of the mother and location of the CM. For those patients with known CMs who are considering pregnancy, obstetric and neurosurgical consultations should be sought prior to pregnancy. Although an exact relationship has not been determined, there appears to be an increased risk for mass expansion and/or hemorrhage during pregnancy. For those women desiring children, surgical intervention may be entertained prior to conception if the CM is in an accessible location. For those patients diagnosed during pregnancy, the indications for surgery must then be tempered by concern for the fetus. Since the vascular dynamics of CMs differ from that of AVMs or aneurysms, unmodified vaginal delivery may not carry the same risk of hemorrhage. Conservative management during pregnancy may be appropriate if the mother is neurologically stable.

Role of Radiosurgery

The role of radiosurgery for the treatment of brain stem CMs as an alternative to surgery has been briefly addressed by Weil et al.[41] Six patients were treated with radiosurgery (23–50 Gy) and all 6 remained unchanged radiologically after 2 years. Three of the patients developed progressive deficits related to radiation effects and have suffered recurrent hemorrhage. The authors concluded that no therapeutic benefit was seen after stereotaxic radiosurgery. Similar results were also determined in 10 patients with supratentorial CMs treated by radiosurgery at the same institution. Thus it appears that neither conventional teletherapy nor stereotaxic radiosurgery has any substantial role as alternative treatments for CMs, although further studies in this area are needed to completely resolve this question.

Role of Surgery

Traditionally, the main indications for surgery were based upon reduction or control of seizures, reversal of symptoms or deficits related to mass effect, and finally, prevention of hemorrhage or recurrent hemorrhage.

Control of seizures related to CMs remains a strong indication for surgical resection. The morbidity related to resection of lesions located near cortical regions is very low and most studies report favorable outcomes with regard to seizure control. Sophisticated preoperative monitoring, such as a grid and/or depth electrodes, may be applied to cases with questionable seizure localization and may further improve postoperative seizure outcome. The extent to which adjacent brain containing hemosiderin deposits should be resected for seizure control has not been formally addressed.

CMs may also produce neurologic deficits secondary to mass expansion. The accessibility to the lesion producing such deficits appears to be the main factor in considering surgical therapy. Reversal of neurologic symptoms has been well documented following surgical resection of symptomatic lesions located in the cerebral hemispheres. In contrast, surgical intervention remains controversial in the management of deep-seated lesions (i.e. thalamus) which have been associated historically with poorer outcomes.[3] With regard to the brain stem, a similar restraint should be applied if a safe surgical approach cannot be determined (Figure 1).[45] However, those patients with progressive neurologic deterioration may eventually become surgical candidates, since conservative management may pose a higher risk than that of surgery. The results of surgical series concerning deep-seated and brain stem lesions have been satisfactory (in select cases) when strict preoperative selection criteria are applied.

The management of CMs with regard to potential for hemorrhage and subsequent effects remains under scrutiny. Comparing the risk of hemorrhage to the risk of surgical intervention has been and remains a difficult preoperative assessment. The morbidity from primary hemorrhage of a CM is undetermined; however, epidemiological data would indicate that this figure is low. As MRI has enhanced the diagnosis of these lesions, hints as to the behavior of the natural history has also been supplied and surgical indications based upon "concern of hemorrhage" may need revision. In two recent studies by Curling et al and Robinson et al, the issue of hemorrhagic risk has been addressed.[6,30] Each was based upon a population of patients with CMs collected from MRI archives. Curling et al found 32 patients with CMs by MRI but only 3 had a history of clinically significant hemorrhage. The risk of bleeding was esti-

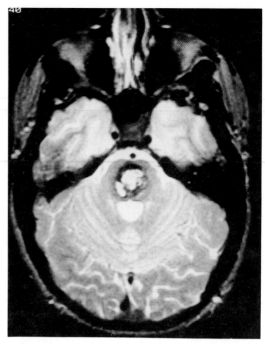

Figure 1. Axial MRI (T2-weighted) revealing a pontine CM in an adult male. The lack of surface presentation precludes safe surgical resection.

mated at 0.25% per person per year, or 0.10% per person per lesion per year. Robinson et al in a similar analysis identified 66 patients, 9 of whom were asymptomatic, and calculated a hemorrhage rate of 0.7% per year per lesion. Thus the estimated risk of hemorrhage from a CM appears to be relatively low. It should be added that data were formulated from a population of patients who had sought MR examinations; therefore it is reasonable to presume that the true incidence of asymptomatic cases is higher and the actual risk of hemorrhage somewhat lower than that calculated. Therefore, surgical resection of CMs solely to prevent primary hemorrhage should be carefully weighed against the neurologic status, age of the patient, location of the lesion, and risk of the operative approach.

Once a clinically significant hemorrhage has been documented, the indications for surgery become more appropriate, but perhaps only insofar as there appears to be an associated progression of neurologic symptoms. Resolution of neurologic symptoms

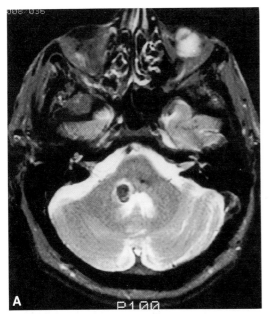 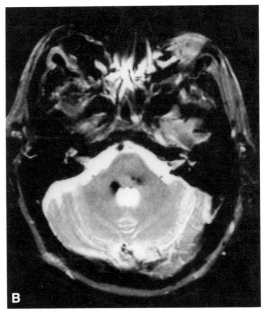

Figure 2. (A) A 65-year-old male was diagnosed with multiple sclerosis at age 35 following an episode of diplopia and right arm and leg hypalgesia. Thirty years later the patient presented with diplopia and right facial hypalgesia. Axial MRI (T2-weighted) revealed a small left pontine CM, probably responsible for the symptoms 30 years prior, and a hemorrhagic right pontine CM accounting for the current presentation. **(B)** Six-month follow-up MRI (T2-weighted) demonstrates resolution of the right pontine hemorrhage coinciding with improvement in the diplopia and facial hypalgesia.

induced by hemorrhage, even within the brain stem, has been well documented (Figure 2). The indications for surgery in those cases of neurologic improvement after a single hemorrhage, then, are based more upon the surgical accessibility of the lesion and the projected ability of that region of the CNS to withstand recurrent hemorrhage (i.e. brain stem or posterior fossa).[45]

Summary

The risk of surgical management of CMs must always be weighed against the risk of conservative therapy. At present, this assessment is an estimate at best in some cases, since the natural history is not well known. However, conservative management may be very appropriate for selected cases of inaccessible lesions and in asymptomatic cases. With a few exceptions, it is evident that as diagnostic capabilities have improved, so has the surgical management of CMs. Surgical success seems less dependent upon location, no doubt as the result of microscopic surgical techniques. The development of selection criteria for surgical resection in order to minimize complications related to epilepsy, mass expansion, and hemorrhage will occur as the results of ongoing investigations of the natural history of this condition become available.

In general, there is no evidence or data to support resection of the asymptomatic CM regardless of location. These patients should probably undergo routine clinical and MRI evaluation at 6–12-month intervals (particularly patients with lesions of the brain stem) in order to detect at an early stage any changes in the lesion that may require surgical intervention.

References

1. Becker DH, Townsend JJ, Kramer RA, et al. Occult cerebrovascular malformations: a series of 18 histologically verified cases with negative angiography. *Brain.* 1979;102:249–287.

2. Bergstrand A, Olivecrona H, Tonnis W. *Gefaberibildungen und Gefabgeschwulste des gehirns.* Leipzig, Germany: Thieme;1936.

3. Bertalanffy H, Gilsbach IM, Eggert HR, et al. Microsurgery of deepseated cavernous angiomas: report of 26 cases. *Acta Neurochir (Wien).* 1991;108:91–99.

4. Cappabianca P, Spaziante R, De Devitiis E. Thalamic cavernous malformations. *J Neurosurg.* 1991;75:169–171. Letter to the editor.

5. Chadduck WM, Binet EF, Farrell FW Jr, et al. Intraventricular cavernous hemangioma: report of three cases and review of the literature. *Neurosurgery.* 1985;16:189–197.

6. Curling OD Jr, Kelly DL Jr, Elster AD, et al. An analysis of the natural history of cavernous angiomas. *J Neurosurg.* 1991;75:702–708.

7. Dandy WE. Venous abnormalities and angiomas of the brain. *Arch Surg.* 1928;17:715–793.

8. Davis DH, Kelly PJ. Stereotactic reduction of occult vascular malformations. *J Neurosurg.* 1990;72:698–702.

9. Englehardt H. Zur Frage der Dauerheilung nach Operativer Behandlung der Traumatischen Jacksonschen Epilepsie. *Dtsch med Wochenschr.* 1904;8:97–99.

10. Fahlbusch R, Strauss C, Huk W, et al. Surgical removal of pontomesencephalic cavernous hemangiomas. *Neurosurgery.* 1990;26:449–457.

11. Fortuna A, Ferrante L, Mastronardi L, et al. Cerebral cavernous angioma in children. *Childs Nerv Svst.* 1989;5:201–207.

12. Gangemi M, Longatti P, Maiuri F, et al. Cerebral cavernous angiomas in the first year of life. *Neurosurgery.* 1989;25:465–469.

13. Giombini S, Morello G. Cavernous angiomas of the brain: account of fourteen personal cases and review of the literature. *Acta Neurochir (Wien).* 1978;40:61–82.

14. Hassler W, Zentner J, Wilhelm H. Cavernous angiomas of the anterior visual pathways. *J Clin Neuro Opthalmol.* 1989;9:160–164.

15. Isla A, Roda J, Alvarez F, et al. Intracranial cavernous angioma in the dura. *Neurosurgery.* 1989;5:657–659.

16. Le Doux MS, Aronin PA, Odrezin GT. Surgically treated cavernous angiomas of the brain stem: report of two cases and review of the literature. *Surg Neurol.* 1991;35:395–399.

17. Little JR, Awad IA, Jones SC, et al. Vascular pressures and cortical blood flow in cavernous angiomas of the brain. *J Neurosurg.* 1990;73:555–559.

18. McCormick WF, Nofzinger JD. "Cryptic" vascular malformations of the central nervous system. *J Neurosurg.* 1966;24:865–875.

19. McCormick WF, Hardman JM, Boulter TR. Vascular malformations ("angiomas") of the brain, with special reference to those occurring in the posterior fossa. *J Neurosurg.* 1968;28:241–251.

20. Mori K, Handa H, Gi H, et al. Cavernomas in the middle fossa. *Surg Neurol.* 1980;14:21–31.

21. Moritake K, Handa H, Nozaki K, et al. Tentorial cavernous angioma with calcification in a neonate. *Neurosurgery.* 1985;16:207–211.

22. Namba S. Extracerebral cavernous hemangioma of the middle cranial fossa. *Surg Neurol.* 1983;19:379–388.

23. Ogawa A, Katakura R, Yoshimoto T. Third ventricle cavernous angioma: report of two cases. *Surg Neurol.* 1990;34:414–420.

24. Ondra SL, Doty JR, Mahla ME, et al. Surgical excision of a cavernous hemangioma of the rostral brain stem: case report. *Neurosurgery.* 1988;23:490–493.

25. Pozzati E, Giuliani G, Nuzzo G, et al. The growth of cerebral cavernous angiomas. *Neurosurgery.* 1989;25:92–97.

26. Pozzati E, Padovani R, Morrone B, et al. Cerebral cavernous angiomas in children. *J Neurosurg.* 1980;53:826–832.

27. Rigamonti D, Drayer BP, Johnson PC, et al. The MRI appearance of cavernous malformations (angiomas). *J Neurosurg.* 1987;67:518–524.

28. Rigamonti D, Spetzler RF. The association of venous and cavernous malformations: report of four cases and discussion of the pathophysiological, diagnostic, and therapeutic implications. *Acta Neurochir (Wien).* 1988;92:100–105.

29. Rigamonti D, Pappas CTE, Spetzler RF, et al. Extracerebral cavernous angiomas of the middle fossa. *Neurosurgery.* 1990;27:306–310.

30. Robinson JR, Awad IA, Little JR. Natural history of the cavernous angioma. *J Neurosurg.* 1991;75:709–714.

31. Roda JM, Alvarez F, Isla A, et al. Thalamic cavernous malformation: case report. *J Neurosurg.* 1990;72:647–649.

32. Russell DS, Rubenstein LJ. *Pathology of Tumours of the Nervous System.* 5th ed. Baltimore, Md: Williams & Wilkins; 1989:730–736.

33. Scott RM, Barnes P, Kupsky W, et al. Cavernous angiomas of the central nervous system in children. *J Neurosurg.* 1992;76:38–46.

34. Seifert V, Gaab MR. Laser-assisted microsurgical extirpation of a brain stem cavernoma: case report. *Neurosurgery.* 1989;25:986–990.

35. Shibata S, Mori K. Effect of radiation therapy on extracerebral cavernous hemangioma in the middle fossa: report of three cases. *J Neurosurg.* 1987;67:919–922.

36. Simard JM, Garcia-Bengochea F, Ballinger WE Jr, et al. Cavernous angioma: a review of 126 collected and 12 new clinical cases. *Neurosurgery.* 1986;18:162–172.

37. Tagle P, Huete I, Mendez J, et al. Intracranial cavernous angioma: presentation and management. *J Neurosurg.* 1986;64:720–723.

38. Vaquero J, Salazar J, Martinez R, et al. Cavernomas of the central nervous system: clinical syndromes, CT scan diagnosis, and prognosis after surgical treatment in 25 cases. *Acta Neurochir (Wien).* 1987;85:29–33.

39. Villani RM, Arianta C, Caroli M. Cavernous angiomas of the central nervous system. *J Neurosurg Sci.* 1989;33:229–252.

40. Voigt K, Yasargil MG. Cerebral cavernous haemangiomas or cavernomas. Incidence, pathology, localization, diagnosis, clinical features and treatment: review of the literature and report of an unusual case. *Neurochirurgia (Stuttg).* 1976;19:59–68.

41. Weil S, Tew JM Jr, Steiner L. Comparison of radiosurgery and microsurgery for treatment of cavernous malformations of the brain stem. *J Neurosurg.* 1990;72:336A. Abstract.

42. Wilkins RH. Natural history of intracranial vascular malformations: a review. *Neurosurgery.* 1985;16:421–430.

43. Yamasaki T, Handa H, Yamshita J, et al. Intracranial and orbital cavernous angiomas: a review of 30 cases. *J Neurosurg.* 1986;64:197–208.

44. Yoshimoto T, Suzuki J. Radical surgery on cavernous angioma of the brain stem. *Surg Neurol.* 1986;26:72–78.

45. Zimmerman RS, Spetzler RF, Lee KS, et al. Cavernous malformations of the brainstem. *J Neurosurg.* 1991;75:32–39.

Chapter 9

Microsurgical Treatment of Supratentorial Lesions

Mitesh V. Shah, MD, and Roberto C. Heros, MD

The distribution of cavernous malformations (CMs) approximates the distribution of nervous tissue along the craniospinal axis.[6] More than 75% of all CMs are located supratentorially.[6,26,36,58] Within the supratentorial compartment these lesions are found mainly in the cortical and subcortical regions.[12,35,43,54] Deeply located lesions in or around the basal ganglia, thalamus, insula, corpus callosum, or paraventricular regions account for about 5% to 20% of all supratentorial lesions.[25,56,58]

The operative management of CMs in accessible areas is relatively straightforward and the risk of removal is quite low.[51,52] This fact, along with numerous reports on the efficacy of operative resection for tissue diagnosis, for prevention or amelioration of seizures or progressive neurologic deficits, and for avoiding the risk of potentially fatal hemorrhage has served as impetus for adopting an aggressive philosophy in the management of most CMs. However, more recent data suggesting a relatively benign natural history of CMs has indicated the need for re-evaluating management decisions.[6,36]

Indications for surgical resection are considered in Chapter 8. The only clear indications for surgical resection of accessible supratentorial lesions include: (1) medically intractable epilepsy; (2) the need to establish a pathologic diagnosis if the magnetic resonance image (MRI) appearance is not classic, particularly in patients without a family history of CMs; (3) documented recurrent hemorrhage; and (4) progressive neurologic deficit.

As the risk of significant hemorrhage is low, the prevention of hemorrhage is not an absolute indication for surgical resection.[6,36] Furthermore, the role of resection in patients with focal neurologic deficit is uncertain, as some of these symptoms may improve spontaneously.[36] Thus, accessibility, certainty of diagnosis, history of recurrent hemorrhage, and the significance of focal neurologic deficit as it relates to the lesion are the main factors weighing in the decision of whether or not to recommend surgical resection.

Our discussion of surgical approaches and techniques applies equally to CMs as well as to angiographically occult arteriovenous malformations. In fact, there is a recognized difficulty in clearly separating these lesions clinically, pathologically, and radiographically.[23,30,32,56] For this reason, the term "angiographically occult vascular malformation" (AOVM) has been suggested to include both CMs and other angiographically occult lesions having a similar appearance on MRI, but pathologically resembling small arteriovenous malformations (AVMs) or having a predominance of venous or capillary vessels.[23,32] The term AOVM specifically excludes venous malformations, which are very different lesions generally having a very benign clinical course and are usually angiographically visible in the late venous phase.[30]

Preoperative Preparation

Once surgical resection of a supratentorial CM has been decided upon, the principal concern is which approach will best provide access to the lesion with the least morbidity. MRI is invaluable in making an accurate preoperative diagnosis in most cases, and its capability of multiplanar imaging for guiding the surgical approach. Angiography is not routinely used to evaluate a lesion with the classic MRI appearance of a CM because the majority of these lesions do not demonstrate any angiographically visible abnormalities, although nonspecific findings such as capillary blush or early-draining veins may be seen in 10% to 20% of the patients.[2,35]

Dural-based CMs are more apt to be hypervascular lesions with enlarged feeding vessels and perhaps arteriovenous shunting, but these abnormalities may also be seen with meningiomas.[3,9,26,28,39] The most reasonable indications for preoperative angiography are extracerebral location, hemorrhagic presentation, or atypical MRI or computed tomography (CT) appearance.[25] While the classic MRI appearance of a central core of mixed signal intensity surrounded by a ring of hypointensity on both T1- and T2-weighted images is fairly specific for cavernous malformations, low-grade glial tumors and hemorrhagic metastatic tumors (especially melanoma) may present with an identical MRI appearance.[32,34,50]

Preoperative localization of lesions relative to functionally important or eloquent cortex is imperative for determining the risk of surgery and planning the surgical approach for subcortical lesions. Careful evaluation of the MRI allows identification of the central sulcus and thus the primary motor cortex. Berger et al established the accuracy of MRI landmarks for motor cortex localization by comparing functional maps from intraoperative stimulation and recording studies in patients with brain tumors.[1]

The deepest sulcus on an axial section of the brain close to the vertex at a 60° to 70° angle from the interhemispheric fissure is reliably identifiable as the central sulcus. The precentral sulcus is not as deep, but can be identified in relation to the superior frontal sulcus which is parallel to the interhemispheric fissure and perpendicular to the precentral sulcus. The sensory-motor cortex can be identified in the parasagittal MRI section by finding the marginal sulcus which extends from the cingulate sulcus to the angle of the hemispheric convexity in the parietal region. The region anterior to the marginal sulcus is the paracentral lobule.

The inferior half of the central sulcus is difficult to identify because it is very shallow, close to the sylvian fissure, and cannot usually be followed from superior to inferior by evaluation of serial, axial MRI slices. Three-dimensional (3-D) images reconstructed from data obtained on routine MRI can be used to identify the precentral gyrus in the perisylvian region.[24] This technique provides good resolution of cortical surface detail, and can be used to obtain axial sections to reveal subcortical features at any given region.

The anatomic identification of essential language cortex on the dominant hemisphere is not as precise as for the motor cortex. This was noted by Ojemann et al based on electrophysiologic studies on 117 awake patients.[31] In this study, essential speech areas were localized to the anterior and posterior superior and middle temporal gyri, the inferior parietal region, and

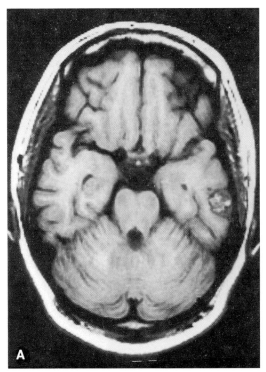

Figure 1A. A 31-year-old woman with an 8-year history of well-controlled partial complex seizures presented with a recent onset of increased seizure frequency. Axial T1-weighted MRI shows a typical cavernous malformation in the left posterior temporal region.

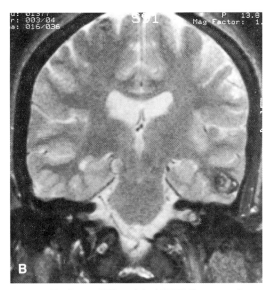

Figure 1B. Coronal T2-weighted MRI illustrates the superficial location in the inferior temporal gyrus. The lesion was resected using a standard temporal craniotomy. Intraoperatively, the cortical surface discoloration helped to localize the lesion.

diffusely in the posterior frontal region. Coronal and parasagittal MRI sections will identify the sylvian fissure and the temporal sulci, allowing an estimation of the risk of language deficits with resection of a lesion of the dominant hemisphere.

In general, it may be desirable to perform intraoperative electrophysiologic functional mapping to supplement and confirm findings of imaging studies if there is any doubt and the lesion is large and deep. Most small superficial lesions can be removed with little risk of neurologic deficit, even from critical areas, as will be discussed.

Preoperative MRI will determine whether deep lesions in the basal ganglia or thalamus are resectable. Only lesions involving the posterolateral aspect of the thalamus and the inferolateral portion of the basal ganglia lateral to the internal cap-

sule can be excised with relative safety. Thalamocaudate lesions on the ventricular surface can be resected with relatively little risk.

General Surgical Techniques

The surgical resection of supratentorial CMs in accessible areas is usually relatively simple because these lesions have no major arterial supply and do not bleed much at surgery. The most difficult task in resection is intraoperative localization. Superficial cortical lesions may be conspicuous because of the presence of overlying discolored cerebral cortex (Figure 1).

Small subcortical lesions that usually result in no surface abnormalities are much more difficult to localize. CT- or MRI-guided stereotaxic craniotomy or intraoperative ultrasonography are major surgical adjuncts that can aid in intraoperative localization. Real-time ultrasonography is particularly useful for lesions that present no surface abnormalities.[4,55] After identifying the most superficial aspect of the lesion with ultrasound, dissection through an overlying gyrus or sulcus can expose the subcortical lesion.

The trans-sulcal approach has been suggested by many because of the ability to save 1–2 cm of cortical dissection and to use a "keyhole" approach to deeper lesions in combination with stereotaxic localization.[7,14,20,57] Whether disruption of the U-fibers of two adjacent gyri is less detrimental than disruption of vertical fibers with a transgyral approach is unclear.[14,16] The trans-sulcal approach must be used with caution, particularly in inexperienced hands, as it may be more traumatic than the transgyral approach, especially if injury to the sulcal vessels occurs during dissection or if one becomes disoriented in locating a relatively superficial lesion.[14] In experienced hands, the trans-sulcal approach is preferable whenever feasible.

Davis and Kelly, and others, described the usefulness of stereotaxis for intraoperative localization with resection of AOVMs, including CMs.[7,26] Using this technique, the surgical approach or trajectory can be planned to avoid functional cortex and major blood vessels.[19,20] Stereoscopic angiography may help to identify sulci that can be used to approach deep lesions and thus minimize transcortical dissection. These lesions can be removed through a 1.5-inch diameter trephine craniotomy. In Davis and Kelly's series of 26 patients with AOVMs, 10 patients suffered morbidity related to location of the lesion and surgical approach used; however, these deficits were transient in 9 and permanent only in 1 patient. There was incomplete removal of the lesion as evident by persistent calcification or contrast enhancement in 3 patients, but none had documented hemorrhage in the followup period. Two patients did well neurologically and 1 died of an unknown cause.[7]

CMs are identified grossly as well-circumscribed, blue or purple, lobulated masses resembling mulberries or grapes.[26,38,58] Although they lack a true cap-

sule, they are usually surrounded by a well-defined, hemosiderin-stained gliotic plane. Histologically, they are composed of dilated, collagenized vascular channels lined with a single layer of endothelial cells and contain no intervening normal neural parenchyma.[38] Calcification within the nodules is common, and there is usually evidence of recent and old hemorrhage.[30,38,58]

As previously mentioned, bleeding is not a major problem during resection of a CM. Occasionally at surgery, small feeding arteries that connect with the sinusoidal spaces may be seen at the lesion periphery.[58] The well-defined gliotic plane allows easy separation of the lesion from surrounding tissue and complete removal of the lesion. Incomplete removal entails future risk of hemorrhage and should be avoided. Excessive coagulation should be avoided since histologic diagnosis may be obscured by cautery artifact. Rarely, initial internal decompression with simple suction or with an ultrasonic aspirator or laser may be necessary for large lesions.[21,32] The hemosiderin-laden gliotic tissue is felt to be the cause of seizures; therefore, the removal of peripheral hemosiderin containing gliotic tissue is recommended for supratentorial lesions that are not located in crucial regions.[56] Obviously, this is to be avoided in lesions of the brain stem or spinal cord.

Once the cavernous malformation has been resected, the cavity wall is gently irrigated and inspected for any additional abnormal vessels. Hemostasis is checked by raising the systolic blood pressure by 10–20 mm Hg above what is normal for the patient and by performing a Valsalva maneuver. The resection cavity can then be lined with a single layer of oxidized regenerated cellulose (Surgicel™, Johnson & Johnson, New Brunswick, NJ).

Surgical Approaches to Deep Lesions in Specific Sites

All adult patients receive 10 mg of dexamethasone and a first-generation cephalosporin on induction of anesthesia. After induction and intubation, central and arterial lines are placed, if necessary. We place central lines in all patients who will be in the sitting or semi-sitting position. Since basal cisterns may not be accessible initially in the subtemporal approach, a lumbar drain should be placed when this approach is planned. We routinely use furosemide, 10–20 mg intravenously, and mannitol, 1 gm/kg intravenously, in adults for obtaining adequate brain relaxation whenever brain retraction is contemplated. Furosemide is given after a Foley catheter has been placed and mannitol started at the time of skin incision.

Even with these adjuncts, there still may not be enough brain relaxation to approach deep lesions, and aggressive retraction in these instances may lead to retraction injury as well as venous occlusion. To avoid this, certain deep lesions may best be exposed by resecting small, noneloquent regions of brain.

Approaches to Callosal, Cingulate, and Subfrontal Lesions

Lesions that involve the anterior corpus callosum near the genu and the cingulate gyrus can be approached through a small frontal craniotomy. The patient is positioned supine, with the head in the neutral position and slightly flexed using a three-point fixation device. An alternative, which we have used particularly for larger lesions, is to position the patient laterally, on the side of the hemisphere to be retracted down, with the head flexed toward the upper shoulder (see Figure 3B). This allows that hemisphere to fall by gravity, with little or no retraction necessary.

If the lesion is large and good brain relaxation may be necessary, a lumbar drain may be placed preoperatively. Using a bicoronal incision, a boneflap is made extending across the midline just in front of the coronal suture (Figure 2A). Another option is to place burrholes and cut the boneflap directly over the sagittal sinus

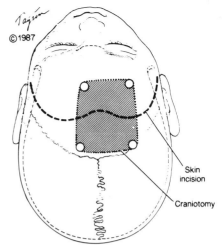

Figure 2A. Right frontal craniotomy is used to approach anterior corpus callosum and cingulate gyrus lesions that do not extend into the deep subfrontal region. Bicoronal incision and a craniotomy that extends across the midline are illustrated. The head should be in the neutral position with the neck slightly flexed.

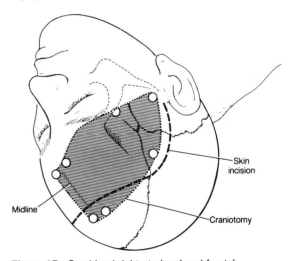

Figure 2B. Combined right pterional and frontal craniotomy extending to the left of the midline is used for approaching lesions that extend into the deep subfrontal region. (Reprinted with permission from Ojemann RG, Heros RC, Crowell RM. *Surgical Management of Cerebrovascular Disease*. Baltimore, Md: Williams & Wilkins; 1988:384.)

where injury to medially draining veins or venous lakes is not likely to occur.[49] A shallow quadrangular dural incision is made with the base close to the superior sagittal sinus. In an anterior or posterior parasagittal approach, the surgeon occasionally encounters large bridging veins in the field that makes such an approach impossible without sacrifice of at least one of these veins. Whether a specific vein can be safely taken is a matter of surgical judgment. A small resection of the brain between such veins may permit entry into the interhemispheric fissure at a depth of about 2–3 cm without endangering the veins. Of course, this can only be undertaken in the anterior or middle frontal regions or in the superior occipital or posterior parietal regions, and absolutely should be avoided in the immediate region of the primary motor, primary sensory, supplementary motor, and primary visual regions.

Once the site of interhemispheric approach has been selected, self-retaining retractors on both the falx and the medial hemisphere may be used to expose the lesions. Care should be taken to avoid direct compression of the sagittal sinus with the retractors. The trajectory is tangential in approaching this type of lesion, and good brain relaxation is important.

Lesions that are more basal in the subfrontal or septal regions will require a lower frontal craniotomy through a bicoronal incision, with the patient supine and the head in the neutral position. Otherwise, the general principles of an interhemispheric approach should be followed. For large lesions that extend medial to lateral in the basal frontal area, it may be necessary to extend the standard pterional craniotomy more anteriorly to reach the medial basal aspect of the lesion (Figure 2B).[30,57] It may be useful to turn the head approximately 30° away from the side of the lesion with this exposure. The subfrontal retraction may stretch and damage the olfactory tract unilaterally if care is not taken.

Posterior parasagittal approaches to lesions in the body and splenium of the corpus callosum, cingulate gyrus, posterior frontal, posterior parietal, or occipital regions are performed with the patient either

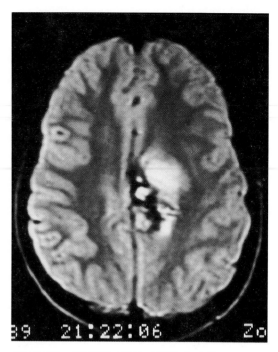

Figure 3A. Axial T2-weighted MRI of a left parasagittal cavernous malformation in the posterior frontal region. The lesion was resected using a parasagittal approach.

in the semi-sitting position with the head flexed and looking straight ahead, or in the lateral position with the ipsilateral side down, as discussed earlier (Figure 3).[30,47,59] If the semi-sitting position is used, precautions should be taken to prevent air embolism. A horseshoe-shaped parieto-occipital scalp incision is made that crosses the midline.

We advocate a broader craniotomy in the anterior posterior dimension (approximately 6–7 cm) than is needed in the lateral dimension.[16,31] This permits inspection of the venous anatomy to select the best approach between draining veins. Again, important bridging veins in the primary motor and sensory regions should not be sacrificed. This approach can be used to reach lesions in the region of the third ventricle, as well as the medial side of the trigone of the lateral ventricle.[30,47] However, for the latter we generally prefer the paramedian posterior parietal incision, as described later.

Skin Incision Craniotomy

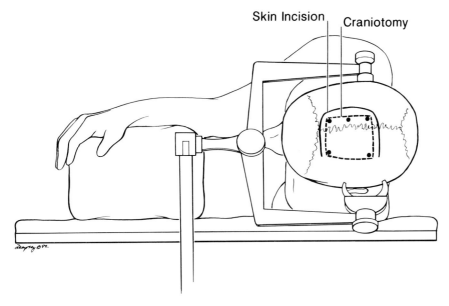

Figure 3B. The parasagittal approach. The lateral position with the head tilted toward the superior shoulder and the lesion side down is illustrated. The semi-sitting position with the same type of boneflap may also be utilized. The craniotomy should extend across the midline.

Approaches to Paratrigonal Lesions

Lesions near the trigone of the lateral ventricle can be approached **(1)** laterally through either the inferior or middle temporal gyrus, **(2)** superiorly either through the superior parietal lobule or the temporoparietal junction on the right side, or **(3)** medially through the parasagittal approach entering the brain in the perisplenial region.[13,18,27,33,46] For lesions that are on the roof or on the medial wall of the trigone or on the dorsal surface of the thalamus, the senior author prefers to use a transverse paramedian brain incision in the posterior parietal region. This approach has been used by others for resecting meningiomas of the trigone.[5,10,13] For this approach, the patient is placed in the semi-sitting position or in the prone position with the head tilted up (Figure 4). The lateral position with the ipsilateral side down should not be used, as the brain shifts laterally and the landmarks to the ventricles are distorted.

The incision should be centered approximately 9 cm up from the inion and 1.5–2 cm lateral to the midline. The bone flap should extend to the midline or across it. Once the dura is opened, the area of cortical incision should be about 7 cm up from the occipital tip along the dorsal convexity. The landmark to reach the ventricle from this incision is simply to aim for the ipsilateral pupil, but this may not always be accurate. Ultrasound may be useful, but this is difficult to perform with the patient in the semi-sitting position. A ventricular needle may be used to identify the ventricle. Another useful landmark is that the trigone is about 2.5 cm off the midline in the plane created by the posterior aspect of the splenium; therefore, we usually identify the splenium with a minimal degree of brain retraction and then direct our transcortical approach in a direction parallel to the plane of the splenium.[40]

The main advantage of this transcortical approach over the parasagittal approach includes the avoidance of prolonged retrac-

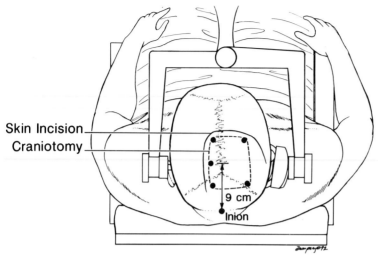

Skin Incision
Craniotomy

Figure 4A. Craniotomy for a parasagittal approach to the splenium or transcortical approach to the atrium of the right ventricle through the posterior parietal lobule. The craniotomy is centered 9 cm above the inion. This will be approximately 7 cm above the tip of the occipital lobe as measured intradurally. The craniotomy should be carried out to the left of the midline to provide parasagittal access, which is useful both for splenial lesions or for the transcortical approach to the ventricle, where exposure of the splenium will help guide the direction of transcortical approach to the atrium.

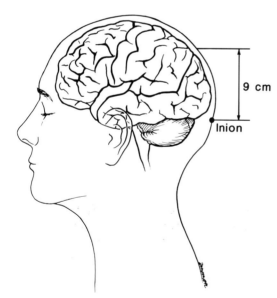

Figure 4B. Transverse paramedian cortical incision centered 9 cm above the inion should result in no major sensory or visual deficits.

tion and a more direct view of the trigone by the transcortical route. Also, since the trajectory of the small transverse cortical incision is between the parietal sensory

association fibers and the occipital visual association fibers, no significant neurologic deficit should be produced. There is a disadvantage to this approach, with AVM surgery and meningioma surgery, in that the body of the lesion is encountered prior to identification of the major blood supply. This disadvantage is not relevant in surgery for CMs, which have no large feeding arteries.

Lesions located lateral to the atrium may be approached using a transcortical incision in the middle temporal or, with nondominant lesions, the superior temporal gyrus. There is risk to the optic radiations with this approach. On the dominant side these approaches should not be performed without cortical mapping. For lesions located more inferiorly, a subtemporal approach to the lesion may be used, as described later.[16] However, one must work in an upward direction toward the atrium, which is relatively awkward. It is possible with this approach to stay below the bulk of the optic radiation, but a superior quadrantanopsia is likely.

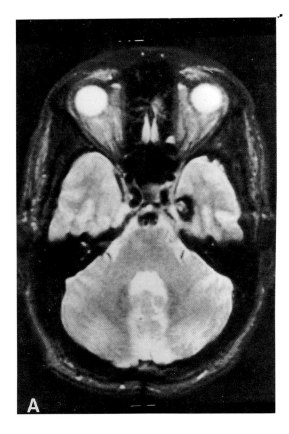

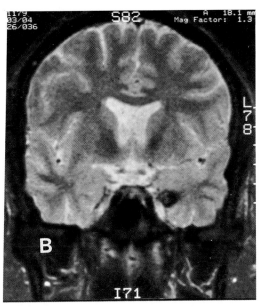

Figure 5. A 32-year-old man who presented with partial complex seizures. **A** and **B** show axial and coronal T2-weighted MRIs, respectively, of an anterior mesial temporal cavernous malformation. Complete resection was accomplished using a standard pterional craniotomy. Cortical surface discoloration was not evident intraoperatively. Ultrasonography could not be utilized for localization.

Approaches to Deep Temporal Lesions

Medial anterior temporal lesions involving the amygdala, the hippocampus, the uncus (Figure 5) or the inferior lateral aspect of the basal ganglia (lateral to the internal capsule) are approached through the sylvian fissure using a standard pterional craniotomy.[30,47,58] Enlarging the craniotomy slightly in the inferior and posterior temporal region may be helpful for the larger lesions (Figure 6). We routinely remove the pterion and the lateral aspect of the lesser wing of the sphenoid. The dura is opened approximately 2.5 cm superior to the temporal fossa in a gently curved manner, with the base toward the temporal fossa.

After CSF is drained from the prechiasmatic cisterns, the draining veins from the anterior temporal tip are taken and self-retaining retractors are placed. Using the microscope, the carotid artery is exposed and the sylvian fissure opened medially.

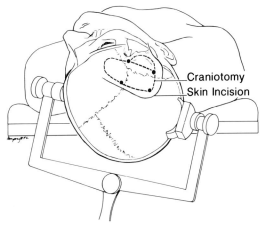

Figure 6. Full frontotemporal craniotomy for approaching large anterior mesial temporal lesions. With the head rotated 30° to 60°, a skin incision is made behind the hairline or about 1–1.5 cm in front of the hairline at the level of the pupil. The key is to have good exposure of the floor of the anterior fossa, which is accomplished by accurate placement of a burrhole at the frontal zygomatic point (keyhole). A smaller craniotomy may be used for lesions as depicted in Figure 5.

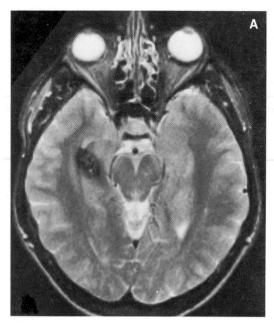

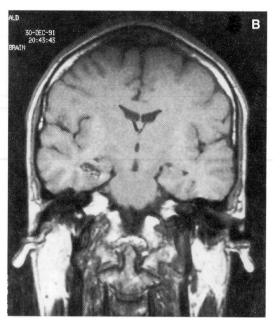

Figure 7A. A 30-year-old white male with intractable seizure disorder. Axial T2-weighted MRI illustrates a mesial temporal lesion situated posterior to the basilar artery.

The fissure is opened widely by posterolateral temporal retraction and microsurgical lysis of the adhesions between the temporal and frontal lobes. Posterolateral temporal retraction is much better tolerated than the upward retraction required for a subtemporal approach.

With the trans-sylvian approach, one can actually see back to the first anterior temporal branch of the posterior cerebral artery. It is very difficult to use an ultrasound probe in determining where to place the cortical incision in the medial temporal region. Careful evaluation of the preoperative MRI may aid in guiding the decision if there is no discoloration on the surface. Lesions in the anterior insular region can be approached readily by the trans-sylvian route.[30,53,58]

Lesions located more posteriorly in the hippocampus, the parahippocampal gyrus, and the posterior inferior thalamus can be approached subtemporally or through an incision or resection of the inferior temporal gyrus (Figures 7 and 8).[16,30,44,47] After

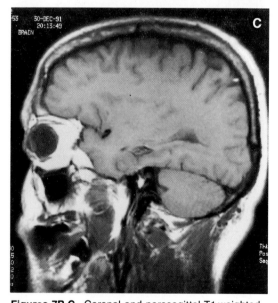

Figures 7B,C. Coronal and parasagittal T1-weighted MRIs. Note the lesion lies inferior to the temporal horn of the lateral ventricle. This lesion was resected using a standard temporal craniotomy. Intraoperatively, the lesion was localized by ultrasound and complete re-section was accomplished through a small corticectomy in the inferior temporal gyrus just behind the vein of Labbé. No postoperative field deficit was apparent.

placement of a lumbar drain, the patient is positioned laterally with the side of the lesion superior. The head is tilted down

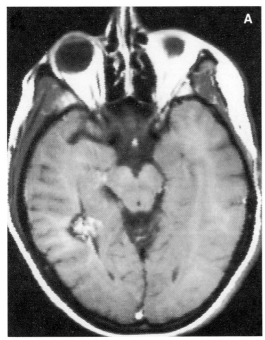

Figure 8A. A 17-year-old female presented with a history of depression and headaches. Axial T1-weighted MRI illustrates the location of the lesion slightly inferior to the temporal horn.

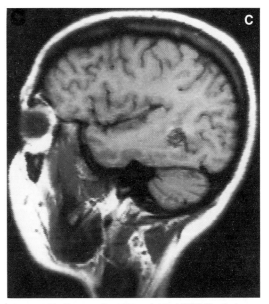

Figure 8C. Parasagittal T1-weighted MRI illustrates the deep posterior temporal location. Using a temporal craniotomy, this lesion was localized intraoperatively with the ultrasound. A corticectomy in the inferior temporal gyrus was used to resect the lesion. A small contralateral superior quadrantanopsia was present postoperatively due to the more posterolateral as opposed to inferior (as in Figure 7) location of the lesion in relation to the temporal horn.

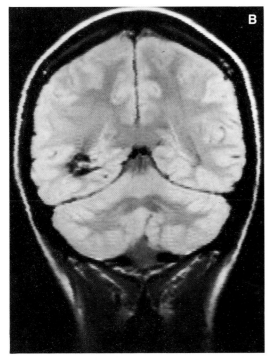

Figure 8B. Coronal T2-weighted MRI. Note the lesion lies not only inferior but also lateral to the temporal horn.

toward the contralateral shoulder to permit the temporal lobe to fall away by gravity.

Using a standard horseshoe skin incision based above the ear, a small temporal craniotomy is turned (Figure 9). It is important to rongeur or drill off bone until the exposure is flush with the floor of the temporal fossa. The dural incision is horseshoe-shaped and based at the floor of the temporal fossa. Care should be taken not to injure the transverse sinus at the back limb of the dural opening. The vein of Labbé should be identified and protected. Using ultrasound, the contours of the lesion may be identified relative to surface veins. Retraction of the temporal lobe in this region carries the risk of injury to the vein of Labbé, which may be devastating, particularly, but not exclusively, in the dominant hemisphere. Even if the vein is not overtly injured, it can thrombose from prolonged stretching.

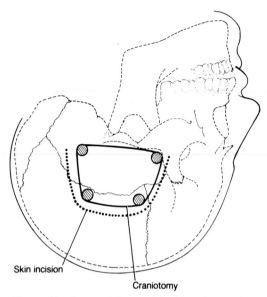

Figure 9A. Approach for mesial mid- and posterior temporal lesions. Horseshoe-shaped skin incision and the craniotomy are outlined. The craniotomy at the inferior margin should be as low as possible. Bone may need to be drilled or ronguered to the floor of the temporal fossa.

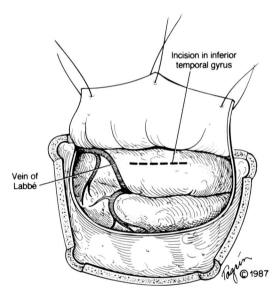

Figure 9B. Incision (or small amount of brain resection) in the inferior temporal gyrus is preferable to elevation of the temporal lobe which incurs risk of injury to the vein of Labbé. If the vein drains more anteriorly, the incision or brain resection can be immediately behind the vein. (Reprinted with permission from Ojemann RG, Heros RC, Crowell RM. *Surgical Management of Cerebrovascular Disease.* Baltimore, Md: Williams & Wilkins; 1988:368.)

When it appears that the vein of Labbé will be at risk from retraction, the senior author prefers to resect a small amount of brain in the inferior temporal gyrus either in front or behind the vein.[15,16,17,30] This can be carried out to a depth of about 2.5 cm, allowing one to enter the subtemporal space about midway between the lateral surface of the temporal lobe and the incisura. The area of brain resected is lateral to the inferior optic radiation, and in the senior author's experience there has been no instance of postoperative visual field deficit that could be attributed to this maneuver.

The other option is to make a small cortical incision in the inferior temporal gyrus over the cavernous malformation located by ultrasound, and approach the lesion directly transcortically. Drake has described the approach of using an incision in the fusiform gyrus, which is medial to the optic radiations.[8] For more superiorly located lesions, an incision in the superior and middle temporal gyri may offer a more direct access, but it will result in injury to the optic radiations, and in the dominant hemisphere it may result in speech deficits.[8]

Posterior insular lesions can be approached by a posterior trans-sylvian route, using the standard temporal horseshoe type of skin incision just described.[30] Inferior exposure is not as critical, and it is not necessary to remove the pterion or to open the medial aspect of the sylvian fissure. Posteriorly, the fissure may be obscured but it can be found by following a medial sylvian fissure vein posteriorly. Minimal subpial dissection may be necessary superficially when the fissure is not well-defined. In a deeper plane the fissure is better defined. Care is taken not to injure branches of the middle cerebral artery once the sylvian fissure is opened.

Approaches to Thalamic and Basal Ganglia Lesions

Deep temporal or trigonal lesions involving the basal ganglia or thalamus have been discussed. This section describes approaches to deep thalamic and basal ganglia lesions that are accessible through the lateral ventricle.[15,30] Intraventricular access can be exposed transcortically or by using an interhemispheric transcallosal approach.[30,42,45,58] Lesions on the posterodorsal aspect of the thalamus can be reached using the posterior parietal transcortical approach to the atrium previously described. Lesions of the anterior dorsal aspect of the thalamus can be reached by a transcortical frontal approach, which may be preferable when there is hydrocephalus, or by an anterior transcallosal approach. The incision in the corpus callosum should be only 1–2 cm; the fornix, which lies deep to the corpus callosum, may need to be resected ipsilaterally for large lesions.[45] The most common postoperative complication may be disturbance of recent memory, but this usually improves with time.[45]

Lesions in the head of the caudate nucleus can be operated on successfully as long as they do not extend to the internal capsule. The senior author prefers the transcortical approach when the ventricles are large, and otherwise prefers the interhemispheric transcallosal approach previously described.[17,30] For the transcortical approach, the patient is supine and the head is in a neutral position, slightly flexed. A small unilateral frontal exposure with the boneflap centered about the coronal suture is made (Figure 10). The dural incision is based toward the superior sagittal sinus. Frequently, a deep middle frontal sulcus can be followed for a good distance toward the ventricle. The lesion is removed microscopically, avoiding injury to the thalamostriate or septal veins.

Approaches to Extracerebral and Pineal Region Lesions

Extracerebral dural-based lesions arise primarily in the middle fossa or parasellar regions.[3,9,26,28,37,39] Extracerebral CMs are rare and have been reported predominantly in females of Oriental descent.[28] In 1983,

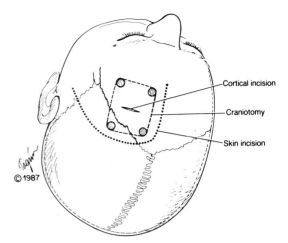

Figure 10. Left frontal craniotomy for a transcortical approach to the anterior aspect of the left lateral ventricle. The patient is supine with the head neutral and the neck slightly flexed. (Reprinted with permission from Ojemann RG, Heros RC, Crowell RM. *Surgical Management of Cerebrovascular Disease.* Baltimore, Md: Williams & Wilkins; 1988:388.)

Namba presented a review of 23 cases reported in the literature.[28] Nearly 50% of the patients had ocular symptoms and signs such as diplopia, anisocoria, and visual acuity or visual field deficits. This was attributed to cavernous sinus involvement in the parasellar lesions.

The preoperative diagnosis in most of the cases was a parasellar or medial sphenoid wing meningioma. The angiographic appearance of these lesions, as previously mentioned, is indistinguishable from that of a meningioma. The meningohypophyseal trunk or middle meningeal artery are usually the primary feeders to the lesion. Similar to a meningioma, exacerbation of the cavernous sinus syndrome may occur during pregnancy. Thus, the dural-based CMs, although pathologically similar to the intracerebral lesions, are much more aggressive clinically.

The surgical management of this lesion is difficult. In two-thirds of the cases reported by Namba, only partial removal was achieved because of profuse intraoperative hemorrhage.[28] These lesions arise within the leaves of the dura of the middle fossa and can completely encase the cavernous segment of the internal carotid artery and cranial nerves III–VI. The use of preoperative embolization through the external carotid artery may or may not be useful in reducing intraoperative bleeding. Preoperative irradiation has been used to decrease intraoperative bleeding but its role in the management of these lesions is inconclusive.

Prior to surgery, balloon test occlusions of the carotid artery along with xenon-CT blood flow determination to assess tolerance to carotid ligation may be helpful.[41,60] The best approach will vary with the extent of the lesion, but frequently an intradural and extradural combined approach to the cavernous sinus may be necessary.[41] The need for proximal carotid control should be anticipated.

Another rare location for a CM is the pineal region.[11] In this region, the preoperative MRI may not contribute to the specific pathologic diagnosis. CMs reported in this region are not as vascular as the dural-based lesions. The presence of CMs in this area again stresses the need for obtaining tissue diagnosis. The standard infratentorial supracerebellar approach in the sitting position probably provides the best surgical exposure for most lesions of this region.[48]

Conclusion

The surgery of supratentorial CMs is relatively straightforward because bleeding is not a problem. The technique of resection resembles that used for metastatic neoplasms rather than that used for cerebral AVMs. There are almost never large feeding arteries or draining veins, and there is almost always a clear gliotic plane surrounding the lesions, although the lesion can be quite irregular with lobules buried in the brain in different directions. Most frequently, a lesion is decompressed internally with suction and bipolar coagulation; only occasionally is the ultrasonic aspirator or laser necessary.

After internal decompression, the lesion is dissected systematically from its surrounding gliotic plane. When working in noneloquent brain, it is preferable to resect this gliotic tissue to reduce the likelihood of postoperative seizures. In general, the morbidity of the surgery is determined by the surgical approach to deep lesions—e.g. by the eloquence of brain that has to be traversed or retracted to reach the lesion. Once the surgeon reaches the lesion, resection should add little or no morbidity, even if the lesion is located in eloquent brain. This is why very large CMs of the brain stem can be resected with little neurologic morbidity, provided they present in either the lateral surface of the brain stem or in the floor of the fourth ventricle.

References

1. Berger M, Choen W, Ojemann G. Correlation of motor cortex brain mapping with magnetic resonance imaging. *J Neurosurg*. 1990;72:383–387.

2. Bogren H, Svalander C, Wickbom I. Angiography in intracranial cavernous hemangiomas. *Acta Radiol Diagn*. 1970;10:81–89.

3. Buonaguidi R, Canapicci R, Mimassi N, et al. Intrasellar cavernous hemangioma. *Neurosurgery*. 1984;14:732–734.

4. Chandler WF, Knake JE, McGillicuddy JE, et al. Intraoperative use of real-time ultrasonography in neurosurgery. *J Neurosurgery*. 1982;57:157–163.

5. Cramer F. The intraventricular meningioma: a note on the neurologic determinants governing the surgical approach. *Arch Neurol*. 1960;3:98. Abstract.

6. Curling OD Jr, Kelly DL Jr, Elster AD, et al. An analysis of the natural history of cavernous angiomas. *J Neurosurg*. 1991;75:702–708.

7. Davis DH, Kelly PJ. Stereotactic resection of occult vascular malformations. *J Neurosurg*. 1990;72:698–702.

8. Drake CG. Cerebral arteriovenous malformations: considerations for and experience with surgical treatment in 166 cases. *Clin Neurosurg*. 1979;26:145–208.

9. Fehlings MG, Tucker WS. Cavernous hemangioma of Meckel's cave: case report. *J Neurosurg*. 1988;68:645–647.

10. Fornari M, Saviaiardo M, Morello G, et al. Meningiomas of the lateral ventricles: neuroradiological and surgical considerations in 18 cases. *J Neurosurg*. 1981;54:64–74.

11. Fukui M, Matsuoka S, Hasuo K, et al. Cavernous hemangioma in the pineal region. *Surg Neurol*. 1983;20:209–215.

12. Giombini S, Morello G. Cavernous angioma of the brain: account of 14 personal cases and review of the literature. *Acta Neurochir*. 1978;40:61–82.

13. Guidetti B, Delfini R, Gagliardi FM, et al. Meningiomas of the lateral ventricles: clinical, neuroradiologic and surgical considerations in 19 cases. *Surg Neurol*. 1985;24:364–370.

14. Harkey HL, Al-Mefty O, Haines DE, et al. The surgical anatomy of the cerebral sulci. *Neurosurgery*. 1989;24:651–654.

15. Heros RC. Arteriovenous malformations of the medial temporal lobe: surgical approach and neuroradiological characterization. *J Neurosurg*. 1982;56:44–52.

16. Heros RC. Brain resection for the exposure of deep extracerebral and paraventricular lesions. *Surg Neurol*. 1990;34:188–195.

17. Heros RC, Korosue K. Surgery of parenchymal cerebral arteriovenous malformations: complications and their avoidance. In: Apuzzo M, ed. *Brain Surgery: Complication, Avoidance and Management*. New York, NY: Churchill Livingstone; 1992. In press.

18. Jun CL, Nutik SL. Surgical approaches to intraventricular meningiomas of the trigone. In: Schmidek HH, Sweet WH, eds. *Operative Neurosurgical Techniques, Indications, Methods and Results*. Orlando, Fla: Grune & Stratton; 1988:596–600.

19. Kelly PJ. Volumetric stereotactic surgical resection of intra-axial brain mass lesions. *Mayo Clin Proc*. 1988;63:1186–1198.

20. Kelly PJ, Goerss SJ, Kall BA. The stereotactic retractor in computer-assisted stereotaxic microsurgery. Technical note. *J Neurosurg*. 1988;69:301–306.

21. Kudo T, Ueki S, Kobayashi H, et al. Experience with the ultrasonic surgical aspirator in a cavernous hemangioma of the cavernous sinus. *Neurosurgery*. 1989;24:628–631.

22. Little JR, Awad IA, Jones SC, et al. Vascular pressures and cortical blood flow in cavernous angioma of the brain. *J Neurosurg*. 1990;73:555–559.

23. Lobato RD, Perez C, Rivas JJ, et al. Clinical, radiological and pathological spectrum of angiographically occult intracranial vascular malformations. *J Neurosurg*. 1988;68:518–531.

24. Martin N, Grafton S, Vinuela F, et al. Imaging for arterial functional localization. In: Selman, ed. *Clinical Neurosurgery*. Baltimore, Md: Williams & Wilkins; 1992:132–165.

25. Maruoka N, Yamakawa Y, Shimauchi M. Cavernous hemangioma of the optic nerve: case report. *J Neurosurg*. 1988;69:292–294.

26. McCormick PC, Michelsen WJ. Management of intracranial cavernous and venous malformations. In: Barrow DL, ed. *Intracranial Vascular Malformations*. Neurosurgical Topics. Park Ridge, Ill: American Association of Neurological Surgeons; 1991:197–217.

27. Nagata S, Rhoton AL Jr, Barry M. Microsurgical anatomy of the choroidal fissure. *Surg Neurol*. 1988;30:3–59.

28. Namba S. Extracerebral cavernous hemangioma of the middle cranial fossa. *Surg Neurol*. 1983;19:379–388.

29. Ojemann G, Ojemann J, Lettich E, et al. Cortical localization in left dominant hemisphere: an electrical stimulation mapping investigation in 117 patients. *J Neurosurg*. 1989;71:316–326.

30. Ojemann RG, Heros RC, Crowell RM. *Surgical Management of Cerebrovascular Disease*. Baltimore, Md: Williams & Wilkins; 1988:347–413.

31. Ondra SL, Doby JR, Mohla ME, et al. Surgical excision of a cavernous hemangioma of the rostral brainstem: case report. *Neurosurgery*. 1988;23:490–493.

32. Ogilvy CS, Heros RC, Ojemann RG, et al. Angiographically occult arteriovenous malformations. *J Neurosurg*. 1988;69:350–355.

33. Rhoton AL Jr, Tamamoto I, Peace DA. Microneurosurgery of the third ventricle: part 2. Operative approaches. *Neurosurgery*. 1981;8:357–372.

34. Rigamonti D, Drayer BP, Johnson PC, et al. The MRI appearance of cavernous malformations (angiomas). *J Neurosurg*. 1987;67:518–524.

35. Rigamonti D, Hadley MN, Drayer BP, et al. Cerebral cavernous malformations: incidence and familial occurrence. *N Eng J Med*. 1988;319:343–347.

36. Robinson JR, Awad IA, Little JR. Natural history of the cavernous angioma. *J Neurosurg*. 1991; 75:709–714.

37. Rosenblum B, Rothman AS, Lanzieri C, et al. A cavernous sinus cavernous hemangioma: case report. *J Neurosurg*. 1986;65:716–718.

38. Russell DS, Rubenstein LJ. *Pathology of Tumors of the Nervous System*. 4th ed. Baltimore, Md: Williams & Wilkins; 1977.

39. Sansone ME, Liurnicz BL, Mandyluir TI. Giant pituitary cavernous hemangioma: case report. *J Neurosurg*. 1980;53:124–126.

40. Seeger W. Supratentorial structures near the ventricles. In: *Atlas of Topographical Anatomy of the Brain and Surrounding Structures*. New York, NY: Springer-Verlag; 1978:368–427.

41. Sekhar LN, Sen LN. Surgical treatment of tumors involving the cavernous sinus. In: Wilkins RH, Rengachary SS, eds. *Neurosurgery: Update I*. New York, NY: McGraw-Hill Inc; 1990:334–345.

42. Shucart W. Anterior transcallosal and transcortical approaches. In: Apuzzo ML, ed. *Surgery of the Third Ventricle*. Baltimore, Md: Williams & Wilkins; 1987:303–325.

43. Simard JM, Garcia-Bengochea F, Ballinger WE, et al. Cavernous angioma: a review of 126 collected and 12 new clinical cases. *Neurosurgery*. 1986;18:162–172.

44. Solomon RA, Stein BM. Surgical management of arteriovenous malformations that follow the tentorial ring. *Neurosurgery*. 1986;18:708–715.

45. Solomon RA, Stein BM. Interhemispheric approach for the surgical removal of thalamo-caudate arteriovenous malformations. *J Neurosurg*. 1987;66:345–351.

46. Spencer DD, Collins W, Sass KJ. Surgical management of lateral intraventricular tumors. In: Schmidek HH, Sweet WH, eds. *Operative Neurosurgical Techniques*. Orlando, Fla: Grune & Stratton; 1988:583–596.

47. Stein BM. Arteriovenous malformations of the medial cerebral hemisphere and the limbic system. *J Neurosurg*. 1984;60:23–31.

48. Stein BM. Infratentorial supracerebellar approach. In: Apuzzo ML, ed. *Surgery of the Third Ventricle*. Baltimore, Md: Williams & Wilkins; 1987:570–590.

49. Sundt TM Jr. Operative techniques for arteriovenous malformations of the brain. In: Barrow DL, ed. *Intracranial Vascular Malformations*. Neurosurgical Topics. Park Ridge, Ill: American Association of Neurological Surgeons; 1990:111–124.

50. Sze G, Krol G, Olson WL, et al. Hemorrhagic neoplasms: MR mimics of occult vascular malformations. *AJR*. 1987;149:1223–1230.

51. Vaquero J, Leunda G, Martinez R, et al. Cavernomas of the brain. *Neurosurgery*. 1983;12:208–210.

52. Vaquero J, Salazar R, Martinez P, et al. Cavernomas of the central nervous system: clinical syndromes, CT scan diagnosis, and prognosis after surgical treatment in 25 cases. *Acta Neurochir*. 1987;85:29–33.

53. Viale GL, Turtas S, Pau A. Surgical removal of striate arteriovenous malformations. *Surg Neurol*. 1980;14:321–324.

54. Voigt K, Yasargil MA. Cerebral cavernous hemangiomas or cavernomas. *Neurochir*. 1986;65:188–193.

55. Voorhies RM, Engel I, Gamache JW Jr, et al. Intraoperative localization of subcortical brain tumors: further experience with B-mode real-time sector scanning. *Neurosurgery*. 1983;12:189–194.

56. Wilson CB. Cryptic vascular malformations: In: Selman, ed. *Clinical Neurosurgery*. Baltimore, Md: Williams & Wilkins; 1992:49–84.

57. Yasargil MG. Microsurgical anatomy of the brain. In: *Microneurosurgery*, Vol I. New York, NY: Thieme Medical Publishers; 1984:284–320.

58. Yasargil MG. Arteriovenous malformations of the brain, history, embryology, pathological considerations, hemodynamics, diagnostic studies, microsurgical anatomy. In: *Microneurosurgery* Vol. IIIA. Stuttgart, West Germany: George Thiems Verlag; 1987.

59. Yasargil MG, Jain KK, Antic J, et al. Arteriovenous malformations of the anterior and the middle portions of the corpus callosum: microsurgical treatment. *Surg Neurol*. 1976;5:67–80.

60. Yonas H, Guvk D, Johnson D, et al. Xenon-CT cerebral blood flow analysis. In: Latchaw R, ed. *MRI and CT Imaging of the Head, Neck and Spine*. St. Louis, Mo: Mosby-Year Book; 1991:109–128.

Chapter 10

Microsurgical Treatment of Infratentorial Cavernous Malformations

Thomas M. Wascher, MD, and Robert F. Spetzler, MD, FACS

Autopsy studies indicate that cavernous malformations (CMs) comprise approximately 13% of all vascular malformations of the posterior fossa.[30] Previously published series indicate that 10% to 30% of all intracranial CMs are located in the infratentorial space and are more frequently symptomatic than their supratentorial counterparts.[29] These lesions of the brain stem and cerebellum have a distinctive clinical presentation and course once they become symptomatic, resulting in progressive cranial nerve deficits, facial pain, hypesthesia, vertigo, headache, nausea and vomiting, ataxia, weakness, and hemisensory deficit.[53] Once patients present with neurologic deficits, signs and symptoms appear to progress as a result of growth of vascular tissue as well as of repetitive micro- and gross hemorrhages, which may eventually be fatal. Surgical resection of infratentorial CMs appears to be the treatment of choice when: **(1)** the patient is symptomatic, **(2)** the lesion is located in the cerebellum or superficially in the brain stem, and **(3)** an operative approach can spare eloquent brain parenchyma.[53] The natural history of and the surgical indications for infratentorial CMs are discussed elsewhere in this text. This chapter briefly reviews the surgical principles and approaches that we have found most useful in the management of symptomatic infratentorial CMs.

General Principles of Preoperative and Intraoperative Management

The cornerstone of successful management of infratentorial CMs, as in all neurosurgical procedures, is the selection of an appropriate approach that optimizes exposure of the offending lesion with an absolute minimum of distortion of normal neurovascular relationships. A detailed and thorough knowledge of the normal neurovascular anatomy of the posterior fossa, tentorial incisura, foramen magnum region, temporal bone, and cerebellum–brain stem is a prerequisite to suitable preoperative planning and appropriate intraoperative decision making. A complete understanding of the relationships of the neurovascular structures as well as readily identifiable reference points in the surgical field (e.g. major arterial branches, cranial nerve entry root zones, mass effect from an underlying CM, residua from previous hemorrhage) provides confidence in relating anatomic and pathologic structures and in formulating a surgical plan after exact intraoperative localization of the lesion. There can be no error in localization because there is no allowance for surgical exploration of the brain stem. Stereotaxically guided craniotomy, although useful for supratentorial lesions, is not as reliable for infratentorial surgery due to the required extra-axial dissection, cerebrospinal fluid (CSF) drainage required for brain relaxation, and the resulting alterations in spatial relationships between brain and skull.

After localizing the lesion, the surgeon usually encounters a cavity containing vascular spaces of the CM and degradation products of prior hemorrhage. Unlike supratentorial malformations, lesions located within the brain stem can be extremely adherent to surrounding normal parenchyma.[53] Initial dissection should concentrate on circumferential separation of the malformation from surrounding gliosis prior to internal decompression of the lesion, if possible. Despite the lack of apparent feeding vessels, bleeding can occasionally be brisk if the center of the malformation is entered before circumferential dissection.[49] Once devascularized, the intracapsular contents of the malformation are removed in a piecemeal fashion; the remaining portions of the capsule are then dissected from the surface of the brain stem and nerves, rather than attempting to deliver the intact malformation through a small opening. All perforating arterial vessels must be dissected meticulously and preserved.

The goal of surgery must be complete extirpation of the lesion (with reasonable attention to minimize injury to normal brain); several authors have reported symptomatic recurrences and hemorrhages after partial or seemingly complete removal.[4,53] While complete resection is a relatively routine endeavor with small lesions (those less than 2 cm in diameter), the degree of resection becomes more difficult to assess

intraoperatively with larger multilobulated lesions. This is particularly true when sizable lesions involve the brain stem and cerebellum, where the complexity of the anatomy makes complete resection difficult without some risk to normal pathways. When the CM can be excised completely, the risk of further neurologic deterioration due to further growth and hemorrhage is eliminated and cure is permanent. Evidence of persistent or recurrent CM on postoperative magnetic resonance imaging (MRI) indicates the need for close followup with consideration of additional surgery to achieve complete resection. However, the natural history of an incompletely resected or recurrent CM has yet to be elucidated.

The association between CMs and venous malformations, which may be as high as 16%,[4,37,53] must be recognized. Although the surgical management of CMs requires that the entire raspberry-like lesion should be removed, interruption of a venous malformation can threaten drainage from normal parenchyma and result in venous infarction.[4] Therefore, when a large venous malformation is encountered in the proximity of a symptomatic CM, the surgical approach must be tailored to permit resection of the CM while maintaining drainage from the venous malformation.

Finally, there is mounting evidence that capillary telangiectases and CMs represent two pathologic extremes within the same spectrum of vascular malformations, termed *cerebral capillary malformations*.[36] It has been suggested that a de novo CM may arise from fusion of the adjacent dilated capillary telangiectasia. Therefore, according to this classification scheme, transitional forms are not separate entities but rather various stages in the development from capillary telangiectases to CMs. This concept is further supported by the MRI similarities of CMs and capillary telangiectases and the fact that these two vascular malformations are frequently identified in the same patient.[36] The surgical significance of this association awaits further confirmation.

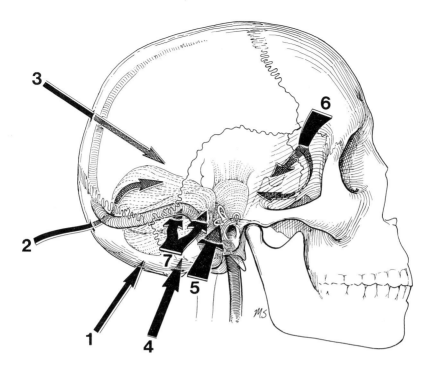

Figure 1. Summary of surgical approaches to CMs involving the brain stem. These include: **(1)** suboccipital; **(2)** infratentorial supracerebellar; **(3)** occipital transtentorial; **(4)** far lateral; **(5)** transtemporal; **(6)** frontotemporal/subtemporal transtentorial; and **(7)** combined petrosal approaches.

Surgical Approaches to Infratentorial Cavernous Malformations

The surgical approaches described below are those we have found most useful for the surgical management of CMs involving the brain stem. These various approaches are summarized in Figure 1.

Suboccipital Approach

Lesions of the cerebellar vermis, medial cerebellar hemispheres, floor of the fourth ventricle, and dorsal medulla are easily approached through a standard suboccipital craniotomy.[6,8] With the patient in the prone or park-bench position (to avoid complications associated with air embolism), a vertical midline or hockey-stick suboccipital incision (depending on the degree of lateral exposure desired) is used. The subcutaneous tissues are separated from the cervical fascia, which is incised in a Y-shaped fashion with the upper arms of the Y beginning 1 cm below the external occipital protuberance. The inferior arm of the Y is extended down the midline to C1–2. The muscular and ligamentous attachments are then freed from the occipital bone and the posterior elements of C1–C2. A unilateral or bilateral craniotomy is performed, extending as high as the transverse sinus and including the foramen magnum, depending on the desired exposure. The dura is opened again in a Y-shaped or hockey-stick fashion, with care to respect the transverse, occipital, and marginal venous sinuses.

Posterior cerebellar malformations may now be approached directly. Intraoperative ultrasonography may be useful to guide dissection when these lesions are located entirely within the cerebellar hemisphere. Malformations involving the floor of the fourth ventricle may require separation of the cerebellar tonsils or division of the vermis. With this approach, CMs as far rostrally as the dorsal pontine tegmentum can be exposed and resected safely after division of the cerebellar vermis.

When CMs involve the dorsal brain stem, it is imperative that the floor of the fourth ventricle be identified as the major regional landmark to avoid unnecessary dissection within the brain stem itself.[8] The branches of the posterior inferior cerebellar artery, as it courses around the tonsil, should not be injured. After the operation is completed, the dura is closed in a watertight fashion (using a fascial graft if required), as is the Y-shaped incision in the cervical fascia. Although providing excellent exposure of midline posterior lesions, the suboccipital approach provides poor access to ventrally located lesions without a significant amount of retraction.

Infratentorial Supracerebellar Approach

Originally described by Krause and popularized by Stein, the infratentorial supracerebellar approach permits exposure of malformations involving the tectum and pineal region.[43-45] Positioning and approach are as described for the suboccipital approach, except that the craniectomy must be extended to expose the transverse sinus-torcular junction. The dura is opened bilaterally to the edges of the transverse sinuses. Bridging veins from the superior aspect of the cerebellum are divided to permit exposure to the incisural region between the anterior vermis and the inferior surface of the tentorium. When dividing the arachnoid over the quadrigeminal cistern, care must be taken to identify and prevent injury to the vein of Galen, the internal cerebral veins, the basal veins of Rosenthal, and the midbrain branches of the posterior choroidal arteries. If necessary, further exposure may be achieved by incising the tentorium 1 cm lateral to the straight sinus.

Small, angled dental mirrors may be useful for inspecting the bed of a resected CM involving the inferior third ventricle or caudal region of the tectal plate. Advantages of this approach include adequate exposure of the dorsal midbrain, avoiding the deep venous system without violation of normal brain parenchyma.[45] Limitations of the approach are defined by superolateral extension of the malformation above the tentorium, which may be difficult to reach from an infratentorial exposure.

Occipital Transtentorial Approach

Originally described by Poppen and later modified by Jamieson, the occipital transtentorial approach provides exposure of the superior cerebellar peduncles and vermis, the anterior medullary velum, the posterior third ventricle, the splenium, and the quadrigeminal plate.[21,34,35] Compared to the infratentorial supracerebellar approach, this approach provides broader exposure in the region of the tentorial incisura, especially for lesions extending dorsally above the incisura, without sacrificing normal neurovascular structures.[35] However, the occipital transtentorial approach may require retraction of the occipitoparietal lobe, resulting in sensory or visual-field deficits.[45]

The patient is positioned on the right side in a three-quarter-prone orientation with the neck slightly flexed and the head rotated 30°–40° to the left. This position allows gravity to assist in deflecting the right occipital pole away from the tentorium, minimizing the need for retraction.[5] A right occipital craniotomy is performed, exposing the superior sagittal and the right transverse sinus. The dura is then opened in a T-shaped fashion, extending to the edge of the torcular Herophili. Bridging veins may be encountered between the lateral occipital lobe and the tentorium or lateral sinus (which must be preserved), but no veins are located between the occipital pole and the sagittal sinus.[5,35] Dissection is continued along the falx to expose the

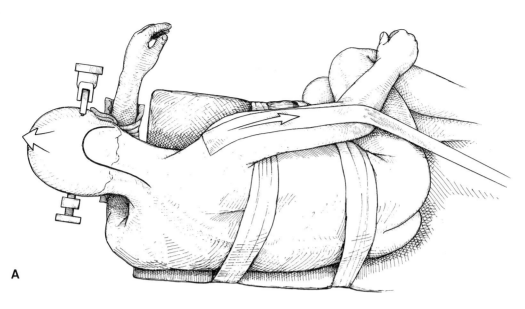

A

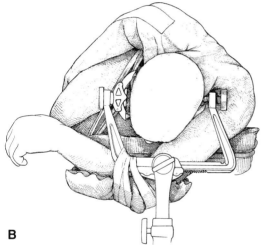

B

Figure 2. Positioning for the far lateral approach. **(A)** View from above (approach for a right-sided lesion). The patient is placed in a modified park-bench position with the cervical spine flexed in the anteroposterior plane, rotated 45° to the left, and flexed laterally 30° to the left. The inverted hockey-stick incision extends along the midline, following the superior nuchal line, and terminates just medial to the mastoid process. **(B)** View from cranial vertex. Note how the dependent arm has been padded carefully and cradled beneath the Mayfield head holder. (Reprinted with permission. From Spetzler RF, Grahm TW. The far-lateral approach to the inferior clivus and the upper cervical region: technical note. *BNI Quart.* 1990;6:35–38.)

falcotentorial junction and the incisural region. The tentorium can then be divided parallel to the straight sinus beginning 1 cm lateral to the sinus at the incisura. The free edges of the tentorium are retracted with sutures, exposing the anterior-superior cerebellar vermis. Arachnoid extending over the pineal region and enveloping the major deep veins is then sharply incised, visualizing the dorsal midbrain. Through this approach, the superior vermis may be divided to enter the superior fourth ventricle and to expose the superior cerebellar peduncles.[5] The precentral cerebellar and other bridging cerebellar veins may be taken, but all other veins in the pineal re-

gion should be spared. Additionally, by dissecting between the major veins and opening the suprapineal recess, exposure of the third ventricle as far forward as the foramen of Monro can be achieved.[5]

Far Lateral Approach

As elaborated by Heros and modified by Spetzler for vertebrobasilar junction aneurysms,[18,42] the far lateral approach provides excellent exposure of the anterior and lateral medulla, cervicomedullary junction, and associated structures. The patient is placed in a modified park-bench position with the cervical spine flexed in the antero-posterior plane, rotated 45° to the contra-lateral side, and laterally flexed 30° toward the opposite shoulder. In this position, the ipsilateral mastoid process is the highest point in the operative field (Figure 2A). The dependent arm is allowed to drop off the end of the table, which is extended several inches with a three-quarter-inch plastic sheet. The arm is cradled underneath the edge of the table where it is attached to the Mayfield head holder with adhesive tape (Figure 2B). Padding is placed beneath the dependent axilla and between the patient's knees. The ipsilateral shoulder is pulled toward the feet and the entire body secured in position with adhesive tape to allow full rotation of the table.

An inverted hockey-stick incision is used, beginning just medial to the mastoid process and extending up to the superior nuchal line. The incision is carried medially along the nuchal line to the midline, at which point it follows the midline down to C3 or C4. A myocutaneous flap is elevated laterally, leaving a 1 cm cuff of cervical fascia attached to the superior nuchal line to allow for a water-tight closure after completion of the procedure. Subperiosteal dissection is used to expose the occipital bone as well as the spinous processes and ipsilateral laminae of C1 and C2.

The vertebral artery surrounded by its venous plexus is identified and dissected from surrounding soft tissues between the sulcus arteriosus of the lateral mass of C1 and the entry of the artery into posterior fossa dura. A C1 hemilaminectomy using the Midas Rex drill with B1 bit and foot-plate (Midas Rex Institute, Inc., Fort Worth, TX) is then performed; the lamina can be replaced after the procedure.

A retrosigmoid craniotomy (extending from the midline to as far laterally as possible, down to the foramen magnum and the dural entry of the vertebral artery) is performed. Further lateral exposure using ron-geurs of various sizes and the Midas Rex drill is achieved by removal of the lateral

foramen magnum as well as the posterior third of the occipital condyle and superior lateral mass and facet of C1. The extradural vertebral artery should be protected at all times with a small dissector during maneu-vers in this region. Entry into the condylar vein indicates sufficient anterior bone re-moval. Because the hypoglossal canal is situated in the anterior third of the occipital condyle, the XIIth nerve is protected if dissection is limited to the posterior third of the condyle. The extreme lateral removal of bone from the occipital condyle and lateral mass of C1 is the key to approaching the anterior brain stem from an inferolat-eral angle with minimal retraction.[18] Even more extensive exposure can be achieved by drilling away the mastoid process and the occipitoatlantal articular facet, but this necessitates bony fusion of the craniocervi-cal junction if postoperative stability is to be maintained.[40]

At this point, the dura is opened in a curvilinear fashion, with its base laterally, and tacked to the edges of the craniotomy. The extensive extradural bone removal allows for lateral retraction of the vertebral artery when the surrounding dura is tented, per-mitting unobstructed exposure of the infe-rior clivus, anterolateral medulla, and cer-vicomedullary junction (Figure 3). Slight elevation of the cerebellar tonsil allows for visualization as far rostrally as the ponto-medullary junction with a minimum of retraction.

Further arachnoidal microdissection will permit approaches to laterally and anteri-orly placed malformations between the VII–VIII, the IX–X–XI, and the XIIth nerve complexes. The XIth cranial nerve can usu-ally be distinguished from and separated from the IX–Xth nerve complex, exposing the region where the posterior inferior cer-ebellar artery originates from the vertebral artery.[18]

The critical anterolateral relationships of the inferior cranial nerves and the associated vasculature are exquisitely displayed with the far lateral approach. Its advantages include the following: **(1)** an extremely flat

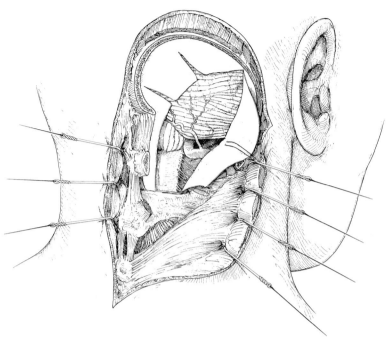

Figure 3. Intraoperative view after durotomy has been performed. Far lateral suboccipital bone removal allows for lateral retraction of the vertebral artery after the dura is tented, exposing the cerebellar hemisphere, inferior clivus, anterolateral medulla, and cervicomedullary junction with minimal retraction. From Spetzler RF, Grahm TW. The far-lateral approach to the inferior clivus and the upper cervical region: technical note. *BNI Quart.* 1990;6:35–38. Reprinted with permission.

approach to the clivus, provided by removal of the occipital condyle, therefore allowing a wide angle of visualization along the skull base; **(2)** proximal and distal control of the vertebral artery and its branches; **(3)** excellent exposure of the inferior cranial nerves and craniovertebral junction; and **(4)** no retraction whatsoever of neurovascular structures. However, it is technically challenging and requires expertise with dissection around the vertebral artery.

Transtemporal (Translabyrinthine, Transcochlear, and Transotic) Approaches

The transtemporal approaches provide direct access to lesions in and around the internal auditory meatus. These exposures would be ideally suited for the patient with a CM involving the pontomedullary junction who has lost serviceable hearing. The exposures are based on bone removal, not

cerebellar retraction, and the course of the facial nerve is identified early in the procedure, ensuring its protection. Additionally, the translabyrinthine exposure can be combined with the transcochlear or transotic approach to permit access to the anterior pons or combined with a retrosigmoid approach to improve exposure of the lateral pontomedullary junction.[14] The translabyrinthine exposure shortens the working distance to the brain stem and provides adequate exposure of the anterolateral pontomedullary junction without brain retraction or transgression of septic spaces. Disadvantages include hearing loss and temporary paralysis of the facial nerve after its transposition, as occurs in the transcochlear approach.

The translabyrinthine procedure is performed with the patient in the supine position and the head turned in a true lateral position.[24] A curved postauricular incision is made 3 cm posterior to the pinna down to the inferior border of the mastoid. The ear is reflected anteriorly, and temporal squama and mastoid processes cleared of overlying pericranium and muscle. Dissection is continued down to the spine of Henle to avoid entry into the external auditory canal. A complete mastoidectomy is performed, and bone overlying the sigmoid sinus and adjacent retrosigmoid region is removed with a high-speed drill.

The operative microscope is used for the remainder of the operation. The remaining air cells of the mastoid process are removed to the level of the lateral semicircular canal. The lateral semicircular canal is an important landmark to the location of the facial nerve, which is situated immediately inferior to the canal itself, paralleling its anterior border.[24] The mastoid portion of the facial nerve is identified and preserved by leaving a thin bony layer over the nerve itself. Drilling is continued to enter the semicircular canals, with care taken to identify the junction of the superior canal ampulla and the posterior canal ampulla. The superior canal ampulla is located just inferior and posterior to the labyrinthine segment of the facial nerve. The descending portion of the facial nerve is skeletonized, delineating the anterior extent of the exposure.[10] Labyrinthectomy is performed, beginning with the lateral semicircular canal. Bone is removed posteriorly until the superior petrosal sinus and the sinodural angle are exposed. The internal auditory canal is skeletonized, identifying the transverse and vertical crests. The posterior wall of the internal auditory canal is followed medially until the lateral lip of the porus is removed. The limits of exposure thus include the middle fossa dura superiorly, the middle ear cavity and descending facial nerve anteriorly, the cochlear aqueduct and jugular bulb inferiorly, the internal auditory canal medially, and the posterior fossa dura posteriorly.[10]

Further exposure can be achieved by the transcochlear approach.[20] As described by House and Hitselberger, a translabyrinthine exposure to the internal auditory canal is performed.[20] The extended facial recess is then entered, and the chorda tympani and the greater superficial petrosal nerves are divided, allowing transposition of the facial nerve from the fallopian canal posteriorly.[15,20] The base of the cochlea is drilled away, and the incus and stapes are removed. This maneuver permits identification of the internal carotid artery anteriorly and the jugular bulb inferiorly, exposing a triangular "window" of dura anterior to the internal auditory canal and adjacent to the anterior petrous tip and clivus.[12,20] This additional bone removal allows exposure of the most anterior extent of the cerebellopontine angle, but postoperative facial paresis results from the transposition (at least transiently).[12]

The translabyrinthine-transotic approach as described by Fisch is similar to the translabyrinthine-transcochlear operation, except that the tympanic and mastoid portions of the fallopian canal are left in situ as a bridge across the surgical field to protect the facial nerve.[10] The cochlea is drilled away and the cochlear aqueduct is followed to its subarachnoid connection between the jugular bulb and the carotid. Dissection is again continued inferiorly to the jugular bulb, superiorly to the superior petrosal sinus, anteriorly to the internal carotid artery, and posteriorly to the sigmoid sinus. This results in the widest possible transtemporal exposure of the cerebellopontine angle, avoiding both cerebellar retraction and facial paresis as a result of transposition.[10]

The dura is incised just inferior and parallel to the superior petrosal sinus and just superior to the jugular bulb. These two dural incisions meet at the sinodural angle and at the porus acusticus. The dura of the internal auditory canal is opened, entering the cerebellopontine angle. Further exposure can be achieved by ligation and division of the superior petrosal sinus and adjacent tentorium.[28] Adequate closure requires obliterating the eustachian tube and packing the dead space created by temporal bone resection with fat to avoid a postoperative CSF leak.

Frontotemporal/Subtemporal Transtentorial Approach

CMs involving the anterior midbrain-interpeduncular fossa region can be approached through a frontotemporal or a subtemporal craniotomy, the details of which have been well described by Yasargil.[50,51] The petrous ridge is followed to the edge of the tentorium, which is folded back to identify the trochlear nerve. The tentorium is coagulated and incised just posterior to the superior petrosal sinus, dividing the tentorial incisura posterior to the entry point of the trochlear nerve into the undersurface of the tentorial leaf.[38] The divided tentorium can be retracted with sutures, allowing entry into the interpeduncular and prepontine cisterns and exposing the anterolateral midbrain and upper half of the pons.[32] Further exposure of this region can be achieved by extradural removal of the petrous apex medial to the petrous internal carotid artery as described by Kawase.[22,23] For medially placed malformations within the interpeduncular cistern, wide splitting of the sylvian fissure through a frontotemporal craniotomy combined with division of the medial tentorium will permit excellent exposure of the bilateral cerebral peduncles, interpeduncular cistern, posterior third ventricular floor, and associated neurovascular structures. Extended exposure of lesions located high in the interpeduncular fossa can be achieved by removal of the zygomatic arch and posterior ridge of the frontal process of the zygoma, as well as by intradural removal of the posterior clinoid process as described by Dolenc.[7,11] Although requiring a certain degree of retraction, these approaches allow delineation of the cranial nerves of the anterolateral upper brain stem and associated blood supply in a direct fashion.

Combined (Petrosal) Approaches

The combined approaches include a combination of subtemporal, transtentorial, and retrosigmoid approaches that provides excellent exposure of the lateral upper two-thirds of the brain stem without brain retraction, sacrifice in hearing, or endangerment of the facial nerve. The approach, as described by Malis, includes division of the sigmoid sinus distal to the vein of Labbé.[26] Therefore, to avoid venous infarction, a prerequisite to this maneuver is good quality bilateral venous phase angiography demonstrating transverse sinuses that communicate through a widely patent torcular as well as through an intact contralateral sigmoid sinus, jugular bulb, and internal jugular vein.

The patient is placed in the supine position and the head rotated away from the side of the lesion and tilted slightly toward the floor. The scalp incision begins inferiorly and medially to the mastoid process and continues above the ear to the anterior hairline above the brow before curving back inferiorly over the temporal root of the zygoma.[26]

The myocutaneous flap is taken down to the level of the external auditory canal, and mastoidectomy is performed. Bone is removed over the transverse sinus, sigmoid sinus, and their junction. A standard subtemporal craniotomy is performed. The dura is opened over the lateral posterior fossa and the floor of the middle cranial fossa to the edges of the transverse-sigmoid junction, allowing for identification and protection of the vein of Labbé. The lateral sinus is ligated between the entrance of the vein of Labbé posteriorly and the sigmoid sinus and petrosal sinus anteriorly.[26] The tentorium is divided, allowing a retractor to be placed beneath the tentorium to elevate it, the lateral sinus, the temporal lobe, and the vein of Labbé together. This maneuver permits the vein of Labbé to drain through

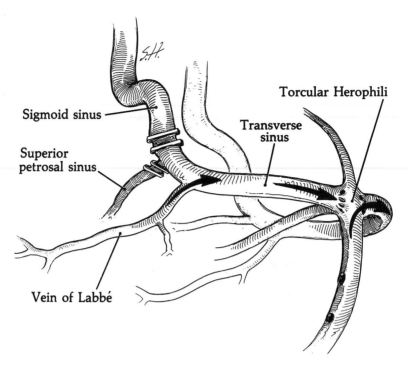

Figure 4. Schematic diagram of the major veins and dural venous sinuses to be considered in the combined (petrosal) approaches. Orientation is as seen by the surgeon; the top of the figure is inferior anatomically and the right of the figure corresponds to posterior anatomically. Before ligating the sigmoid sinus, a widely patent torcular and contralateral jugular venous system must be demonstrated angiographically. This allows the vein of Labbé to drain through the medial lateral sinus and across the torcular through the opposite jugular vein. (Reprinted with permission of the Barrow Neurological Institute.)

the medial portion of the lateral sinus and across the torcular through the opposite jugular vein (Figure 4). Incision of the tentorium from the superior petrosal sinus to the hiatus allows for excellent exposure of the lateral brain stem as well as the anterior and superior surfaces of the cerebellum.

The petrosal approach, as described by Al-Mefty,[1,2] involves more extensive drilling of the temporal bone. Positioning is again with the patient supine such that the petrous base is the highest point in the operative field. A curvilinear skin incision extends from the temporal root of the zygoma over the pinna to just medial to the mastoid process. A myocutaneous flap is developed down to the level of the external canal and retracted inferiorly. A single bone flap is elevated over the posterior temporal and lateral suboccipital regions, as well as over the intervening lateral and sigmoid

sinuses. A high-speed drill is used to perform a mastoidectomy and to skeletonize the sigmoid sinus down to the jugular bulb and the sinodural angle. As in the initial labyrinthine exposure, the superficial air cells posterior to the external canal are drilled away, exposing the fallopian canal and the lateral and superior semicircular canals. Bone removal continues medially to thin the petrous bone toward its apex, with care taken to preserve the middle and inner ear cavities. The dura is opened just anteriorly to the sigmoid sinus from the jugular bulb to the sinodural angle and along the floor of the middle cranial fossa (Figure 5). The superior petrosal sinus can be clipped and divided, allowing the dural incision to be extended through the tentorium (posterior to the fourth nerve) to the hiatus. Dura can also be opened posterior to the sigmoid sinus, allowing the surgeon to alter the field of view between the supra- and infra-

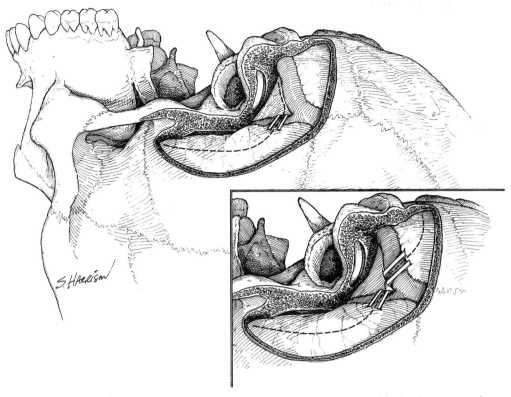

Figure 5. Right combined (petrosal) approach. After completion of craniotomy and further bone removal, durotomy is performed along the floor of the middle cranial fossa and the superior petrosal sinus is ligated and divided. As described by Al-Mefty,[1,2] the dural opening is continued just anterior to the sigmoid sinus from the jugular bulb to the sinodural angle, preserving the sigmoid sinus. (Inset) Alternatively, as described by Spetzler et al,[42] if adequate collateral venous drainage can be demonstrated, the sigmoid sinus can be divided inferiorly to the sinodural angle. (Reprinted with permission of the Barrow Neurological Institute.)

tentorial routes without transecting the sinus itself. Care must be taken to minimize retraction of the temporal lobe, stretching the vein of Labbé; this structure can be mobilized by dissection from the cortical surface to minimize tension on the venous wall.[1] Alternately, as described by Spetzler,[41] the superior petrosal sinus is ligated, and the sigmoid sinus can then be divided inferiorly to the sinodural angle. This allows the vein of Labbé to be safely retracted superiorly with the divided tentorium similar to that described above in Malis's approach (Figure 5, inset). Again, division of the sigmoid sinus requires preoperative angiographic documentation of adequate collateral venous drainage. This approach affords excellent exposure of the anterolateral brain stem down to the level of the foramen magnum (Figure 6). The advantages to this approach, especially suited for large malformations involving extensive areas of the anterolateral brain stem are as follows: **(1)** minimal retraction is required; **(2)** the operative distance to the brain stem is shortened by extensive bone removal; **(3)** the approach permits a direct line of sight to the anterolateral brain stem; **(4)** the vestibular and auditory apparati are preserved; **(5)** the vein of Labbé is preserved; and **(6)** multiple axes for dissection between the cranial nerves are provided.[1]

Other Combined Approaches

Limitations of exposure associated with any one of the preceding approaches can easily

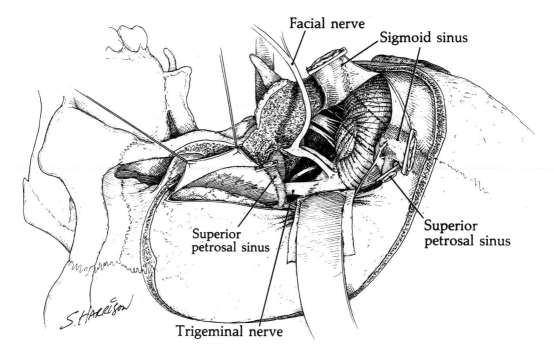

Figure 6. Right combined (petrosal) approach, after durotomy with ligation of the superior petrosal and sigmoid sinuses. Division of the tentorium allows the vein of Labbé to be retracted superiorly with the tentorial leaflets. This affords excellent exposure of the anterolateral brain stem down to the foramen magnum with protection of the vein of Labbé and a minimum of brain retraction. (Reprinted with permission of the Barrow Neurological Institute.)

be overcome by using a combination of approaches. Combined suboccipital-petrosal retroauricular and preauricular transpetrosal-transtentorial, anterior transpetrosal-transtentorial, and suboccipital-translabyrinthine approaches, which have all been described for resection of cerebellopontine angle and clival tumors to maximize exposure and to minimize brain retraction, are also applicable to CMs of the anterolateral brain stem.[13,15,16,19,22] Using a combination of far lateral suboccipital, translabyrinthine, subtemporal, and transtentorial approaches (referred to as the *extensive combined* or the *far lateral-combined* approach), the entire anterior and lateral brain stem and craniovertebral junction, with excellent exposure of the cranial nerves and associated vascular structures, can be visualized.

Selection of the Appropriate Surgical Approach

Surgical management of CMs involving the deep cerebellum and brain stem remains a formidable challenge. The myriad of approaches described in the literature emphasize that no one approach is perfect for all cases. Therefore, each approach or combination of approaches has its own advantages and disadvantages that necessitate individualization of every case.

MRI in the axial, coronal, and sagittal planes, and (most recently) three-dimensional reconstructions utilizing computer-assisted parallel processing have proven invaluable in preoperative localization and in selection of the most advantageous surgical route. Individual evaluation must be performed to determine if a corridor to the malformation through noneloquent brain is available, if the potential resulting neurologic deficits would be acceptable, and if the risks preclude operative intervention. Finally, factors such as pre-existing neurologic deficits, the presence of co-existing cerebrovascular malformations, and the presence of existing bone defects as a result of previous procedures (as well as location, size, and relationship of the CM to the brain stem surface) must all be considered in choosing the appropriate avenue of surgical attack.

Results of Surgical Management of Infratentorial Cavernous Malformations

Previously published reports have suggested that an aggressive surgical approach to the treatment of symptomatic CMs of the infratentorial space can provide favorable results.* Since 1985, the senior author (Spetzler) has operated on 64 intracranial CMs, of which 22 (34%) involved the cerebellum or brain stem. Operative indications for this series of patients included: **(1)** progressive symptomatology, **(2)** superficial location of the malformation within the brain stem, and **(3)** an operative approach that could spare eloquent brain tissue.[53]

The average age of these 15 females and 7 males was 37.9 ± 13.5 years (range, 14–71 years). Of the 22 patients, 19 (86%) described acute onset of symptomatology suggestive of an apoplectic event. Neurologic deficits at the time of operation are delineated in Table 1. Nine of these patients had at least one additional lesion scattered elsewhere throughout the neuraxis; 6 of these patients had other family members with CMs in accordance with a familial inheritance pattern.

The location of the malformations and the surgical approaches employed to effect their resection are shown in Table 2. The average size of the lesion in this series was 1.6 ± 1.0 cm (range, 0.4–4.0 cm). Three patients also had an associated venous malformation, requiring modification of the surgical approach in 1 case. An arachnoid

*References 3,4,9,17,25,27,30,31,33,39,46–49,52,53

Table 1. Preoperative Neurologic Signs and Symptoms in 22 Patients with Infratentorial CMs

Signs and Symptoms*	Number (%)
Facial pain/hypesthesia	11 (50)
Hemiparesis	10 (45)
Disorder of ocular motility	10 (45)
Severe headaches	10 (45)
Hemisensory deficit/dysesthesias	8 (36)
VII, VIII CN neuropathies	5 (23)
IX, X, XI, XII CN neuropathies	5 (23)
Ataxia, dysmetria	4 (18)
Parinaud's syndrome	2 (9)

*A patient may display more than one sign and/or symptom.
CN = cranial nerve

cyst and an AVM unrelated to the CM were observed in 1 patient each. Complete resection (as judged by intraoperative findings as well as postoperative MRI) was possible in 19 of the 22 cases (86%); an estimated 90% to 95% resection was achieved in the remaining 3 cases. Histopathologic examination revealed acute or subacute thrombus in 64% and hemosiderin in 91% of the surgical specimens, indicating the propensity of these lesions to hemorrhage and rehemorrhage.

Median followup was 27 ± 22 months. Table 3 lists the neurologic deficits appearing after or exacerbated by surgery. Transient complications resolved completely on follow-up examinations. Overall, there was no mortality, no major morbidity, and a permanent minor morbidity related to surgery of 23%. At the time of last followup, all 22 patients were significantly improved compared to their preoperative neurologic status. Using appropriate individualized planning and case selection and employing the surgical approaches and principles described above, symptomatic superficial CMs of the infratentorial space can be removed completely with minimal morbidity and mortality.

Table 2. Location and Surgical Approach Used in 22 Patients with Infratentorial CMs

Location		Number (%)
Midbrain Tectum:		3 (14)
Suprecerebellar infratentorial approach	2	
Occipital transtentorial approach	1	
Midbrain Tegmentum:		1 (5)
Combined approach		
Midbrain Crura Cerebri:		1 (5)
Fronto-subtemporal transtentorial approach		
Pontomesencephalic Junction:		2 (9)
Supracerebellar infratentorial approach	1	
Fronto-subtemporal transtentorial approach	1	
Pontine Tegmentum:		
A) Midline:		5 (23)
Suboccipital splitting of vermis		
B) Lateral:		2 (9)
Combined approach		
Basis Pontis:		2 (9)
Subtemporal transtentorial approach	1	
Frontosubtemporal transtentorial approach	1	
Pontomedullary Junction:		1 (5)
Combined approach		
Medulla:		1 (5)
Far lateral approach		
Cerebellum:		2 (9)
Suboccipital approach		
Cervicomedullary Junction:		2 (9)
Suboccipital approach + C1–2 Laminectomies		

Table 3. Complications Related to Surgical Management of 22 Patients with Infratentorial CMs

Complications	Number (%)
Transient	
Hemiparesis	5 (23)
Diplopia, disorder of ocular motility	4 (18)
CN VI, VII neuropathies	4 (18)
Hydrocephalus, shunt failure	3 (14)
Meningitis	2 (9)
Lower extremity deep venous thrombosis	2 (9)
Gait ataxia	1 (5)
CN IX, X, XI, XII neuropathies	1 (5)
Cerebrospinal fluid leak	1 (5)
Permanent	
Dysmetria + internuclear ophthalmoplegia	2 (9)
Partial CN III neuropathy	1 (5)
Mild upper and lower extremity dysmetria	1 (5)
Mild internuclear ophthalmoplegia	1 (5)

References

1. Al-Mefty O. Surgical exposure of petroclival tumors. In: Wilkins RH, Rengachary SS, eds. *Neurosurgery Update I. Diagnosis, Operative Technique, and Neuro-Oncology*. New York, NY: McGraw-Hill; 1990:409–414.

2. Al-Mefty O, Fox JL, Smith RR. Petrosal approach for petroclival meningiomas. *Neurosurgery*. 1988;22:510–517.

3. Bellotti C, Medina M, Oliveri G, et al. Cystic cavernous angiomas of the posterior fossa: report of three cases. *J Neurosurg*. 1985;63:797–799.

4. Bertalanffy H, Gilsbach JM, Eggert HR, et al. Microsurgery of deepseated cavernous angiomas: report of 26 cases. *Acta Neurochir (Wien)*. 1991;-108:91–99.

5. Clark K. The occipital transtentorial approach to the pineal region. In: Schmidek NH, Sweet WH, eds. *Operative Neurosurgical Techniques. Indications, Methods, and Results*. 2nd ed. Orlando, Fla: Grune & Stratton; 1988;1:411–422.

6. De Oliveira E, Rhoton AL Jr, Peace D. Microsurgical anatomy of the region of the foramen magnum. *Surg Neurol*. 1985;24:293–352.

7. Dolenc VV, Skrap M, Sustersic J, et al. A transcavernous-transsellar approach to the basilar tip aneurysms. *Br J Neurosurg*. 1987;1:251–259.

8. Duckworth J, Schmidek NH. Surgical management of posterior fossa tumors. In: Schmidek NH, Sweet WH, eds. *Operative Neurosurgical Techniques: Indications, Methods, and Results*. 2nd ed. Orlando, Fla: Grune & Stratton; 1988;1:653–664.

9. Fahlbusch R, Strauss C, Huk W, et al. Surgical removal of pontomesencephalic cavernous hemangiomas. *Neurosurgery*. 1990;26:449–457.

10. Fisch U, Mattox D. *Microsurgery of the Skull Base*. New York, NY: Thieme; 1988:74–131, 546–577.

11. Fujitsu K, Kuwabara T. Zygomatic approach for lesions in the interpeduncular cistern. *J Neurosurg*. 1985;62:340–343.

12. Gardner G, Robertson JH, Clark WC. Transtemporal approaches to the posterior cranial fossa. In: Schmidek HH, Sweet WH, eds. *Operative Neurosurqical Techniques: Indications, Methods and Results*. 2nd ed. Orlando, Fla: Grune & Stratton; 1988:665–672.

13. Glasscock ME III, Gulya AJ, Pensak ML. Surgery of the posterior fossa. *Otolaryngol Clin North Am*. 1984;17:483–497.

14. Glasscock ME III, Hays JW, Jackson CG, et al. A one-stage combined approach for the management of large cerebellopontine angle tumors. *Laryngoscope*. 1978;88:1563–1576.

15. Glasscock ME III, Miller GW, Drake FD, et al. Surgery of the skull base. *Laryngoscope*. 1978;88:905–923.

16. Hakuba A, Nishimura S, Jang BJ. A combined retroauricular and preauricular transpetrosal-transtentorial approach to clivus meningiomas. *Surg Neurol*. 1988;30:108–116.

17. Heffez DS, Zinreich SJ, Long DM. Surgical resection of intrinsic brain stem lesions: an overview. *Neurosurgery*. 1990;27:789–798.

18. Heros RC. Lateral suboccipital approach for vertebral and vertebrobasilar artery lesions. *J Neurosurg*. 1986;64:559–562.

19. Hitselberger WE, House WF. A combined approach to the cerebellopontine angle: a suboccipital petrosal approach. *Arch Otolaryngol*. 1966;84:267–285.

20. House WF, Hitselberger WE. The transcochlear approach to the skull base. *Arch Otolaryngol*. 1976;102:334–342.

21. Jamieson KG. Excision of pineal tumors. *J Neurosurg*. 1971;35:550–553.

22. Kawase T, Shiobara R, Toya S. Anterior transpetrosal-transtentorial approach for sphenopetroclival meningiomas: surgical method and results in 10 patients. *Neurosurgery*. 1991;28:869–876.

23. Kawase T, Toya S, Shiobara R, et al. Transpetrosal approach for aneurysms of the lower basilar artery. *J Neurosurg*. 1985;63:857–861.

24. King TT, Morrison AW. Translabyrinthine operation for the removal of acoustic nerve tumors. In: Schmidek HH, Sweet WH, eds. *Operative Neurosurgical Techniques: Indications, Methods, and Results*. 2nd ed. Orlando, Fla: Grune & Stratton; 1988;1:685–704.

25. LeDoux MS, Aronin PA, Odrezin GT. Surgically treated cavernous angiomas of the brain stem: report of two cases and review of the literature. *Surg Neurol*. 1991;35:395–399.

26. Malis LI. Surgical resection of tumors of the skull base. In: Wilkins RH, Rengachary SS, eds. *Neurosurgery*. New York, NY: McGraw Hill; 1985:1011–1021.

27. Mangiardi JR. The surgical management of brainstem hematomas. *Perspect Neurolog Surg*. 1991;2:33–48.

28. Mayberg MR, Symon L. Meningiomas of the clivus and apical petrous bone: report of 35 cases. *J Neurosurg*. 1986;65:160–167.

29. McCormick PC, Michelsen WJ. Management of intracranial cavernous and venous malformations. In: Barrow DL, ed. *Intracranial Vascular Malformations*. Park Ridge, Ill: American Association of Neurological Surgeons; 1990:197–217.

30. McCormick WF, Hardman JM, Boulter TR. Vascular malformations ("angiomas") of the brain, with special reference to those occurring in the posterior fossa. *J Neurosurg*. 1968;28:241–251.

31. Ondra SL, Doty JR, Mahla ME, et al. Surgical excision of a cavernous hemangioma of the rostral brain stem: case report. *Neurosurgery*. 1988;23:490–493.

32. Ono M, Ono M, Rhoton AL Jr, et al. Microsurgical anatomy of the region of the tentorial incisura. *J Neurosurg*. 1984;60:365–399.

33. Pendl G, Vorkapic P, Koniyama M. Microsurgery of midbrain lesions. *Neurosurgery*. 1990;26:641–648.

34. Poppen JL. The right occipital approach to a pinealoma. *J Neurosurg*. 1966;25:706–710.

35. Reid WS, Clark WK. Comparison of the infratentorial and transtentorial approaches to the pineal region. *Neurosurgery*. 1978;3:1–8.

36. Rigamonti D, Johnson PC, Spetzler RF, et al.

Cavernous malformations and capillary telangiectasia: a spectrum within a single pathological entity. *Neurosurgery.* 1991;28:60–64.

37. Rigamonti D, Spetzler RF. The association of venous and CMs: report of four cases and discussion of the pathophysiological, diagnostic, therapeutic implications. *Acta Neurochir (Wien).* 1988;92:100–105.

38. Rosomoff HL. The subtemporal transtentorial approach to the cerebellopontine angle. *Laryngoscope.* 1971;81:1448–1454.

39. Saito N, Yamakawa K, Sasaki T, et al. Intramedullary cavernous angioma with trigeminal neuralgia: a case report and review of the literature. *Neurosurgery.* 1989;25:97–101.

40. Sen CN, Sekhar LN. Surgical management of anteriorly placed lesions at the craniocervical junction: an alternative approach. *Acta Neurochir (Wien).* 1991;108:70–77.

41. Spetzler RF, Daspit CP, Pappas CTE. The combined supra- and infratentorial approach for lesions of the petrous and clival region: experience with 46 cases. *J Neurosurg.* 1992;76:588–599.

42. Spetzler RF, Grahm TW. The far-lateral approach to the inferior clivus and the upper cervical region: technical note. *BNI Quart.* 1990;6:35–38.

43. Stein BM. The infratentorial supracerebellar approach to pineal lesions. *J Neurosurg.* 1971;35:197–202.

44. Stein BM. Supracerebellar approach for pineal region neoplasms. In: Schmidek HH, Sweet WH, eds. *Operative Neurosurgical Techniques: Indications, Methods and Results.* 2nd ed. Orlando, Fla: Grune & Stratton; 1988;1:401–409.

45. Stein BM, Bruce JN, Fetell MR. Surgical approaches to pineal tumors. In: Wilkins RH, Rengachary SS, eds. *Neurosurgery Update I: Diagnosis, Operative Technique and Neuro-Oncology.* New York, NY: McGraw-Hill; 1990:389–398.

46. Vaquero J, Carrillo R, Cabezudo J, et al. Cavernous angiomas of the pineal region: report of two cases. *J Neurosurg.* 1980;53:833–835.

47. Voight K, Yasargil MG. Cerebral cavernous haemangiomas or cavernomas: incidence, pathology, localization, diagnosis, clinical features and treatment: review of the literature and report of an unusual case. *Neurochirurgia.* 1976;19:59–68.

48. Well SM, Tew JM Jr. Surgical management of brain stem vascular malformations. *Acta Neurochir (Wien).* 1990;105:14–23.

49. Yasargil MG with Curcic M, Kis M, Teddy PJ, et al. *Microneurosurgery, IIIB: AVM of the Brain, Clinical Considerations, General and Special Operative Techniques, Surgical Results, Nonoperated Cases, Cavernous and Venous Angiomas, Neuroanesthesia.* New York, NY: Thieme; 1988:415–429.

50. Yasargil MG with Smith RD, Young PH, Teddy PJ. *Microneurosurgery, I: Microsurgical Anatomy of the Basal Cisterns and Vessels of the Brain, Diagnostic Studies, General Operative Techniques and Pathological Considerations of the Intracranial Aneurysms.* New York, NY: Thieme; 1984:215–233.

51. Yasargil MG, Mortara RW, Curcic M. Meningiomas of basal posterior cranial fossa. In: Krayenbuhl H, Brihaye J, Loew F, et al, eds. *Advances and Technical Standards in Neurosurgery.* New York, NY: Springer Verlag; 1980;7:4–115.

52. Yoshimoto T, Suzuki J. Radical surgery on cavernous angioma of the brainstem. *Surg Neurol.* 1986;26:72–78.

53. Zimmerman RS, Spetzler RF, Lee KS, et al. Cavernous malformations of the brain stem. *J Neurosurg.* 1991;75:32–39.

Chapter 11

Extra-Axial Cavernous Malformations

Joseph M. Zabramski, MD, and Deepak Awasthi, MD

Extra-axial cavernous malformations (CMs) share the distinct histologic appearance common to all CMs: abnormally dilated, thin-walled, vascular channels, with walls composed of collagen, lined by an endothelial layer without elastic or muscle fibers or intervening parenchyma. These lesions represent a distinct category of CMs because of their site of origin, radiologic appearance, clinical manifestations, and management. Extra-axial CMs are most commonly found in the middle fossa region (Table 1).* The cavernous sinus is the presumed site of origin of middle fossa lesions.[14,26] Middle fossa lesions tend to extend outward from the cavernous sinus, but they can be entirely intracavernous.** Less commonly, these lesions have been reported in other intracranial extra-axial locations (see Table 1): tentorium cerebelli (6 cases)[16,19,25]; cerebellopontine angle (4 cases)[37]; tegmen tympani (1 case)[24]; cerebral convexity (1 case)[8,9,31]; Meckel's cave (1 case)[5]; torcula (1 case)[17]; petrosal sinus (1 case)[17]; and foramen magnum (1 case).[15] In addition, these lesions have been rarely described in the spinal extra-axial space.[27]

One case of a midthoracic epidural CM has also been seen at Barrow Neurological Institute (BNI). This chapter will concentrate on the major clinical features and management of the more common middle fossa CMs.

Terminology

Extra-axial CMs have been referred to as extra-axial cavernous hemangiomas, angiomas, and cavernomas. In addition, different authors have attempted to separate the more common middle fossa lesions into "middle fossa" cavernous hemangiomas and "intracavernous" cavernous hemangiomas.[11,12,18,21,34] Such distinctions do not seem valid as these lesions all appear to originate from the dural walls of the cavernous sinus and then grow to preferentially involve either the intra- or extracavernous space. Meyer et al observed that extra-axial lesions commonly originate in the dural sinuses, and proposed that the term "sinus cavernoma" should be used to distinguish them from the more common intra-axial lesions.[17] These lesions can, however, arise from other dural sites. Thus, the term "extra-axial CMs" seems more appropriate.

---

*References 11,12,14,17,18,21,24,29,30,32,34,37,38
**References 11,12,14,17,29,30,32,34

Table 1. **Location of Intracranial Extra-Axial Cavernous Malformations**

Site	Number of Reported Cases	Percentage
Middle fossa/cavernous sinus	46	73
Tentorium cerebelli	6	9
Cerebellopontine angle	4	6
Meckel's cave	1	2
Cerebral convexity	3	5
Torcula	1	2
Petrosal sinus	1	2
Foramen magnum	1	2
Total	63	100

Epidemiology

The true incidence of extra-axial CMs is difficult to assess but is clearly rare compared to other vascular malformations. In 1966, McCormick and Boulter found only two extra-axial CMs among almost 500 vascular malformations of the central nervous system that they reviewed (0.4%, of all vascular malformations).[16] More recently, Simard et al included 18 cases of extra-axial CMs among 138 symptomatic, histologically verified cases of CMs (13% of all CMs).[37] Yamasaki et al reported 4 cases of extra-axial CMs in their series of 30 cases treated between 1965 and 1984 (13% of all CMs).[38] Based on these estimates, extra-axial CMs make up no more than 0.4% to 2% of all vascular malformations.

Forty-six cases of middle fossa CMs have been described in the literature (73% of the reported cases of intracranial extra-axial CMs including 3 cases from BNI.* In addition, 13 patients with middle fossa/cavernous sinus CMs have been briefly mentioned by commenting authors.[3,13,23,33] These lesions have an overwhelming female predominance. At least 33 of the 36 reported cases of middle fossa CMs have occurred in females (11:1). The most common age of presentation for middle fossa lesions is the fifth decade (16 of 36 cases) with the overall range between ages 14 and 72.

---

*References 7,11,12,14,17,18,20–22,24,29,30,32,34–36

Although reports of intra-axial CMs are relatively rare in the Japanese literature, 22 of the 42 extra-axial middle fossa cases have been reported in this population (52.5%). There have been no reports of multiplicity or familial occurrence with extra-axial CMs.

Pathology

The histopathology of extra-axial CMs is similar to CMs found elsewhere in the body. It consists of abnormally dilated, thin-walled, vascular channels with walls composed of collagen, lined by a single layer of endothelium and without intervening parenchyma. The internal elastic membrane as well as muscle fibers and stromal cells are absent in these lesions.

Clinical Presentation

Clinical presentation varies with the location and size of the lesion (Table 2). Headache is common because of mass effect and stretching of the dura as well as erosion of the bone. Headache may be associated with nausea and vomiting, but is not of localizing value. Papilledema may rarely be seen with very large lesions and increased intracranial pressure (ICP).

Middle fossa extra-axial CMs tend to attain a large size before producing signs or symptoms. They are usually located extradurally with the dura forming a pseudocapsule of the mass. These lesions are thought

Table 2. Clinical Presentation of 46 Patients with Extra-Axial Cavernous Malformations of the Middle Fossa Reported in the Literature

Symptoms	Number of Patients	Percentage
Headache	14	30
Visual acuity decrease	20	43
Visual field deficits	4	9
CN III palsy	27	59
CN IV palsy	8	17
CN V palsy	12	26
CN VI palsy	12	26
CN VII palsy	6	13
Hemiparesis	4	9
Papilledema	4	9
Optic atrophy	5	11
Exophthalmos	10	22
Retro-orbital pain	3	6
Vertigo	1	2
Tinnitus	1	2
Seizure	2	4
Sensory disturbance	1	2
Amenorrhea/obesity	4	9
Galactorrhea	1	2

to arise from within the cavernous sinus, producing symptoms as they grow and compress cranial nerves III, IV, V_1, V_2, and VI. As these masses enlarge, they frequently encase the internal carotid artery. They may extend into the orbit through the superior orbital fissure and may even erode into the sella turcica.[7,21,29] They can also compress and stretch the optic nerve and/or chiasm.[7] This growth pattern accounts for the common presentation of these lesions with ocular/visual signs and symptoms (see Table 2). Third and sixth nerve palsies are especially common and were reported in 59% and 26% of the patients, respectively. Other ocular/visual signs and symptoms include exophthalmos (22% of cases), decreased visual acuity (43% of cases), and visual field deficits (9% of cases). Increasing compression of the optic nerve may lead to optic atrophy (11% of cases).

Some form of the cavernous sinus syndrome (involvement of cranial nerves III, IV, V_1, V_2, and/or VI) is invariably present in patients with symptomatic middle fossa CMs. The ophthalmoplegia may or may not be associated with retro-orbital pain and/or proptosis.[21,32]

Other less common signs and symptoms of middle fossa lesions have included a peripheral seventh cranial nerve palsy (6 cases), hemiparesis (5 cases), amenorrhea/obesity (4 cases), galactorrhea (1 case), vertigo (1 case), tinnitus (1 case,) sensory disturbances in the extremity (1 case), and seizures (2 cases). It is important to remember that the symptoms may precipitate or worsen during pregnancy (presumably secondary to vascular engorgement of the CM) with resultant increase in size.[8,11,21]

Radiologic Evaluation

Plain Skull X-Rays

Bony erosion involving the dorsum sella, posterior or anterior clinoid processes, superior orbital fissure, and floor of the middle cranial fossa is a typical finding on plain skull x-rays.[7,10,11,21,29] Hyperostosis on plain skull x-rays has not been reported in association with these lesions. Calcifications of extra-axial CMs are also rare and have been reported in only one case on plain x-rays.[10]

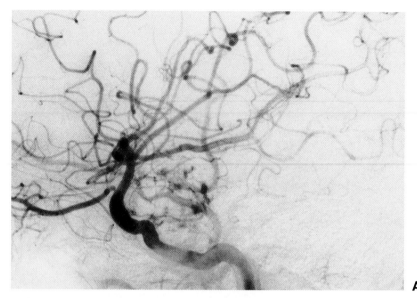

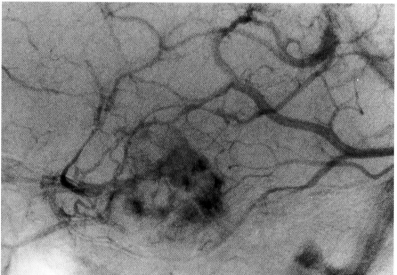

Figure 1. Lateral views of a right common carotid artery angiogram in a 42-year-old male who presented with a history of progressive ocular palsy and retro-orbital pain. **(A)** Early arterial phase film demonstrates a mass arising in the area of the cavernous sinus, supplied by branches of the meningo-hypophyseal trunk. **(B)** Late venous phase film shows tumor staining and pooling of contrast in the area of the cavernous sinus with draining veins.

Angiography

In contrast to intra-axial CMs, extra-axial CMs are highly vascular and well visualized on cerebral angiography (Figure 1). Middle fossa lesions are often fed by branches of the external carotid artery (especially the middle meningeal artery) and the intracavernous portion of the internal carotid artery, particularly the meningohypophyseal trunk (see Figure 1).[17,18,21,29] More rarely, these lesions will present as an avascular mass.[11,29] Cerebral angiography may

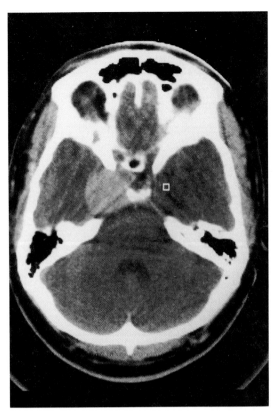

Figure 2. Preoperative CT scan in the same patient as described in Figure 1. This contrasted scan reveals a homogeneously enhancing mass in the right cavernous sinus region. The appearance of this lesion is consistent with meningioma or extra-axial CM. Hyperostosis, if present, would favor meningioma.

also show the displacement of vessels and sinuses by the enlarging mass.[12]

Computed Tomography (CT)

The appearance of middle fossa extra-axial CMs on CT is readily confused with that of meningiomas (Figure 2). The bony erosion and remodeling on plain skull films described above are well visualized on CT. Unlike meningiomas, however, hyperostosis is only rarely associated with these lesions and has been reported in only one case on CT.[7] The CT appearance of extra-axial CMs is usually hyperdense on uncontrasted images[18,21,35] but can be iso-[12,18,20] or hypodense.[6] After intravenous contrast administration, there is usually dense, homogenous enhancement.

Magnetic Resonance Imaging (MRI)

The MRI appearance of extra-axial CMs does not have the characteristic features described for intra-axial lesions.[28] Nevertheless, MRI is still the most useful preoperative diagnostic study and is particularly helpful for differentiating between extra-axial CMs and meningiomas in the cavernous sinus region.[29] Extra-axial CMs are usually iso- or slightly hyperintense on T1-weighted images but markedly hyperintense on T2-weighted images (Figure 3). On the other hand, approximately 80% of meningiomas are isointense or hypointense on both T1-weighted and T2-weighted images.[1,4] The only regular exception to this rule is an angioblastic meningioma, which may be markedly hyperintense on T2-weighted images.[4] Thus, MRI can regularly distinguish extra-axial CMs from about 80% of cavernous sinus meningiomas.

Differential Diagnosis

Because of their radiologic and clinical manifestations, extra-axial CMs are frequently misdiagnosed as meningiomas before surgery. The possibility of an extra-axial CM should always be considered when investigating a suspected meningioma in the middle fossa or parasellar region, especially in middle-aged females. As mentioned, spin-echo MR images may help in differentiating the two lesions (Figure 3). In addition, bony radiographic changes (hyperostosis vs. erosion) as well as the angiographic findings may lead to a clinical impression of the diagnosis, but biopsy of the lesion is the only way to distinguish between the two entities accurately. Intraoperatively, extra-axial CMs have a notorious tendency to hemorrhage profusely upon incision into the tumor capsule. Because bleeding is difficult to control, it becomes apparent that the lesion is not likely a meningioma, and histopathology supports diagnosis of a CM.

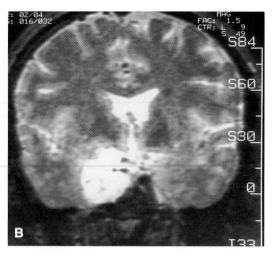

Figure 3. Preoperative MRI in the patient described in Figures 1 and 2. The T1-weighted axial image **(A)** reveals a well-demarcated mass in the region of the cavernous sinus. While the T1-weighted image would be consistent with both extra-axial cavernous malformation and meningioma, the intense signal seen on the T2-weighted coronal image **(B)** argues in favor of an extra-axial cavernous malformation.

Other parasellar and intracavernous lesions can usually be differentiated from CMs by clinical and radiologic evaluations. One case, however, has been reported in which a lesion with the preoperative diagnosis of a pituitary adenoma was a middle fossa CM.[17]

From a clinical perspective, Dolenc stresses that the symptoms and signs associated with CMs arising from the cavernous sinus tend to fluctuate, becoming more pronounced with physical exertion and decreasing in severity with rest.[3] This fluctuation, he states, can be explained by the engorgement of the CM during exercise.

Comparison to Intra-Axial CMs

Despite their similar histopathology, extra-axial lesions differ significantly from their intra-axial counterparts with respect to clinical presentation, radiographic features and management. For intra-axial lesions, symptoms and growth appear to be related to recurrent hemorrhage: seizures secondary to the irritative effects of hemorrhage

are the most common presentation for supratentorial lesions, while in the brain stem and spinal cord the presentation usually involves a stuttering progression of focal neurologic deficits associated with changes in mass effect produced by recurrent hemorrhage.[39] The presence of hemorrhages of varying age also accounts for the highly characteristic MRI appearance of intra-axial CMs.[37,38] Finally, despite their propensity for hemorrhage, intra-axial CMs are relatively avascular and simple to resect. In contrast, hemorrhage from extra-axial CMs is exceedingly rare. Only two reported cases mention the possibility of intralesional hemorrhage in association with onset of symptoms.[11] There is no mention of subdural, epidural, or subarachnoid hemorrhage in association with these extra-axial lesions. Extra-axial CMs appear to produce signs and symptoms by compressing and distorting surrounding structures as they slowly enlarge. As a result, they frequently are quite large when initially discovered. In addition, unlike their intra-axial counterparts, extra-axial CMs are highly vascular and difficult for the surgeon to remove completely.

Natural History

As noted above, extra-axial middle fossa CMs cause symptoms by slow growth and enlargement of the tumor mass, with resulting compression of the cranial nerves in the cavernous sinus and superior orbital fissure, as well as in the optic nerves and the pituitary gland. Thus, these extra-axial lesions tend to attain a large size before they manifest clinically; smaller lesions may be incidental findings at autopsy.[16,19,26] Symptoms tend to worsen during pregnancy due to congestion of the vascular spaces in the malformation.

Once completely excised, extra-axial lesions have not been reported to recur. Total resection, however, is difficult because of the tendency of these CMs to bleed intraoperatively and because of the intimate relationship of these lesions to surrounding neurovascular structures. There are only a few reported cases of a successful initial total removal.[7,14,17,22,34] In cases of subtotal removal, external beam radiation therapy has been useful in decreasing the size and vascularity of these lesions.[17,29,35,36]

CMs are hamartomas of the vascular system. Thus, if completely and successfully excised, the patient is expected to have a normal life expectancy. The preoperative ophthalmoplegia, however, usually does not resolve completely even after total excision of the lesion. Visual dysfunction has only rarely been reported to improve postoperatively.[11,17]

Management

The difficulty in differentiating an extra-axial CM from a meningioma necessitates an open surgical biopsy of the lesion. The highly vascular nature of this lesion and the surrounding anatomy underlie the difficulty in surgical management. Prior case reports have repeatedly mentioned the profuse hemorrhage from these lesions after incising the capsule.[11,18,21,29] Indeed, of the 46 reported cases of middle fossa lesions, 8 patients (17%) died intraoperatively

of uncontrollable hemorrhage. This outcome has led to strategies of preoperative embolization and radiation therapy to reduce the vascularity of these lesions.

Role of Preoperative Embolization

Preoperative embolization has the potential to reduce intraoperative blood loss in these lesions but has been reported in only three cases.[14,21] In one case, the authors found it helpful.[14] However, Namba reported profuse hemorrhage despite preoperative embolization and thought that alternative methods should be taken to reduce vascularity of the tumor.[21] He suggested preoperative radiation.

Role of Radiation Therapy

Shibata et al were, to our knowledge, the first authors to discuss the role of radiation therapy in the management of middle fossa extra-axial CMs.[35] In 1987 Shibata and Mori published their follow-up study of three cases initially reported in the early 1980s.[36] All three of their patients showed a significant decrease in the size and vascularity of the lesion following radiation therapy. One patient had a two-stage total resection of the lesion after an initial partial resection followed by radiation therapy (5,000 rads). The second patient received preoperative radiation therapy (3,000 rads) followed by partial resection of the tumor. The third patient received only radiation (3,000 rads), and her symptoms improved and the mass was reduced. These authors concluded that a radiation dose of 3,000 rads was adequate for increasing the probability of total malformation removal and may even eliminate the need for surgery.[36]

In 1990, Rigamonti et al[29] reported three cases of middle fossa extra-axial CMs treated at BNI. In two of the patients, initial attempts at resection were limited to biopsy by the extreme vascularity of the

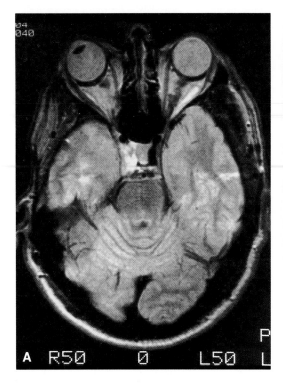

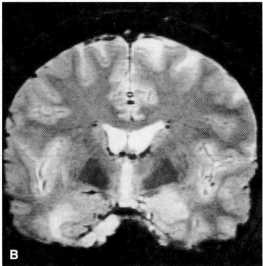

Figure 4. Follow-up MRI 6 months after external-beam radiation therapy (5,000 rads over 5 weeks) in the same patient described in Figures 1, 2, and 3. **(A)** T1-weighted axial image; **(B)** T2-weighted coronal image. Note the marked reduction in the size of the lesion compared to the images in Figure 3.

lesions. One of the patients received a course of standard radiation therapy (5,000 rads over 5 weeks) followed 6 months later by total resection of the lesion. At the time of the second procedure, the vascularity of the lesion was markedly reduced and it was readily resectable. Repeat CT scan and MRI before the second surgery demonstrated substantial reduction in the size of the mass (Figure 4). The patient has remained free of recurrence more than 4 years after resection (Figure 5). The second patient underwent proton-beam therapy in 1977 after her initial surgery was halted by profuse intraoperative hemorrhage. Despite this treatment, the tumor continued to grow as demonstrated radiographically. A second attempt at resection in 1983, 6 years after proton-beam therapy, was again halted by profuse bleeding. Progression of visual symptoms led to a third and successful attempt at gross total resection in 1984. Iridium-125 implants were left in the mal-

formation cavity to reduce the risk of recurrence. The patient has had no evidence of recurrence in more than 5 years of follow-up. The third patient presented with headaches and intermittent episodes of double vision. She underwent an open biopsy to verify the clinical impression of extra-axial CM and was referred for standard radiation therapy (5,000 rads over 5 weeks). A follow-up CT scan at 4 months revealed a decrease in the size of the tumor mass. The patient declined further surgical intervention. Clinically, she has remained stable with no progression of her visual symptoms for more than 4 years.

These reports emphasize the usefulness of standard external-beam radiation therapy in decreasing the vascularity and size of these lesions. We have recommended radiation therapy as an adjunct to aid in total resection of the lesion; however, the marked response observed to radiation alone in our one patient and in the one case reported by Shibata et al[35] argues for further evaluation

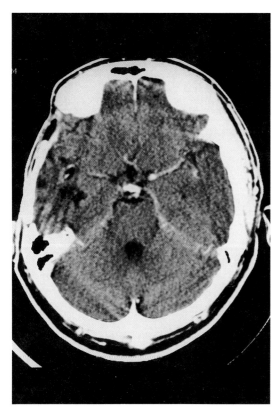

Figure 5. Follow-up contrast-enhanced CT scan 4 years after complete resection of the right middle fossa extra-axial cavernous malformation presented in Figures 1–5, shows no evidence of tumor recurrence.

of this form of therapy as the primary treatment after biopsy. Assuming the lesion is small enough for safe treatment, stereotaxic radiosurgery with the gamma knife or linac scalpel could theoretically be of benefit, although it has not yet been reported. The role of proton-beam therapy is uncertain: our experience with one patient suggests that it did not significantly affect continued growth or the vascularity of the tumor.

Surgical Management

The indications for surgery are the establishment of the diagnosis and decompression of the surrounding structures. The decision to stage the resection with preoperative radiation therapy or to perform a total resection during the initial operation remains a matter of debate.

In patients with suspected middle fossa extra-axial CMs, we prefer to plan a staged resection combined with radiation therapy. The lesion is exposed using a standard fronto-temporal approach, and the clinical diagnosis is verified with open biopsy. The intraoperative appearance is a dark red pulsatile mass with the dura of the cavernous sinus forming a pseudocapsule over all or at least a portion of the lesion. The mass at times can be seen under the microscope to contain minute blood vessels and cavities.[11] Incision for biopsy normally results in profuse bleeding that can be difficult to control. After pathologic confirmation of the diagnosis, the surgeon can decide whether to attempt further resection or to close and refer the patient for radiation therapy. Treatment of the lesion with 3,000–5,000 rads of external-beam radiation over 5 weeks is recommended.

Postradiation follow-up studies demonstrate a reduction in the size of the lesion in as little as 4–6 months. Following radiation, the lesion is much less vascular and can be readily separated from the surrounding neurovascular structures. Cranial nerves III, IV, and V, which run within the dural leaves of the lateral cavernous sinus wall, are normally found stretched over the surface of the tumor and are readily preserved. In contrast, cranial nerve VI and the internal carotid artery, which passes through the cavernous sinus proper, are frequently encased by tumor and may be difficult or impossible to protect without leaving residual tumor. Intraoperative implantation of Iridium-125 seeds is a useful adjunct for the treatment of any residual tumor.

Meyer and colleagues at Mayo Clinic advocate total resection of middle fossa extra-axial CMs during the initial operation.[17] In the majority of their cases, the authors combined an extensive extradural bone dissection (as advocated by Dolenc[2]) including the lesser wing of the sphenoid, the medial aspect of the greater sphenoid wing, and the anterior clinoid process. This bony dissection facilitates early exposure of the neurovascular structures within the cavernous sinus. After the bony dissection, the dura was incised and the sylvian fissure opened widely. The dura overlying the superior orbital fissure was also incised to identify the cranial nerves early in the course of the dissection. This incision was carried posteriorly over the roof of the cavernous sinus as well as to the dural ring of the carotid artery. The malformation was then removed piece-meal. Venous sinus bleeding from the cavernous sinus was controlled with avitene pledgets. In addition, the authors found that early coagulation of the meningohypophyseal trunk helped control intraoperative bleeding.[17] Early access to the feeding arteries from the intracavernous internal carotid artery, however, can be quite difficult.[18,21,32] Of note, the authors reported using 2–8 units of blood per patient to maintain hemodynamic stability. They also recommended that the ipsilateral neck and lower extremity be draped should a saphenous vein interposition graft be needed.[17]

Results and Complications

Of the 46 patients with middle fossa extra-axial CMs reported in the literature, 8 died intraoperatively producing an operative mortality of 17%.[21,29] The majority of these deaths, however, occurred prior to the introduction of modern microsurgical techniques. Meyer et al[17] reported no mortality in their series of eight middle fossa extra-axial cavernous formations. Two patients in their series awoke from surgery with new deficits, representing a neurologic morbidity rate of 25%. One patient awoke with a complete ophthalmoplegia, while in a second case there was new onset of facial numbness. Although ocular motility and visual acuity often improve, oculomotor function rarely returns to normal. Harper et al reported a case with complete resolution of third, fourth, and sixth cranial

nerve palsies within 2 months after resection of a middle fossa extra-axial CM.[7]

Postoperative hematomas (extra- or intra-axial) are potential complications of these highly vascular lesions. Shibata et al reported a fatal postoperative intracerebral hematoma in a patient with a two-stage operation after preoperative radiation.[35] Diffuse intravascular coagulopathy is a potential risk mentioned in the literature after removal of larger middle fossa CMs.[26] No recurrences have been reported after total resection.

In the cases at BNI, two patients had a staged procedure—one with preoperative external radiation and the other with proton-beam treatment. Both patients are currently free of recurrences with no change in their preoperative ocular deficits.

Conclusion

Extra-axial CMs represent a distinct subgroup of CMs originating primarily in the middle fossa, within the cavernous sinus, most commonly found in middle-aged women. They have also been reported in the tentorium cerebelli, cerebellopontine angle, cerebral convexity, Meckel's cave, torcula, petrosal sinus, foramen magnum, and spinal extra-axial space. Pathologically, these lesions are similar to CMs elsewhere in the body.

Unlike intra-axial lesions, however, there is no characteristic radiologic appearance for extra-axial lesions. Middle fossa extra-axial CMs may be seen on cerebral angiography as a stain with a feeding artery and draining vein but without arteriovenous shunting. Visual/ocular symptoms predominate secondary to compression and stretching of the oculomotor and optic nerves by the increasing mass. Patients may also present with headaches, facial dysesthesias, hemiparesis, and amenorrhea. The signs and symptoms have a tendency to worsen during pregnancy and in some cases they may be precipitated during this period secondary to engorgement of the vascular spaces. Management of extra-axial CMs must account for the highly vascular nature of these lesions. External-beam radiation treatment after an initial biopsy reduces the size and vascularity of this lesion, decreasing the risks of total resection at a later date. Safe and total resection during the initial operation (without radiation therapy) using extradural bone dissection has also been shown to be a reasonable management option for middle fossa CMs. The diagnosis of an extra-axial CM must be considered in the differential when investigating a suspected meningioma in the parasellar or sphenoid wing regions.

References

1. Bradac GB, Riva A, Schörner W, et al. Cavernous sinus meningiomas: an MRI study. *Neuroradiology*. 1987;29:578–581.

2. Dolenc VV. A combined epi- and subdural direct approach to carotid-ophthalmic artery aneurysms. *J Neurosurg*. 1985;62:667–672.

3. Dolenc VV. In discussion: Sepehrnia A, Tatagiba M, Brandis A, et al. Cavernous angioma of the cavernous sinus: case report. *Neurosurgery*. 1990;27:151–155.

4. Elster AD, Challa VR, Gilbert TH, et al. Meningiomas: MR and histopathologic features. *Radiology*. 1989;170:857–862.

5. Fehlings MG, Tucker WS. Cavernous hemangioma of Meckel's cave: case report. *J Neurosurg*. 1988;68:645–647.

6. Glasscock ME III, Smith PG, Schwaber MK, et al. Clinical aspects of osseous hemangiomas of the skull base. *Laryngoscope*. 1984;94:869–873.

7. Harper DG, Buck DR, Early CB. Visual loss from cavernous hemangiomas of the middle cranial fossa. *Arch Neurol*. 1982;39:252–254.

8. Isla A, Roda JM, Alvarez F, et al. Intracranial cavernous angioma in the dura. *Neurosurgery*. 1989;25:657–659.

9. Ito J, Konno K, Sato I, et al. Convexity cavernous hemangioma, its angiographic and CT findings: report of a case (in Japanese). *No To Shinkei*. 1978;30:737–747. English abstract.

10. Kamrin RB, Buchsbaum HW. Large vascular malformations of the brain not visualized by serial angiography. *Arch Neurol*. 1965;13:413–420.

11. Kawai K, Fukui M, Tanaka A, et al. Extra-cerebral cavernous hemangioma of the middle fossa. *Surg Neurol*. 1978;9:19–25.

12. Kudo T, Ueki S, Kobayashi H, et al. Experience with the ultrasonic surgical aspirator in a cavernous hemangioma of the cavernous sinus. *Neurosurgery*. 1989;24:628–631.

13. Laws ER Jr. Editorial note in: Sepehrnia A, Tatagiba M, Brandis A, et al. Cavernous angioma of the cavernous sinus: case report. *Neurosurgery*. 1990;27:155.

14. Linskey ME, Sekhar LN. Cavernous sinus hemangiomas: a series, a review, and an hypothesis. *Neurosurgery*. 1992;30:101–107.

15. MacCarty CS, Lougheed LE, Brown JR. Unusual benign tumor at the foramen magnum: report of a case. *J Neurosurg*. 1959;16:463–467.

16. McCormick WF, Boulter TR. Vascular malformations ("angiomas") of the dura mater: report of two cases. *J Neurosurg*. 1966;25:309–311.

17. Meyer FB, Lombardi D, Scheithauer B, et al. Extra-axial cavernous hemangiomas involving the dural sinuses. *J Neurosurg*. 1990;73:187–192.

18. Mori K, Handa H, Gi H, et al. Cavernomas in the middle fossa. *Surg Neurol*. 1980;14:21–31.

19. Moritake K, Handa H, Nozaki K, et al. Tentorial cavernous angioma with calcification in a neonate. *Neurosurgery*. 1985;16:207–211.

20. Nakasu Y, Handa J, Matsuda M, et al. Cavernous angioma of the middle cranial fossa: report of two cases and a review. *Nippon Geka Hokan*. 1985;54:364–371.

21. Namba S. Extracerebral cavernous hemangioma of the middle cranial fossa. *Surg Neurol*. 1983;19:379–388.

22. Pásztor E, Szabó G, Slowik F, et al. Cavernous hemangioma of the base of the skull: report of a case treated surgically. *J Neurosurg*. 1964;21:582–585.

23. Piepgras DG. In discussion: Sawamura Y, de Tribolet N. Cavernous hemangioma in the cavernous sinus: case report. *Neurosurgery*. 1990;26:126–128.

24. Pozzati E, Giuliani G, Ferracini R, et al. Facial nerve palsy secondary to a dural cavernous angioma of the middle cranial fossa eroding the tegmen tympani. *Neurosurgery*. 1988;23:245–247.

25. Quatrocchi KB, Kissel P, Ellis WG, et al. Cavernous angioma of the tentorium cerebelli: case report. *J Neurosurg*. 1989;71:935–937.

26. Rengachary SS, Kalyan-Raman UP. Other cranial intradural angiomas. In: Wilkins RH, Rengachary SS, eds. *Neurosurgery*. New York, NY: McGraw-Hill; 1985;2:1465–1473.

27. Richardson RR, Cerullo LJ. Spinal epidural cavernous hemangioma. *Surg Neurol*. 1979;12:266–268.

28. Rigamonti D, Drayer BP, Johnson PC, et al. The MRI appearance of cavernous malformations (angiomas). *J Neurosurg*. 1987;67:518–524.

29. Rigamonti D, Pappas CTE, Spetzler RF, et al. Extracerebral cavernous angiomas of the middle fossa. *Neurosurgery*. 1990;27:306–310.

30. Rosenblum B, Rothman AS, Lanzieri C, et al. A cavernous sinus cavernous hemangioma: case report. *J Neurosurg*. 1986;65:716–718.

31. Saldaña CJ, Zimman H, Alonso P, et al. Neonatal cavernous hemangioma of the dura mater: case report. *Neurosurgery*. 1991;29:602–605.

32. Sawamura Y, de Tribolet N. Cavernous hemangioma in the cavernous sinus: case report. *Neurosurgery*. 1990;26:126–128.

33. Sehkar LN. In discussion: Sepehrnia A, Tatagiba M, Brandis A, et al. Cavernous angioma of the cavernous sinus: case report. *Neurosurgery.* 1990;27:154–155.

34. Sepehrnia A, Tatagiba M, Brandis A, et al. Cavernous angioma of the cavernous sinus: case report. *Neurosurgery.* 1990;27:151–155.

35. Shibata S, Kurihara M, Mori K, et al. Preoperative irradiation of an extracerebral cavernous hemangioma in the middle fossa: follow-up study with computed tomography (in Japanese). *No Shinkei Geka.* 1981;9:211–215. English abstract.

36. Shibata S, Mori K. Effect of radiation therapy on extracerebral cavernous hemangioma in the middle fossa: report of three cases. *J Neurosurg.* 1987;67:919–922.

37. Simard JM, Garcia-Bengochea F, Ballinger WE Jr, et al. Cavernous angioma: a review of 126 collected and 12 new clinical cases. *Neurosurgery.* 1986;18:162–172.

38. Yamasaki T, Handa H, Yamashita J, et al. Intracranial and orbital cavernous angiomas: a review of 30 cases. *J Neurosurg.* 1986;64:197–208.

39. Zimmerman RS, Spetzler RF, Lee KS, et al. Cavernous malformations of the brain stem. *J Neurosurg.* 1991;75:32–39.

Chapter 12

Spinal Cavernous Malformations

Paul C. McCormick, MD, and Bennett M. Stein, MD

Intramedullary cavernous malformations (CMs) of the spinal cord are a rare but treatable cause of acute, recurrent, or progressive myelopathy. Like their intracranial counterparts, the widespread use and availability of magnetic resonance imaging (MRI) has resulted in an observed increased incidence of spinal lesions.[1-4,6,9] Prior to the availability of MRI, it is likely that many patients harboring spinal CMs were erroneously diagnosed as having multiple sclerosis, transverse myelitis, or other types of medical myelopathies.[4]

The true incidence of spinal CMs is difficult to establish because of the sparse number of spinal cord autopsy studies. The reported incidence of central nervous system (CNS) CMs is quite variable and ranges between 0.02% and 4%.[3] Based on spinal component weight and volume, it is reasonable to assume that 3% to 5% of CNS CMs arise within the spinal canal. These lesions occur proportionally throughout the spinal cord. Malformations of the filum terminale and cauda equina are rare but have been reported.[7] Most CMs are totally intramedullary, although we have encountered one lesion with an exophytic component (Figure 1). While epidural malformations have been described, we have found no examples of intradural extramedullary lesions not related to the nerve roots. A familial occurrence, associated metameric cutaneous vascular nevi, and the coexistence of intracranial CMs have been described.[2,4]

Clinical Features

Like other congenital CNS vascular malformations, the initial presentation may occur at any age. In our series of 12 patients, the age of symptom onset ranged from 13–62 years (mean, 35 years). The clinical features associated with intramedullary CMs are variable. An acute, progressive, or episodic course has been described. The acute presentation is probably secondary to hemorrhage, which may be confined within the sinusoidal spaces of the malformation and cause its acute expansion. Frank hemorrhage into the surrounding spinal cord (i.e. hematomyelia) may also occur. The onset of hemorrhage is usually heralded by back pain that typically approximates the level of the malformation. A recent history of trauma is noted in some, particularly young patients, but it is unclear whether this trauma is causative or coincidental.

The appearance of neurologic deficit, if it occurs, usually begins several hours after the onset of pain. Although the initial onset of symptoms is sudden, neurologic deterioration may evolve over several hours to a few days, which tends to differentiate these lesions from the acute course associated with hemorrhage from spinal arteriovenous malformations (AVMs). While hemorrhage may result in complete and permanent paraplegia or tetraplegia, it is more common that the initial deficit is incomplete and followed by some degree of recovery. Repeat hemorrhage has been described several months or years following the initial presentation.[4] The annual risk of rebleeding for spinal malformations, however, has not been established.

A progressive spinal cord syndrome may be produced by intramedullary CMs. This course may be punctuated by episodic deterioration. These recurrent events may lead to the erroneous diagnosis of a demyelinating myelopathy (e.g. multiple sclerosis).

The progressive course seen with these malformations reflects their dynamic nature. Although these lesions are presumably congenital in nature, their potential for growth and enlargement has been well documented.[4] Capillary proliferation and budding, vessel dilation, and repeated hemorrhage followed by organization and canalization are possible mechanisms of growth. Osmotically active products of red blood cell degradation may result in progressive enlargement in a manner similar to chronic subdural hematomas.[10] A neurotoxic effect of hemosiderin or compromise of the surrounding microcirculation are additional possible mechanisms of progressive deterioration in lesions showing no evidence of interval growth.

Pathology

CMs usually appear as a dark blue or purple lobulated mass frequently described as "mulberry-like" in appearance. Although usually unencapsulated, they are generally well circumscribed and clearly demarcated from the hemosiderin-stained surrounding neural parenchyma. Tiny punctate lesions, clearly separate from the malformation, occasionally may be seen.

The microscopic appearance of CMs generally consists of sinusoidal vascular spaces arranged in a back-to-back or honeycomb orientation without intervening neural tissue. The vessels are of capillary structure, staining negative for elastic or smooth muscle tissue, and usually thick-walled; but greatly thickened, hyalinized vessels are a common find, irrespective of the patient's age. Tongues of gliotic parenchyma may appear within the malformation near its peripheral margin. In addition, disorganized elastic tissue rarely has been noted.

Radiology

As with most other intramedullary pathology, MRI is the imaging procedure of choice for CMs. The characteristic appearance of a central core of mixed-signal intensity from various stages of red blood cell degradation surrounded by a hypointense hemosiderin ring is well known (Figure 2). Enhancement is variable but usually minimal. While this appearance is highly suggestive for CM, it is not pathognomonic. Hemorrhagic neoplasms or a resolving hematoma of any etiology may mimic this appearance. Conversely, variations in MRI appearance occasionally do not allow a confident preoperative diagnosis of CM. This is due primarily to the small volume of spinal cord tissue and variable resolution of MRI equipment. Additionally, a small lesion may be obscured by hemorrhage or edema.

Myelography is frequently normal or may demonstrate only subtle widening despite the presence of significant neurologic deficit. Postmyelographic CT increases sensitivity but may also be normal or nonspecific. Angiography is usually nonrevealing.

Management

The management of intramedullary CMs is dependent on the patient's age, clinical features, and characteristics of the malformation. Because symptomatic lesions are quite rare, no treatment is currently advised for asymptomatic lesions. This situation may be encountered in patients, or their family members, harboring associated intracranial CMs. Surgical exploration is favored in most patients with symptomatic lesions because of the potential morbidity of a future neurologic event. This "effective" natural history of spinal CM is similar to brain stem lesions and certainly much more treacherous than most supratentorial malformations. In some cases, however, visual inspection may influence the surgical objective. In one patient, a clearly diffuse intramedullary CM with an exophytic component was encountered (see Figure 1). Only the extramedullary portion was removed. Another patient was a 55-year-old woman with a 3-year history of arm and leg pain with minimal objective deficit. Exploration was performed following a nondiagnostic MRI, which demonstrated only widening of the spinal cord. At operation, a large CM was seen to occupy the right lateral funiculus (Figure 3). Because of the patient's age, relatively minor symptoms, and potential surgical morbidity, no attempt at removal was made.

Surgical Technique

The spinal cord is exposed through a standard laminectomy with the patient in a prone position. The malformation can frequently be seen as a bluish discoloration within the spinal cord (Figure 4). This appearance is fairly typical, but we have encountered this in one patient harboring an intramedullary melanoma (Figure 5). Occasionally, abnormal surface vasculature related to the malformation is found. These are usually small draining veins, although a rare feeding artery can be seen with the aid of a microscope. We have encountered a small aneurysm on a posterior spinal artery, adjacent to an intramedullary malformation (see Figure 3A). While these associations with an otherwise radiologic, gross, and microscopically typical malformation may raise questions as to the etiology and classification of these and other vascular malformations, they do not alter treatment. Exposure of the malformation is generally through a standard midline myelotomy as described for tumors. For small, eccentrically located lesions with a pial presentation, a small longitudinal myelotomy may be placed at either end of the apex of the lesion. Gentle rotation of the spinal cord with suture retraction on a divided dentate ligament may improve visualization of these lesions (see Figure 3B).

The technique of removal is similar to intramedullary tumors.[5] Gentle traction and cauterization of the malformation surface against the countertraction provided by pial sutures allow the development of a cleavage plane (see Figure 5). Internal decompression with an ultrasonic aspirator or laser can be performed with larger lesions because bleeding from within the malformation is minimal and easily controlled. Occasionally, the malformation may be partially or totally obscured by a hematoma within or surrounding the lesion. Piecemeal evacuation of the clot precedes lesion removal in these cases. Following evacuation of the hematoma, some small malformations may not be readily apparent. Before assuming that the hemorrhage has destroyed the malformation, the walls of the hematomyelic cavity must be carefully inspected under high magnification.

The friable nature and lobulated architecture may pose some problems with removal. Traction on the malformation frequently ruptures the delicate sinusoidal spaces and results in piece-meal removal. Small lobulations of the malformations may extend into and appear buried within adjacent spinal cord tissue. Since the critical surrounding spinal cord tissue requires a

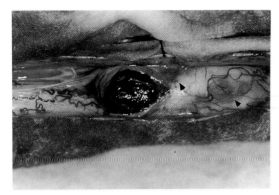

Figure 1. Operative photograph shows a large exophytic mass producing compression and displacement of the spinal cord. Multiple areas of bluish discoloration represent the diffuse intramedullary portion of the cavernous malformation (arrows).

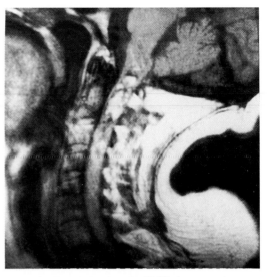

Figure 2. T1-weighted sagittal MRI demonstrates an intramedullary mass of the upper cervical cord. The appearance is characteristic of a cavernous malformation.

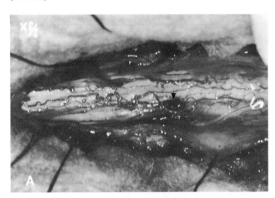

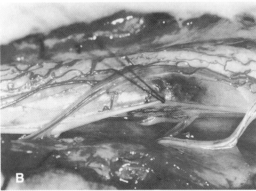

Figure 3. (A) Operative photograph demonstrates a small posterior spinal artery aneurysm (arrow) overlying an intramedullary cavernous malformation. **(B)** A cavernous malformation is seen to occupy the lateral funiculus of the spinal cord. Visualization of lateral cord surface through the posterior laminectomy approach is achieved by suture retraction on divided dentate ligament.

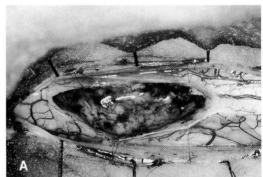

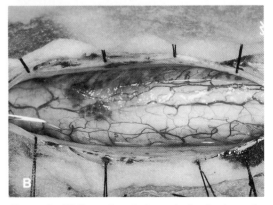

Figure 4. (A) Operative photograph clearly shows the cavernous malformation through the dorsal cord surface. **(B)** Operative photograph after complete resection of the malformation.

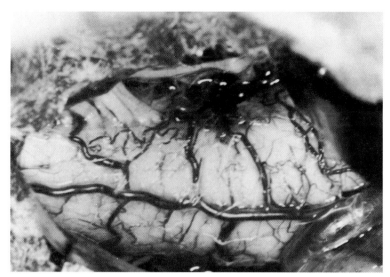

Figure 5. Operative photograph of intramedullary melanoma demonstrates bluish discoloration usually associated with cavernous malformations (arrows).

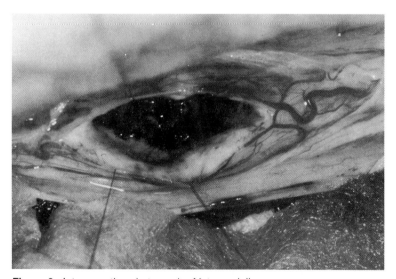

Figure 6. Intraoperative photograph of intramedullary cavernous malformation after midline myelotomy and partially completed dissection from the surrounding spinal cord. Countertraction is achieved with 6–0 silk sutures suspended by mosquito clamps.

precise surface dissection with limited spinal cord retraction (like brain stem malformations), it can be difficult to accurately assess the completeness of removal. Careful inspection of the walls of the resection cavity under high magnification is performed in all cases prior to closure.

Results

It has become clear that the majority of spinal CMs may be safely removed with acceptable morbidity utilizing contemporary microsurgical techniques.[2,4,6] While minor sensory deficits almost invariably occur following midline myelotomy, most patients demonstrate either improvement or stabilization of neurologic function after removal. Follow-up MRI is performed at 6 months and a few years postoperatively to ensure the completeness of removal. It may be difficult to differentiate residual malformations from postoperative changes and hemosiderin. One patient in whom a gross total resection was accomplished and confirmed on 6-month MRI had a recurrence demonstrated on MRI 6 years later. We speculate that enlargement of peripheral residual malformation is responsible for this late recurrence. We have witnessed this in two of our cases of brain stem CMs. It is also possible that the recurrence may arise from residual peripheral telangiectases which cannot be seen at operation. This would support the theory which suggests that telangiectasia and CM represent different developmental forms of the same congenital pathologic entity.[8]

References

1. Cosgrove GR, Bertrand G, Fontaine S, et al. Cavernous angiomas of the spinal cord. *J Neurosurg.* 1988;68:31–36.

2. Lee KS, Spetzler RF. Spinal cord cavernous malformation in a patient with familial intracranial cavernous malformations. *Neurosurgery.* 1990;26:877–880.

3. McCormick PC, Michelsen WJ. Management of intracranial cavernous and venous malformations. In: Barrow DL, ed. *Intracranial Vascular Malformations.* Park Ridge,Ill: American Association of Neurological Surgeons; 1990:197–217.

4. McCormick PC, Michelsen WJ, Post KD, et al. Cavernous malformations of the spinal cord. *Neurosurgery.* 1988;23:459–463.

5. McCormick PC, Torres R, Post KD, et al. Intramedullary ependymoma of the spinal cord. *J Neurosurg.* 1990;72:523–533.

6. Ogilvy CS, Louis DN, Ojemann RG. Intramedullary cavernous angiomas of the spinal cord: clinical presentation, pathologic features and surgical management. *Neurosurgery.* 1992;31:219–230.

7. Ramos F Jr, de Toffol B, Aesch B, et al. Hydrocephalus and cavernoma of the cauda equina. *Neurosurgery.* 1990;27:139–142.

8. Rigamonti D, Johnson PC, Spetzler RF, et al. Cavernous malformations and capillary telangiectasia: a spectrum within a single pathological entity. *Neurosurgery.* 1991;28:60–64.

9. Saito N, Yamakawa K, Sasaki T, et al. Intramedullary cavernous angioma with trigeminal neuralgia: a case report and review of the literature. *Neurosurgery.* 1989;25:97–101.

10. Scott RM, Barnes P, Kupsky W, et al. Cavernous angiomas of the central nervous system in children. *J Neurosurg.* 1992;76:38–46.

Chapter 13

Lesions Mimicking Cavernous Malformations

Gary K. Steinberg, MD, PhD, and Michael P. Marks, MD

Cavernous malformations (CMs) were difficult to diagnose without a surgical or autopsy specimen until the advent of computed tomography (CT) scanning and, more recently, magnetic resonance imaging (MRI).[6,12,18,28] Although usually not demonstrable with angiography, these "angiographically occult" malformations have a characteristic MRI appearance. However, these typical radiologic findings are not pathognomonic for CMs and may also be present with other vascular malformations ("cryptic" arteriovenous malformations [AVMs], capillary malformations [telangiectases], mixed or transitional vascular malformations), hematomas, hemorrhagic tumors, or inflammatory lesions of the central nervous system (CNS).[1,4-6,12,16-18,28] In addition, the clinical presentation and course cannot always differentiate CMs from these other pathologic entities.

Cavernous Malformations

MRI is the most sensitive and specific imaging modality for detecting CMs.[6,11,15,18,25,28] These lesions characteristically are well demarcated, with areas of mixed (high and low) signal attenuation on both T1- and T2-weighted images bounded by a peripheral rim of hypointensity best visualized on the T2-weighted images (Figure 1). This appearance is related to multiple episodes of remote and recent focal hemorrhage in the lesion. The high intensity areas on the T1- and T2-weighted images represent subacute blood in the form of extracellular methemoglobin. Peripheral hypointensity on T1 and T2 images represents hemosiderin and ferritin (chronic hemorrhage); and this area of low signal increases in size with progressive T2-weighting. The MRI appearance is also related to magnetic field strength with higher field strength imaging showing more magnetic susceptibility phenomenon than lower field strength imaging.[6,11,15,18] Hypointensity seen in a more central location may be due to dense calcium deposits, flow voids, or regions of subacute or chronic hemorrhage (intracellular deoxyhemoglobin, hemosiderin, or ferritin). Calcium deposits tend to accumulate centrally in lesions and often have irregular margins.[6]

CMs are usually relatively small (0.2–3.0 cm diameter) but can reach large dimensions (greater than 6 cm diameter) (Figure 2). They may be located anywhere in the CNS—either in the brain or spinal cord.[12,18,22,25] Supratentorial CMs are more common (75% to 85%)

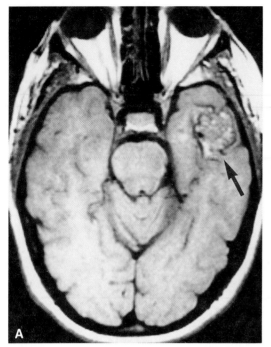 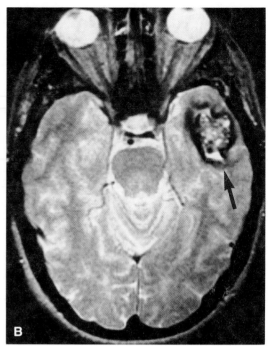

Figure 1. Axial MRI through the temporal lobes demonstrating a left temporal CM (arrow). **(A)** T1-weighted image demonstrates mixed signal within the lesion. Central components of high and intermediate signal are noted and there is a peripheral margin of low signal. **(B)** T2-weighted image at the same level demonstrates mixed signal centrally. The margin of low signal is more prominent due to magnetic susceptibility effect from hemosiderin and ferritin at the periphery of the lesion.

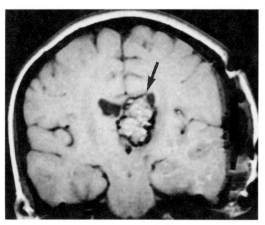

Figure 2. Coronal T1-weighted MRI through a large intraventricular CM (arrow) measuring approximately 2.5 × 4 × 4 cm.

than infratentorial ones.[12,22,25,26] Multiple lesions are found in 13% to 50% of patients.[3,18,22,25,27,32] They are familial in up to 50% of cases, being inherited as an autosomal dominant trait.[19] These vascular lesions may present most frequently with seizures (35% to 50%), gradual progressive neurologic impairment (particularly when located in the brain stem, basal ganglia, or thalamus), rapid clinical deterioration, or headaches. Repeated hemorrhagic events usually occur within CM margins and can cause progressive enlargement of lesion boundaries. Sometimes hemorrhages extend outside the hemosiderin ring, presenting as acute intraparenchymal hemorrhages (20% to 30% of cases). These bleeds may be quite large and clinically symptomatic (Figure 3).[18,22,25,26] CMs are not accompanied by significant surrounding edema unless recent bleeding has occurred. In this case, follow-up imaging should show resolution of the edema.

CT is not as sensitive or specific as MRI for detecting CMs.[6,12,15,18,28] Typically, they are slightly hyperdense but may be isodense, hypodense, or mixed on CT, sometimes with punctate areas of calcification (Figure 4).

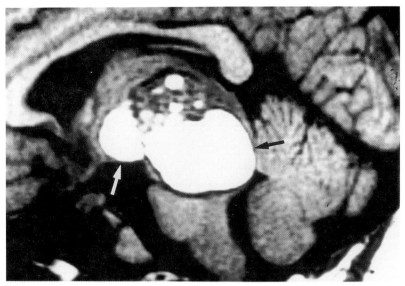

Figure 3. Sagittal T1-weighted MRI through the midline of the brain stem demonstrates a pontomesencephalic CM. Large regions of uniform high signal in the tegmentum and tectum (arrows) are consistent with subacute hemorrhage (methemoglobin). This extensive brain stem hemorrhage caused significant neurologic deterioration.

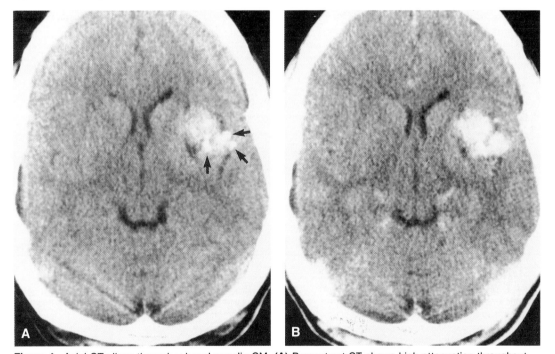

Figure 4. Axial CT slices through a basal ganglia CM. **(A)** Precontrast CT shows high attenuation throughout much of the lesion and a few focal regions of dense calcification are noted (arrows). **(B)** Post-contrast CT scan shows homogenous enhancement throughout the lesion.

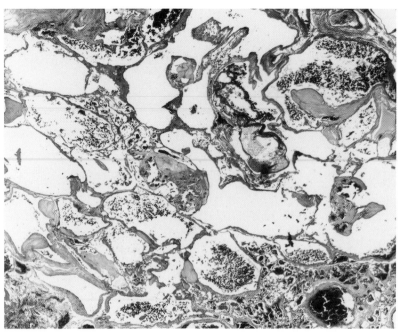

Figure 5. Typical CM surgically resected from frontal region. Malformation is composed of thin-walled, sinusoidal channels closely apposed to one another. Little intervening brain parenchyma is present between the vessels. (H & E, × 30).

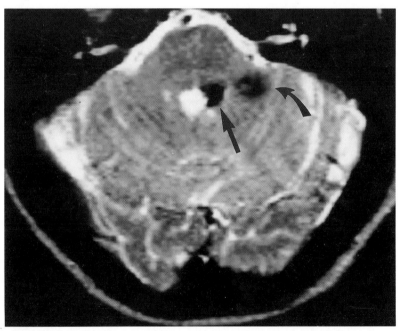

Figure 6. Axial T2-weighted MRI through the posterior fossa at the level of the pons demonstrates two regions of low signal (arrows) consistent with chronic hemorrhage. Pathologic evaluation of the subependymal lesion (straight arrow) after surgical removal demonstrated an angiographically occult AVM.

Mild enhancement is often noted after intravenous contrast infusion. Angiography is usually negative. However, CMs (especially the larger ones) may occasionally show a contrast "blush" during late capillary or venous phases of the angiogram.[6,12,15,18,25] We have encountered several CMs that were associated with developmental venous anomalies, or venous malformations, and this has been previously reported.[1,17,21,24]

Using traditional, strict pathologic criteria, CMs appear well circumscribed and are composed of numerous, thin-walled vascular channels lined by a single layer of endothelial cells, closely apposed to one another, with little or no intervening brain parenchyma (Figure 5). Arteries, arterialized veins, or vessels with elastic fibers or smooth muscle are not found. Hyalinization of the vessel walls and thrombosis may occur. Calcification may be present. Hemosiderin-laden macrophages are usually abundant in the brain parenchyma immediately surrounding the malformation.[12,14,23,25,26,27]

Angiographically Occult ("Cryptic") Arteriovenous Malformations

Angiographically occult ("cryptic", partially thrombosed) AVMs may have an identical radiological appearance to that of CMs (Figure 6).[4,12,16,18,22,25] Pathologically, AVMs have distinct arteries recognized by the presence of an internal elastic lamina (sometimes interrupted or duplicated) and smooth muscle in the media that may vary in thickness (Figure 7). Veins may have extremely thick walls and may demonstrate hyperplasia of smooth muscle (arterialization). Calcification of the AVM vessel media and fibrosis of the intima may occur. Gliotic brain parenchyma is present between the abnormal AVM blood vessels. Hemosiderin is found in macrophages within the intervening and surrounding brain. Despite having a histologic arterial component, they are not angiographically demonstrable due to low flow, small size, partial thrombosis, or

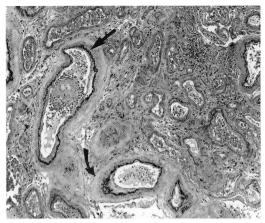

Figure 7. Angiographically occult ("cryptic") AVM surgically removed from occipital lobe. Distinct arteries are characterized by the presence of an internal elastic lamina (straight arrow) and smooth muscle in the media (curved arrow). Vessels vary considerably in size. Gliotic brain parenchyma is present between the abnormal AVM vessels. (EVG, × 100)

compression by a hematoma.[4,12,16,18,22,25] Wakai et al suggest that up to 25% of "spontaneous" lobar hemorrhages with normal initial angiograms are secondary to AVMs compressed by adjacent hematoma.[33,34]

In our series of 49 angiographically occult AVMs resected between 1988 and 1992, a few lesions had pathologic features of AVMs only, including arterialized veins or vessels with elastic tissue and some with smooth muscle. The MRI and CT characteristics of these lesions were similar to those of CMs. Some authors have suggested that angiographically occult AVMs, in distinction to CMs, may present more often with clinical hemorrhage, and a large hematoma, or an intraventricular hemorrhage secondary to bleeding from arterialized blood under higher pressure.[16,33,34,35] However, this is difficult to document and CMs may have an identical presentation.[1,4,12,16,17,18,22,30,31]

Capillary Malformations (Telangiectasias)

Vascular malformations with MRI and CT characteristics typical of CM, but with

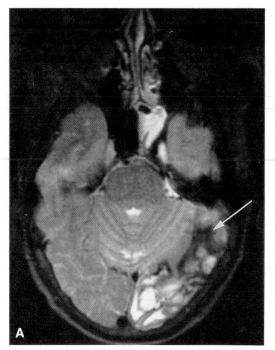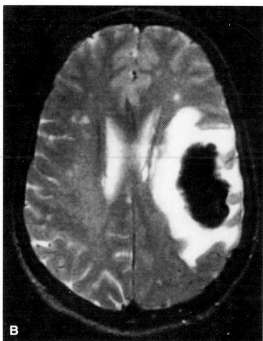

Figure 8. Axial T2-weighted MRI in a patient with proven amyloid angiopathy. The patient had at least 2 clinically separate hemorrhagic events. **(A)** Image through posterior temporal and occipital lobes shows the region of older chronic hemorrhage. Low-signal margins (arrow) are noted surrounding areas of higher signal. This is consistent with hemosiderin and ferritin surrounding regions of gliosis and/or methemoglobin. **(B)** Higher slice through the parietal lobe demonstrates acute hemorrhage (3 days old). Region of uniform low signal consistent with deoxyhemoglobin is seen centrally. A margin of high signal is noted, which is consistent with edema following an acute hemorrhage.

pathologic features of a capillary malformation have also been reported.[20] Capillary malformations are characterized by abnormal, dilated, thin-walled capillaries devoid of smooth muscle and elastic fibers, separated by normal brain parenchyma. The vessel size may vary and ectatic, dilated groups of capillaries may be observed. Microscopic evidence of previous hemorrhage is not usually seen.[14,20,23,27] Rigamonti et al have also described capillary malformations which presented clinically and radiologically like CMs.[20] Capillary malformations are usually punctate lesions located in the pons but can be found anywhere in the brain. They do not usually cause neurologic symptoms or signs, and rarely bleed.

Mixed (Transitional) Vascular Malformations

In our series of 64 angiographically occult vascular malformations, the majority were mixed (transitional) forms with elements of both classic CMs and AVMs or capillary malformations. These pathologic features included substantial gliotic intervening brain tissue between the vascular channels and significant vessel wall thickening with hyalinization, fibrosis, and calcification. Occasionally, vessels with elastic tissue or smooth muscle, or regions of classical telangiectasia were also noted. Other authors have described similar angiographically occult vascular malformations with mixed or transitional pathologic characteristics in-

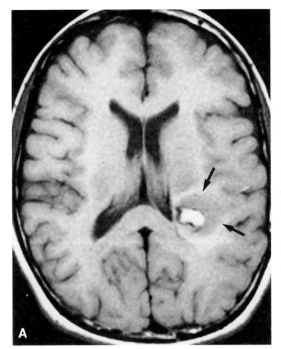 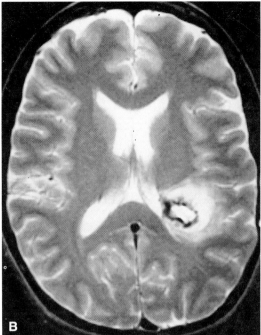

Figure 9. Axial MRI of a patient with a hemorrhagic ependymoma. **(A)** T1-weighted image demonstrates a high-signal central region (consistent with methemoglobin) surrounded by a thin low-signal margin (consistent with hemosiderin and ferritin). Outside of the hemosiderin/ferritin ring is a broader area which appears isointense with gray matter (arrows). This represents surrounding edema. **(B)** Again seen is a central area of high signal (methemoglobin) surrounded by a thin margin of low signal (hemosiderin/ferritin). Outside this margin is the broader area of high signal representative of edema. On the T2-weighted image, this edema is more easily identified due to the greater contrast between edema and surrounding brain parenchyma. This larger region of edema surrounding an area of chronic hemorrhage makes the diagnosis of hemorrhagic neoplasm much more likely than vascular malformation.

cluding CM, AVM, and capillary malformation.[1,4,12,16,17,20,22] Imaging features and clinical presentation of these transitional vascular malformations are indistinguishable from those of classic CMs. It may be more appropriate to consider all angiographically occult vascular lesions as a pathologic continuum between CMs, capillary malformations, and AVMs. Since these various vascular malformations share similar radiologic features and clinical behavior independent of specific pathologic type, the classic distinction between different types of angiographically occult vascular malformations may not be important.[1,4,12,16,17,20,25]

Spontaneous Hemorrhage

Spontaneous intraparenchymal hematoma secondary to hypertension, amyloid angiopathy, or other causes may appear similar to CMs on MRI and CT; however, simple hematomas from a single hemorrhage usually are absorbed relatively uniformly.[5,6,33,34] Consequently, they often form a solitary cavity with blood products of a more uniform age (Figure 8). Although they eventually collapse to form areas of encephalomalacia lined by hemosiderin, they do not usually demonstrate a nidus of heterogeneous signal on MRI surrounded by a rim

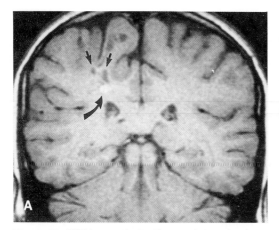

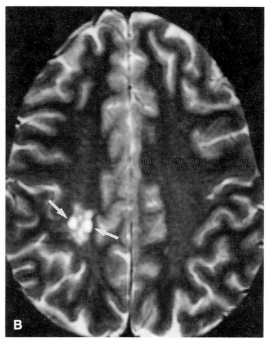

Figure 10. MRI in a patient with a nonhemorrhagic oligodendroglioma. **(A)** Coronal T1-weighted image demonstrates an area of high signal in the posterior parietal white matter (curved arrow). A few areas of lower signal are noted cephalad to this (straight arrows). **(B)** T2-weighted axial image through the lesion shows focal areas of high signal within the lesion (arrows). A margin of surrounding higher signal in the white matter is noted. This represents edema and it was also seen on adjacent slices. The lack of low signal at the margins of this lesion make this unlikely to be a region of chronic hemorrhage. The surrounding edema, although slight, makes this far more likely to be a nonhemorrhagic neoplasm. The area of high signal seen on the T1-weighted image (curved arrow, **A**) can be seen in cystic regions of tumors with higher protein content.

of hypodensity, which would suggest recurrent small bleeds from a vascular malformation. Any acute hemorrhage (including those from CMs) may be associated with surrounding edema and mass effect. In contradistinction to CMs or other angiographically occult vascular malformations, spontaneous intraparenchymal hematomas do not usually recur at the same site.[5,6]

Tumors

Hemorrhagic neoplasms may mimic the radiologic and clinical pattern of CMs (Figure 9).[5,29] According to various series, 3% to 14% of brain metastases and 1% to 3% of gliomas demonstrate intratumoral hemorrhage.[7] Sze et al found 18 of 24 patients with MRl lesions initially diagnosed as occult vascular malformations to have hemorrhagic neoplasms.[29] These included primary brain tumors (astrocytoma, oligodendroglioma, meningioma) or metastatic tumor (melanoma, choriocarcinoma). Other hemorrhagic tumors that may be misdiagnosed as CMs include ependymoma, glioblastoma, renal cell carcinoma, thyroid carcinoma, bronchogenic carcinoma, and pinealoma.[5,7] Brain stem occult vascular malformations are particularly prone to misdiagnoses of brain stem tumors.[9] Features that may distinguish tumors from occult vascular malformations include significant edema persisting over weeks or months despite resolution of the acute hemorrhage and the presence of multiple lesions.[13] With hemorrhagic tumors, the mass effect is often much greater than expected from hemorrhage alone and the low signal surrounding ring may be incomplete due to inconsistent deposition of hemosiderin.[7] Evidence of systemic malignancy would obviously suggest the diagnosis of neoplasm.[10] Gliomas associated with hemorrhage may carry a higher morbidity than CMs. However, none of these radiologic features is completely reliable and the clini-

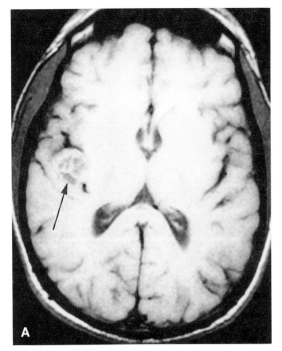 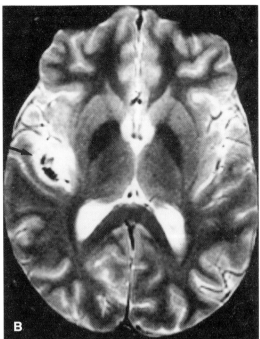

Figure 11. Axial MRI in a patient with a nonhemorrhagic astrocytoma. CT scan (not shown) demonstrated regions of dense calcification within the lesion. **(A)** T1-weighted image through the lesion demonstrates focal areas of lower signal (arrow) in the right parietal lobe. These corresponded to the areas of calcification seen on the CT scan. **(B)** T2-weighted image at the same level demonstrates low signal centrally in the areas of calcification. A surrounding margin of higher signal (arrow) corresponds to edema surrounding the tumor. This appearance of low signal centrally surrounded by higher signal may be seen in a more acute hemorrhage with surrounding edema and central deoxyhemoglobin (as shown in Figure 8). The patient did not have symptoms of an acute episode of hemorrhage, however. These MRI results, coupled with the clinical presentation and the CT findings, are most consistent with a tumor.

cal presentation may also be similar. Occasionally, a nonhemorrhagic tumor will have radiologic features that make it difficult to distinguish from an occult vascular malformation on CT or MRI (Figures 10 and 11). Melanin and fat are high intensity on T1 images and low intensity on T2 images, which may be confused with intracellular methemoglobin (Figure 12). However, melanin is not as hypointense as intracellular methemoglobin, and only intracellular methemoglobin becomes more hypointense as T2-weighting increases.[6,7] Proteinaceous tumor material and calcification may mimic the MRI characteristics of subacute and chronic blood within the lesion.[6] However,

evidence of surrounding edema and signal characteristics at the margins of the lesion usually suggest the correct diagnosis (Figures 10 and 11).

Inflammatory Lesions

Occasionally, intracerebral infection or chronic inflammatory lesions may present clinically and radiologically in a similar fashion to occult vascular malformations.[2,8] We have encountered this in a patient with cysticercosis (Figure 13) and in another with a chronic granuloma. No blood products were found pathologically in the re-

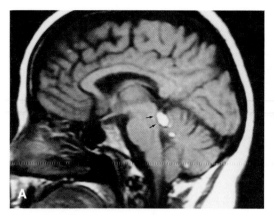

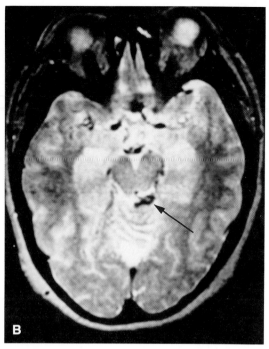

Figure 12. MRI of a patient with a quadrigeminal plate lipoma. **(A)** Sagittal image demonstrates a region of high signal in the region of the quadrigeminal plate. A few additional foci of high signal are noted in the cerebellar hemisphere. Chemical shift artifact is also noted with a rim of low signal along the anterior margin of the lesion (small arrows). **(B)** T2-weighted axial images through the upper portion of the lesion. A region of low signal is noted (arrow). The fatty nature of this lesion is shown by the signal change between the two MR sequences. Chemical shift artifact is commonly seen in fatty lesions. The other two areas of high signal seen on the sagittal image were not diagnosed at surgery but were thought to represent additional lipomas.

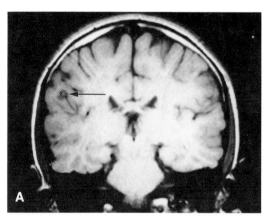

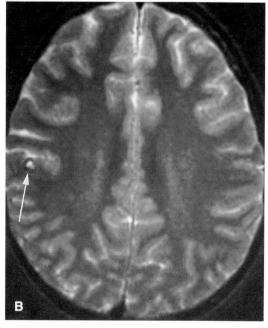

Figure 13. MRI in a patient with cysticercosis. **(A)** T1-weighted coronal image shows an area isointense in signal with gray matter and with a surrounding margin of low signal (arrow). **(B)** T2-weighted axial image through the lesion demonstrates a central region of high signal and surrounding lower signal margin (arrow). These findings are typical of the later stages of parenchymal cysticercosis when the larval contents have often mineralized and the inflammatory capsule is thick and collagenous. The hypointensity seen on T2-weighted images may reflect calcification, collagen, or free radical from macrophages in the inflammatory capsule.

sected lesions. In these cases, calcification and other contents of the granuloma appeared on the MRI similar to the blood products in an angiographically occult malformation. Multiplicity of lesions and the clinical setting might help differentiate inflammatory intracerebral lesions from CMs, but this distinction is not absolute.

References

1. Ahmadi J, Miller CA, Segall HD, et al. CT patterns in histopathologically complex cavernous hemangiomas. *AJNR.* 1985;6:389–393.

2. Chang KH, Cho SY, Hesselink JR, et al. Parasitic diseases of the central nervous system. *Neuroimaging Clin of NA.* 1991;1:159–178.

3. Curling OD Jr, Kelly DL Jr, Elster AD, et al. An analysis of the natural history of cavernous angiomas. *J Neurosurg.* 1991;75:702–708.

4. Ebeling JD, Tranmer BI, Davis KA, et al. Thrombosed arteriovenous malformations: a type of occult vascular malformation. *Neurosurgery.* 1988;23:605–610.

5. Feldmann E. Intracerebral hemorrhage. *Stroke.* 1991;22:684–691.

6. Gomori JM, Grossman RI, Goldberg HI, et al. Occult cerebral vascular malformations: high-field MRI imaging. *Radiology.* 1986;158:707–713.

7. Grossman RI. Intracerebral hemorrhage. In: Latchaw RE, ed. *MR and CT Imaging of the Head, Neck and Spine.* 2nd ed. St. Louis, Mo: Mosby Year Book; 1991:171–202.

8. Jungreis CA, Grossman RI. Intracranial infections and inflammatory disease. In: Latchaw RE, ed. *MR and CT Imaging of the Head, Neck and Spine.* 2nd ed. St. Louis, Mo: Mosby Year Book; 1991:303–346.

9. Kashiwagi S, van Loveren HR, Tew JM Jr, et al. Diagnosis and treatment of vascular brain-stem malformations. *J Neurosurg.* 1990;72:27–34.

10. Kase CS. lntracerebral hemorrhage: non-hypertensive causes. *Stroke.* 1986;17:590–595.

11. Lemme-Plaghos L, Kucharczyk W, Brant-Zawadzki M, et al. MRI of angiographically occult vascular malformations. *AJR.* 1986;146:1223–1228.

12. Lobato RD, Perez C, Rivas JJ, et al. Clinical, radiological, and pathological spectrum of angiographically occult intracranial vascular malformations. *J Neurosurg.* 1988;68:518–531.

13. Martin N, Dion JE. Imaging of intracranial vascular malformations. In: Barrow DL, ed. *Intracranial Vascular Malformations.* Park Ridge, Ill: American Association of Neurological Surgeons; 1990:63–89.

14. McCormick WF. Pathology of vascular malformations in the brain. In: Wilson CB, Stein BM, eds. *Intracranial Arteriovenous Malformations.* Baltimore, Md: Williams & Wilkins; 1984:44–63.

15. New PFJ, Ojemann RG, Davis KR, et al. MR and CT of occult vascular malformations of the brain. *AJNR.* 1986;7:771–779.

16. Ogilvy CS, Heros RC, Ojemann RG, et al. Angiographically occult arteriovenous malformations. *J Neurosurg.* 1988;69:350–355.

17. Rapacki TFX, Brantley MJ, Furlow TW Jr, et al. Heterogeneity of cerebral cavernous hemangiomas diagnosed by MR imaging. *J Comput Assist Tomogr.* 1990;14:18–25.

18. Rigamonti D, Drayer BP, Johnson PC, et al. The MRI appearance of cavernous malformations (angiomas). *J Neurosurg.* 1987;67:518–524.

19. Rigamonti D, Hadley MN, Drayer BP, et al. Cerebral cavernous malformations: incidence and familial occurrence. *N Engl J Med.* 1988;319:343–347.

20. Rigamonti D, Johnson PC, Spetzler RF, et al. Cavernous malformations and capillary telangiectasia: a spectrum within a single pathological entity. *Neurosurgery.* 1991;28:60–64.

21. Rigamonti D, Spetzler RF. The association of venous and cavernous malformations: report of four cases and discussion of the pathophysiological diagnostic, and therapeutic implications. *Acta Neurochir (Wien).* 1988;92:100–105.

22. Robinson JR, Awad IA, Little JR. Natural history of the cavernous angioma. *J Neurosurg.* 1991;75:709–714.

23. Russell DS, Rubinstein LJ. *Pathology of Tumours of the Nervous System.* 4th ed. London: E Arnold; 1977:127–145.

24. Sasaki O, Tanaka R, Koike T, et al. Excision of cavernous angioma with preservation of coexisting venous angioma: case report. *J Neurosurg.* 1991;75:461–464.

25. Scott, RM, Barnes P, Kupsky W, et al. Cavernous angiomas of the central nervous system in children. *J Neurosurg.* 1992;76:38–46.

26. Simard JM, Garcia-Bengochea F, Ballinger WE Jr, et al. Cavernous angioma: a review of 126 collected and 12 new clinical cases. *Neurosurgery.* 1986;18:162–172.

27. Stehbens WE. *Pathology of the Cerebral Blood Vessels.* St Louis, Mo: CV Mosby; 1972:471–558.

28. Steinberg GK, Marks MP, Shuer LM, et al. Occult vascular malformations of the optic chiasm: magnetic resonance imaging diagnosis and surgical laser resection. *Neurosurgery.* 1990;27:466–470.

29. Sze G, Krol G, Olsen WL, et al. Hemorrhagic neoplasms: MR mimics of occult vascular malformations. *AJR.* 1987;149:1223–1230.

30. Tatagiba M, Schonmayr R, Samii M. Intra-ventricular cavernous angioma: a survey. *Acta Neurochir (Wien).* 1991;110:140–145.

31. Tung H, Giannotta SL, Chandrasoma PT, et al. Recurrent intraparenchymal hemorrhages from angiographically occult vascular malformations. *J Neurosurg.* 1990;73:174–180.

32. Villani RM, Arienta C, Caroli M. Cavernous angiomas of the central nervous system. *J Neurosurg Sci.* 1989;33:229–252.

33. Wakai S, Kumakura N, Nagai M. Lobar intracerebral hemorrhage: a clinical, radiographic, and pathological study of 29 consecutive operated cases with negative angiography. *J Neurosurg.* 1992;76:231–238.

34. Wakai S, Ueda Y, lnoh S, et al. Angiographically occult angiomas: a report of thirteen cases with an analysis of the cases documented in the literature. *Neurosurgery.* 1985;17:549–556.

35. Zimmerman RS, Spetzler RF, Lee KS, et al. Cavernous malformations of the brain stem. *J Neurosurg.* 1991;75:32–39.

Cavernous and Other Cryptic Vascular Malformations in the Pediatric Age Group

Michael S. B. Edwards, MD, James E. Baumgartner, MD, and Charles B. Wilson, MD

The term "cryptic vascular malformation" was popularized nearly 40 years ago by Crawford and Russell.[2,9] They used the term to describe small (less than 2 cm) cerebrovascular malformations which, due to hemodynamic or pathologic factors, were not opacified on cerebral angiography, nor clinically significant until they presented with hemorrhage. These lesions share several characteristics in common, including angiographic invisibility, a tendency to bleed, an ability to provoke seizures, and an ability to expand. The pathology of cryptic vascular malformations includes cavernous malformations (CMs), occult arteriovenous malformations (AVMs), venous malformations, and capillary malformations (telangiectases).[47] Before magnetic resonance imaging (MRI) became available, such lesions were considered rare, but with more widespread use of high-field strength MRI, clinical reports of angiographically occult vascular malformations have increased dramatically. The exact pathologic relationship between lesions found via MRI with characteristic findings of cryptic vascular malformation and those reported prior to the use of MRI is uncertain.

The majority of patients with CMs and other cryptic vascular malformations present in the third or fourth decade of life and their presentation in childhood is infrequent. Fortuna et al found only 50 cases of pathologically proven cryptic vascular malformations reported in patients 16 years or younger in the world's literature prior to 1988.[17]

The natural history of these lesions in the adult and pediatric populations is poorly characterized and the treatment is controversial. In this chapter we will review the history, presentation, pathophysiology, radiology, and treatment of CMs and other cryptic vascular malformations in the pediatric population. Whenever possible, we analyze separately cases of proven CMs, while in other instances there is not sufficient pathologic information to distinguish CMs from other cryptic vascular malformations.

Current Controversies

Cryptic vascular malformations in children are controversial in regard to their incidence, pathology, prognosis, and treatment. Although there is no definite proof, the experience at the University of California at San Francisco (UCSF) suggests they are more common than previously reported in the literature. This does not appear to be solely the result of better diagnostic capabilities. Although our increased experience with such lesions may be due to referral patterns, it is just as likely that the incidence is increased and that some of this increase may be due to an acquired rather than congenital etiology.

What is the incidence of cryptic vascular malformations in children? The occurrence of a nontraumatic intracranial hemorrhage in children is most often due to a vascular malformation; and cerebral angiography is usually performed to evaluate such occurrences. One might assume that prior to the advent of computed tomography (CT) or MRI many lesions would be missed because angiography would not visualize them. However, cerebral angiography most often would demonstrate an "avascular" mass lesion, leading to surgical intervention at which time a hematoma would be found and in many instances a vascular malformation identified on pathologic examination. It is also likely that most of these children underwent surgical exploration since hypertension, metastatic melanoma, and cerebral amyloid angiopathy as causes of intracranial hemorrhage were not a consideration. Therefore, it is surprising that cryptic vascular malformations were not reported, nor recognized to be so frequent as they are today. Clearly, lesions within the brain stem and spinal cord were the ones most likely to be missed prior to the era of CT and MRI. It is only since the advent of MRI that these small vascular malformations have been diagnosed prior to surgery.

History

Traditionally, cryptic vascular malformations have been divided into angiographically occult AVMs, CMs, venous malformations, and capillary malformations.[32,42] Venous and capillary malformations are rarely clinically significant per se, but can be found in association with the more clinically significant CM and AVM.[12,32,42,58,59] Although these pathologic entities have been described as discrete forms, they have frequently been reported together in single lesions[32,42,54,59] and may represent a more-or-less continuous spectrum of disease. The classification system recently proposed by Wilson incorporates this concept.[59] In other instances, pathologic information is not complete or precise enough to distinguish lesion types.

Cavernous Malformations

CM is the best characterized of the cryptic vascular malformations. Luschka is credited with the first pathologic description of a CM in 1853,[27] but Virchow gave a more definitive description in 1863.[57] The earliest reported successful operation on a CM was that of Bremer and Carson in 1890.[2] The first attempt at surgical removal of a CM in a child was reported by Finkelnburg in 1905. The patient was 2.5 years old and expired after a partial removal of a fourth ventricular lesion.[16] In 1940, a left lateral ventricular CM was successfully removed in a 16-year-old, but the patient was significantly worse postoperatively.[28] In 1958, Schneider and Liss reported the total removal of a right temporal CM in a 2-year-old, with subsequent neurologic improvement.[50] Up to the era of CT, the literature consists of case reports. Pozatti et al reported the first pediatric series of five supratentorial CMs in 1980.[38] Since MRI has become widely available, the number of pediatric series reported has increased dramatically.[3,17,18,21,30,48,63,64]

Other Cryptic Vascular Malformations

Large series suggest that a significant proportion of cryptic vascular malformations may be AVMs.[7,12,26,35,58] Of the pediatric cases reported in these series, 9 of 14 were described as AVMs. In Lobato and colleagues' review of the literature prior to 1987, 35 of

67 cryptic vascular malformations, which presented before the age of 20, were classified as AVMs. Historic accounts of the resection of "cryptic" AVMs begin with Russell and Crawford's definition in 1954,[9,46] but descriptions of these lesions in the pediatric population are curiously infrequent. Pathologic criteria for a lesion defined as an "AVM" are frequently vague in such series, and it is possible that many angiographically occult "AVMs" are actually CMs or other pathologic types of cryptic vascular malformations.

Venous malformations of the brain are usually considered benign incidental findings.[42,54] Prior to the development of modern imaging techniques, they were only described in autopsy and surgical pathology reports and were not diagnosed clinically.[22,32] More recent reports have implicated venous malformations as a source of intracranial hemorrhage and a variety of neurologic conditions.[15,36,53] Venous malformations have a characteristic appearance on angiography, described as "caput medusa" and are rarely cryptic on angiography.[4] In the Lobato et al literature review, 7 of 67 cryptic vascular malformations that presented before the age of 20 were said to be venous.[26] One of 14 pediatric lesions reported in recent large series was a venous malformation.[7,12,26,35,58] Surgical removal of posterior fossa venous malformations has been associated with significant morbidity and mortality. These lesions are thought to be anomalies of venous drainage that may serve vital hemodynamic functions.[54] In addition, venous malformations are frequently associated with CMs, which are much more likely to be symptomatic.[43,49,59] The recent report of Sasake et al describes removal of a CM with preservation of the associated venous malformation.[49] Some supratentorial venous malformations can be resected without significant morbidity as long as associated brain tissue which they drain is also resected; however, the indications and benefits of surgery for these lesions are questionable.[46]

Capillary malformations are described as small, solitary lesions that occur commonly, usually as autopsy findings.[31] In the Lobato et al literature review, 2 of 67 cases presenting before the age of 20 were capillary malformations, while 1 of the 14 more recently reported pediatric cases of cryptic vascular malformation was a capillary malformation.[7,12,26,35,58] Russell, in 1931, suggested that capillary malformations might be precursors of CMs,[45] although this was not generally accepted. Transitional forms have since been reported and may explain the rare clinically significant form of this lesion.[42]

Epidemiology

Cavernous Malformations

Fortuna et al have reviewed the 50 pediatric cases in the literature prior to 1988 and added six of their own.[17] Subsequent reports have added an additional 57 pathologically proven lesions in 56 children, which are summarized in Table 1.[3,13,14,17,18,21,30,48,52,66] Seven of the 56 children were reported to have multifocal lesions, but the location of the second lesion was reported in only one case. No radiation induced CMs were reported in the children described in the literature since 1988. A family history of CM was reported in 6 patients, three of whom had multiple lesions.[52] Unlike previous descriptions, the families were not Mexican-American.[20,29,41] Although the average age at presentation was 7.7 years, there is a bimodal distribution in the ages at presentation, with peaks below 3 years of age and at 11 years of age. Supratentorial lesions were more likely to present with seizures and were more frequent in the younger children, while focal neurologic deficits were most commonly associated with brain stem lesions and were found most often in older children.

The average duration of symptoms was 20.5 months, but patients could be divided into those with very long and very short clinical histories. Twenty of 56 children presented with chronic histories including

Table 1. **Clinical Features of 56 Pediatric Cases of Cavernous Malformation**

Mean Age at Presentation	7.7 years
Mean Duration of Symptoms	20.5 months

Presenting Symptoms	
Seizures	39.2%
Focal Deficit	39.2%
Headache	14.3%
Hemorrhagic Syndrome	3.7%
Increasing Head Size	1.8%
Incidental	1.8%

Location	
Frontal	29.5%
Parietal	24.7%
Temporal	14.9%
Occipital	3.4%
Ventricular	1.7%
Pineal	1.7%
Cerebellar	3.4%
Pontine	14.9%
Medulla	1.7%
Midbrain	1.7%

Table 2. **Clinical Features of 9 Pediatric Cases of Angiographically Occult AVM**

Mean Age at Presentation	12.4 years
Mean Duration of Symptoms	21 months

Presenting Symptoms	
Seizure, new onset	22.2%
Seizure, chronic	22.2%
Hemorrhagic Syndrome	22.2%
Focal Deficit	33.4%

Location	
Frontal	22.2%
Parietal	22.2%
Temporal	33.3%
Intraventricular	11.1%
Medulla	11.1%

chronic seizures (12 cases), episodic brain stem insults which gradually resolved (5 cases), or as incidental findings with a history of chronic headache or irritability (3 cases). Clinical evidence of prior hemorrhage was found in 7 of the 20 children with a chronic clinical history. Thirty-seven children presented with short clinical histories including a hemorrhagic syndrome (23 cases), or new onset seizure (14 cases).[3,13,14,17,18,21,30,48,52,66]

Four cases of CMs had clinical evidence of lesion enlargement and were usually found in young children. The histories included rapid head enlargement without hydrocephalus (1 case),[18] a progressively worsening seizure disorder (1 case),[4] a seizure disorder with a secondary and progressive focal deficit (1 case)[4] and a progressive focal deficit (1 case).[30]

Other Cryptic Vascular Malformations

Nine cases of histopathologically proven angiographically occult AVMs have been reported in series of cryptic vascular mal-

formations in children. Clinical data are summarized in Table 2.[7,12,26,58] The average age at presentation is considerably older than that for CM, and no cases were reported below the age of 8 years. Clinical histories could be divided into acute (4 cases) and chronic onset (5 cases). While 24% of pediatric CMs are infratentorial, only 1 of 9 occult AVMs occurred in the posterior fossa in children. No positive family histories for vascular malformations were reported. Three of 9 patients had clinical histories consistent with prior hemorrhage, 2 with episodic focal deficits, and a third with 2 episodes of sudden onset of stupor over 2 years.[12,26,58] The hemorrhages associated with occult AVMs tended to be more devastating clinically than those associated with CMs.

A single case of pediatric venous malformation was reported in the series of Lobato et al. The patient was a 16-year-old female who presented with a 1-year history of headaches. Her lesion was located along the third ventricle.[26]

Lobato et al also reported a single case of a symptomatic capillary malformation in a child. The patient presented with a 6-month history of grand mal seizures and was found to have a lesion in the left caudate.[26]

No glial tumors were found in association with any of the cryptic vascular malformations reported in children.* An association between CMs and other vascular malformations with glial tumors (particularly oligodendrogliomas) has been noted previously.[4,27,52]

Radiation Therapy

No prior history of brain irradiation was found in children with vascular malformations reviewed in this chapter.** Wilson reported the appearance of cryptic vascular malformations in irradiated brains after a delay of a few to many years.[59] These have been implicated in an apoplectic intracerebral hemorrhage that occurred 7.5 years following irradiation for a nasopharyngeal tumor.[61] We have seen MRI changes consistent with such lesions in 5 children who received radiation therapy for medulloblastoma or brain stem tumors (see Figures 6 and 7). Two children suffered hemorrhage in the region of these lesions, but the pathology was only of clot (see Figure 7). It is therefore not clear if angiographically occult vascular lesions which are induced by radiation and which are predisposed to hemorrhage are CMs, another type of cryptic vascular malformation, or a different lesion unique to such a scenario. Further pathologic studies are clearly needed.

Diagnostic Imaging

Angiography

Angiography was performed in 22 of the 56 cases of CM reported in children since 1988. The studies were "normal" in 7 cases, demonstrated an avascular mass in 12 cases, and showed a delayed and weak venous blush in 2 cases.*** In the 9 reported occult AVMs, the single venous malformation and the capillary malformation, angiography was "normal".[7,12,26,58] A 15-month-old child who developed projectile

vomiting followed shortly by a generalized seizure and coma was found on CT to have a right frontal, high-density lesion with mass effect. Angiography was performed and revealed a venous malformation. The lesion was resected, and the pathology was typical for CM.[62]

Computed Tomography

CT findings have been summarized with pathologic correlation by Wakai et al and Lobato et al. In both series most lesions appeared hyperdense and were directly visualized without contrast (92% and 71%, respectively). The remaining cryptic vascular malformations were either isodense, hypodense, or of mixed density in roughly equal proportions. Contrast enhancement was variable, being diffuse and weak in 26% to 63% of cases, nodular in 26%, patchy in 18%, and absent in 28%. Surrounding edema was found only in association with associated hematoma.[26,58] CT appearance was not specific for pathologic subtype (Figure 1A).

Magnetic Resonance Imaging

The characteristic MRI findings of cryptic vascular malformations have been extensively described.[1,13,40,58,59] The typical findings include a complete or partial rim of low-to-absent–signal surrounding an isointense-to-high–signal nidus on T1- and T2-weighted images as illustrated in this chapter's figures. The hemosiderin rim becomes thicker and less intense on T2-weighted images. The nidus can have a complex appearance with intermingled areas of high- and low-signal intensity (Figure 1B, C, & D). Hemorrhages of various sizes and intensities (and presumably various ages) can be seen within and adjacent to the nidus capsule (Figure 2). With gadolinium enhancement, associated venous malformations can be visualized. MRI findings do not reliably distinguish between the pathologic subtypes of cryptic vascular

---

*References 3,7,12–14,17,18,21,26,30,48,52,58,66
**References 3,7,12–14,17,18,21,26,30,48,52,58,66
***References 3,7,13,14,18,21,30,48,52,66

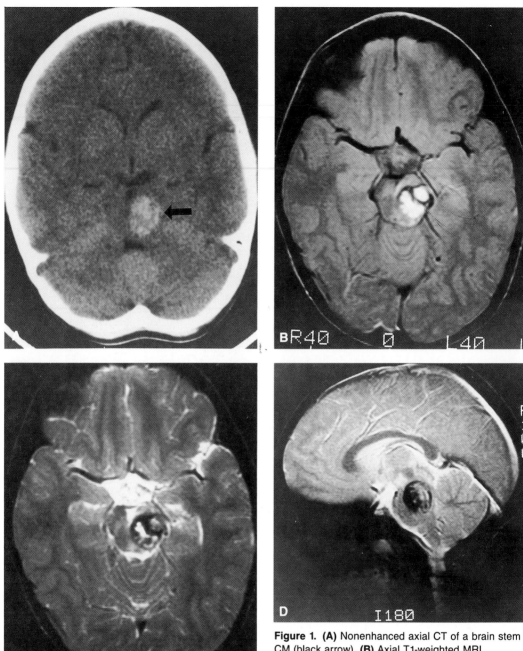

Figure 1. (A) Nonenhanced axial CT of a brain stem CM (black arrow). **(B)** Axial T1-weighted MRI demonstrates encysted areas of blood and mass effect in the left cerebral peduncle. **(C)** Axial T2-weighted MRI demonstrates hemosiderin staining of the brain stem (black areas within the malformation). **(D)** Sagittal T2-weighted MRI of the same lesion also demonstrates hemosiderin deposition within the malformation and surrounding brain stem. MRI gives superior definition and anatomy compared to CT scanning.

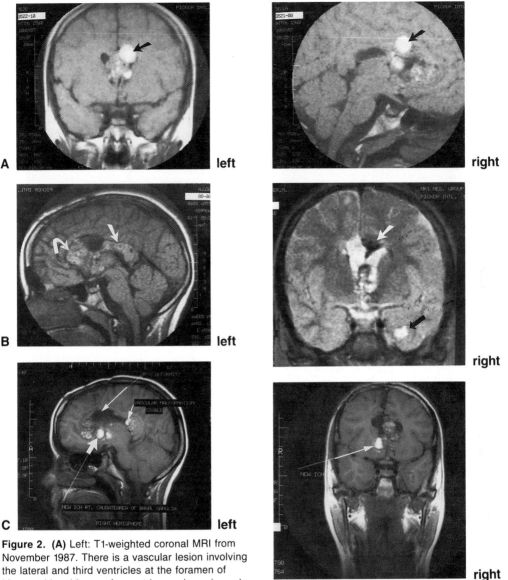

Figure 2. **(A)** Left: T1-weighted coronal MRI from November 1987. There is a vascular lesion involving the lateral and third ventricles at the foramen of Monro, with evidence of recent hemorrhage (arrow). Right: Sagittal MRI on the same date. Arrow points to the recent hemorrhage in the superior portion of the malformation. **(B)** Right: T2-weighted MRI from April 1989, 17 months following subtotal resection of the area of hemorrhage and vascular malformation. The prior area of hemorrhage appears as only a region of hemosiderin-stained brain (white arrow). However, there has been the interval development of a new area of hemorrhage in the temporal lobe (black arrow), presumably from a second hemorrhage. Left: Sagittal T1-weighted MRI from April 1989. There has been interval growth of the lesion anteriorly into the hypothalamus (curved arrow) and posteriorly into the splenium of the corpus callosum (straight arrow). **(C)** Right: T1-weighted coronal MRI from October 1991

demonstrates new hemorrhage into the hypothalamus (white arrow). Left: T1 sagittal MRI on same date demonstrates multiple new hemorrhages (short arrows). However the region of the lesion previously resected in November 1987 remains free of recurrent hemorrhage or regrowth (long arrow). The patient's symptoms consisted of serial hemorrhages beginning at 8 years old. Each hemorrhage was associated with the sudden onset of severe headache. The subtotal resection of her vascular malformation in 1987 reduced the severity and frequency of her hemorrhages. However, as the lesion grew posteriorly, she developed a progressive memory deficit.

Table 3. **Surgical and Clinical Results for 67 Children with Cryptic Vascular Malformations**

Lesion Type	Surgical Results	
	Total Resection	Subtotal Resection
Cavernous Malformation	52/57 (91%)	5/57 (9%)
Occult AVM	9/9 (100%)	
Venous Malformation	1/1 (100%)	
Capillary Malformation	1/1 (100%)	

Lesion Type	Clinical Outcome				
	Symptom Free	Better	Stable	Worse	Dead
Cavernous Malformation	28.7%	55.4%	8.9%	7.2%	1.8%
Occult AVM		88.8%		11.2%	
Venous Malformation				100.0%	
Capillary Malformation		100.0%			

malformations. In addition, lesions other than vascular malformations can have similar characteristics on MRI.[6] Series that are based heavily on MRI findings without pathologic confirmation should be considered with some suspicion with regard to specific pathology of lesions studied.[10,44] Yet, in these series, every lesion considered on MRI to be suspicious for CM that was subsequently resected proved to be a CM.[10,44]

Treatment

The surgical results and clinical outcomes of the children reviewed for this series are summarized in Table 3. The single death occurred in an 8-month-old boy with multiple, giant cystic CMs and an associated hemorrhage. The patient developed signs of uncal herniation, underwent emergent and total resection of both lesions, but never recovered.[48] The patients who were neurologically worse postoperatively presented with a significant focal deficit preoperatively and had lesions which were either deep-seated or located in eloquent cortex.[30,52] The only poor outcome in the occult AVM experience followed the total resection of a medullary lesion. The patient developed severe lower cranial nerve deficits and required a tracheostomy.[7] The single venous malformation patient had a third ventricular lesion that was approached transcallosally. Postoperatively, she was found to have "short term memory deficit and slowed mental processes."[26]

Surgical Indications

Total obliteration or excision is the goal of treatment for all vascular malformations. However, what are the indications to proceed with surgical intervention? The most obvious is when a lesion has produced an intracerebral hemorrhage. The vast majority of vascular malformations that have bled can be removed surgically, even those in eloquent brain. MRI in multiple planes, in conjunction with T2-weighted images, helps define the lesion versus the surrounding hemosiderin-stained brain and allows one to plan the safest surgical approach. The use of brain mapping, intraoperative electrophysiologic monitoring (evoked potentials, electrocorticography, and electroencephalography [EEG]), or awake surgery under local anesthesia has allowed us to remove vascular malformations from eloquent cortex, deep-brain structures, including brain stem and spinal cord, with minimal morbidity and no mortality. In our experience, only extensive size or multiplicity of lesions has prevented total removal.

Second, symptomatic lesions in noncritical, accessible areas of the brain (e.g. anterior frontal and temporal cortex) should be removed even without evidence of recent or prior hemorrhage. Those lesions producing mass effect and neurologic dysfunction or obstructing CSF pathways, such as the foramen of Monro, should be removed irrespective of evidence of hemorrhage. With the advent of MRI, it is unlikely that a CM or other vascular malformation would be mistaken for a tumor, but if the diagnosis is uncertain and there is neurologic dysfunction,[55] an exploration is probably the most reasonable course of action. All patients should have MRIs performed with and without contrast enhancement to detect venous malformations in association with CMs. The long-term outcome for those CMs in association with venous anomalies is very uncertain. If venous outflow restriction plays a role in the pathogenesis of the CM, then resection of the CM alone would not treat the primary pathology, and the lesion would likely recur despite an initial total resection. Lesions diagnosed incidentally, particularly those without evidence of prior hemorrhage (excluding accessible lesions in nondominant brain) probably can be followed with sequential MRI and intervention considered at a later date if hemorrhage or growth occurs.

Seizures

Patients presenting with seizures as the major manifestation of their lesion (Figure 3) should be evaluated using the same techniques used in patients having seizures of other etiologies. The cause of seizures in children with CMs is unknown but may relate to the epileptogenic effect of iron pigments deposited in the cortex surrounding these lesions following hemorrhage.[6,14] If the seizure disorder is refractory to medical management, the need for surgical intervention is even more imperative. We perform a preoperative electroencephalogram and/or videotape/EEG analysis in conjunction with neuropsychologic testing to determine if the seizures are localized to the site of the lesion. If the seizures suggest that language cortex may be involved, or the vascular malformation is in the dom-

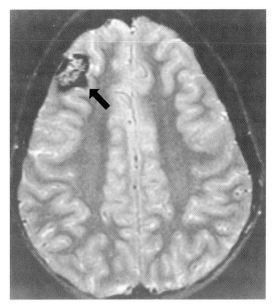

Figure 3. T2-weighted axial MRI of a 14-year-old male presenting with generalized seizure activity secondary to a CM in the right frontal cortex (black arrow).

inant cortex, a Wada test is also performed. In some instances a superselective Wada test is utilized to better define the function of the brain surrounding the lesion. Surgery is carried out using intraoperative electrocorticography and brain mapping. If the child is mature enough and the lesion is in eloquent or language cortex, surgery is performed under local anesthesia. In our experience this is feasible after age 16, and can sometimes be performed in patients as young as age 12, if the child is determined to be mature during the preoperative neuropsychologic evaluation. Although not yet required in the authors' experiences, the use of a subdural or epidural grid should be considered in the young child who would not tolerate local anesthesia and has a vascular malformation involving language cortex.

Multiple and Familial Lesions

Children with familial CMs usually have multiple lesions.[52] In our experience, sporadic multiple CMs are identified more frequently in children than in adults.[59] Scott found multiple lesions in 2 of 19 children without a family history of vascular malformation, while Wilson reported 2 cases of sporadic multiple lesions in a series of 89 adults.[52,59] We have identified multiple lesions in 6 of our 26 cases of pediatric cryptic vascular malformations, and Scott reports multiple lesions in 5 of 19 children.[52] Prolonged T2- or gradient-spin-echo sequences from a high-field strength MRI are best for identifying multiple lesions. When multiple lesions are found, the dilemma is which one(s) to treat. As a general rule, we only treat the symptomatic lesions. If only one has hemorrhaged, the decision is often simple. However, in one of our patients, 2 separate CMs bled at the same time, necessitating multiple surgeries. If one is the source of the child's seizure disorder, the decision is also straightforward. However, what if one is symptomatic, but the others are accessible in silent areas of the brain? Careful observation with sequential MRIs should be considered, and the other lesions treated if they become symptomatic or if the follow-up study reveals evidence of silent hemorrhage or growth.

Giant Cavernous Malformations

Giant CMs require special mention. Some are so extensive that total excision is not possible without the risk of producing significant neurologic deficit. In addition, lesions may grow to giant proportions over a period of only a few years (Figures 2, 4, and 5). These malformations tend to lie along the lateral or third ventricles. While total resection is sometimes possible (Figure 5A-C), the size and complexity of the lesions may necessitate subtotal and staged resections. Usually, one area of the malformation has been the offender, producing recurrent hemorrhage, mass effect, or obstruction of the CSF pathways. This portion should be resected first. This approach has been anecdotally effective in reducing the

frequency and severity of hemorrhage (see Figure 2). The remainder of the lesion is observed and intervention undertaken if new hemorrhage or lesion enlargement is found on serial MRI (see Figures 2 and 4). The long-term prognosis for this group of patients is guarded unless the entire lesion can be resected.

Lesions mimicking CMs on MRI can be seen following radiation therapy to the brain (Figures 6 and 7).[59,61] Surgery is reserved for lesions with gross hemorrhage in our experience. We have not seen seizures as a symptom in this group of children.

Spinal Cord Cavernous Malformations

Spinal cord CMs have also been diagnosed on MRI, usually following the acute onset of spinal cord dysfunction secondary to hemorrhage.[1,8,36,39,52] CMs of the cauda equina have been found in association with hydrocephalus in adults, which resolves after resection of the lesion.[36,39] Lesions producing hemorrhage should be removed surgically (Figure 8). The natural history of spinal cord CMs without hemorrhage is unknown. For the present, a conservative approach using sequential MRIs is the recommended course of action, reserving surgical intervention for those lesions that progress on MRI or produce clinical symptoms.

Radiosurgery

Radiosurgery has been employed in the treatment of CMs and other cryptic vascular malformations in children and adolescents who sustained two or more hemorrhages and whose lesions were deemed to be unresectable with acceptable morbidity and mortality.[25] In general, these were lesions in the dominant hemisphere or in deep-brain structures such as the brain stem (Figure 9). Because the lesions are not visualized on angiography, the effectiveness of radiation therapy is difficult to eval-

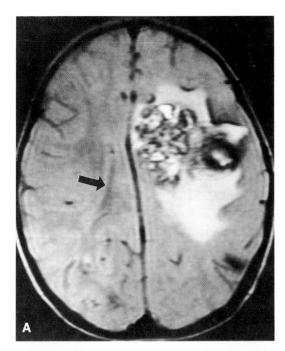

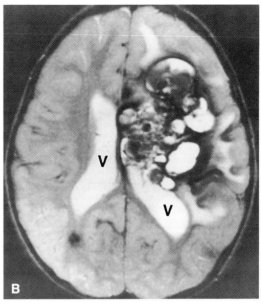

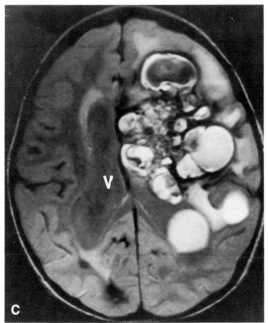

Figure 4. (A) Axial T2-weighted MRI from February 25, 1986, demonstrating a large CM in the left hemisphere with surrounding edema in a 12-year-old female. The ventricle is compressed with a left-to-right shift; the black arrow points to the contralateral ventricle. **(B)** Progressive enlargement of this lesion has occurred over 22 months (through December 1987) due to recurrent hemorrhages. There is evidence of hydrocephalus (V = ventricle) as compared to 1986, due to increased mass effect on the third ventricle. **(C)** Over the next 2 months (through January 28, 1988) the lesion continued to enlarge with recurrent hemorrhage and progressive hydrocephalus (V = ventricle). The malformation has actually enlarged within the ventricular system as well as within the hemisphere. A near gross total excision of the lesion was carried out.

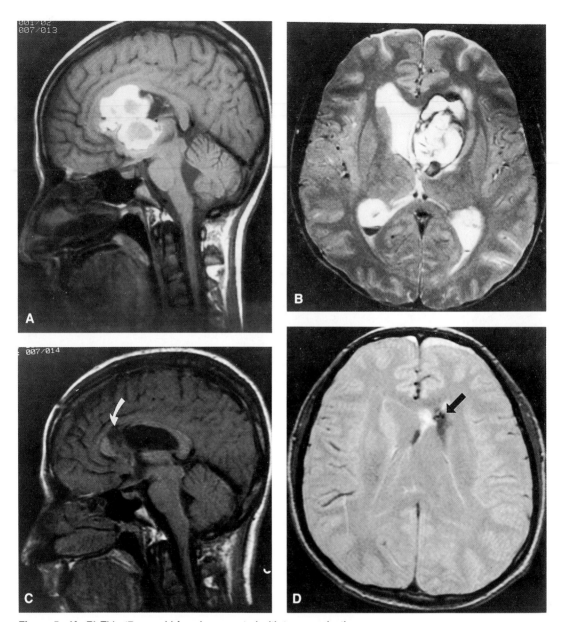

Figure 5. (A, B) This 17-year-old female presented with two apoplectic events, most likely due to hemorrhage. T1-weighted sagittal and T2-weighted axial MRIs performed prior to surgery demonstrates a giant CM with recent hemorrhage filling the lateral and third ventricles and compressing the hypothalamus. In addition, there is unilateral hydrocephalus due to blockage of cerebrospinal fluid flow at the foramen of Monro. **(C, D)** T1-weighted sagittal and T2-weighted axial MRIs following total resection of the lesion. The white arrow points to the defect in the corpus callosum through which the malformation was removed. The black arrow points to hemosiderin staining in the frontal white matter, a residual of previous hemorrhages.

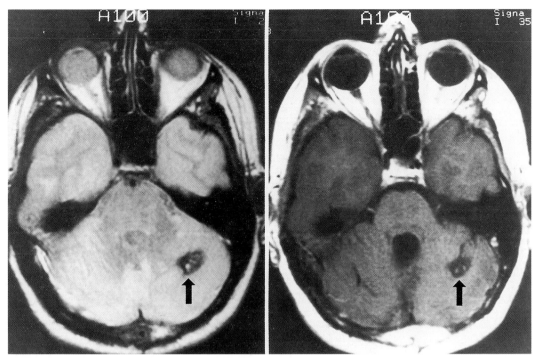

Figure 6. T2-weighted (left) and T1-weighted (right) axial MRIs demonstrating a "radiation induced" cryptic vascular malformation in the left cerebellar hemisphere (black arrows). The lesion was first noted 4 years following 5500 cGy external beam megavoltage radiation therapy for a cervicomedullary glioma.

uate. Only sequential MRI and long-term clinical follow-up studies will help answer this question. Using the incidence of re-bleeding to assess treatment is difficult, especially in light of how little we understand the natural history of this disorder.

We are reluctant to consider radiosurgery for three reasons. First, having seen lesions similar to CMs appear on MRI following radiation therapy (see Figures 6 and 7), and having seen these lesions produce significant intracranial hemorrhage in two children, we are concerned about the long-term effects of radiation. Second, we have seen three children treated with radiosurgery, two of whom continued to have multiple hemorrhages into their brain stem lesions and have required surgical resection at 2 and 3 years postradiosurgery (see Figure 9). Both children were significantly worse neurologically by the time surgery was undertaken. In each child, we were able to completely resect the vascular mal-

formation from within the brain stem, but the lesions were unusually adherent to surrounding tissue and the brain stem tolerated surgical intervention less well than if radiation had not been administered. The third patient was seen in consultation two years following radiosurgery for a medullary lesion. Although there had been no further hemorrhage, radiation necrosis of the cervicomedullary junction had produced severe quadriparesis and the patient had become wheelchair bound. Finally, the surgical experience with deep-seated and brain stem lesions has been surprisingly encouraging in our experience and that of others (Figure 10).[13,23,29,51,59,63,65,66] However, removal of some vascular malformations in the medulla can be devastating.

In summary, for the present, the goal of treatment is gross total resection of symptomatic or accessible CMs. No other therapy has been effective in the prevention of

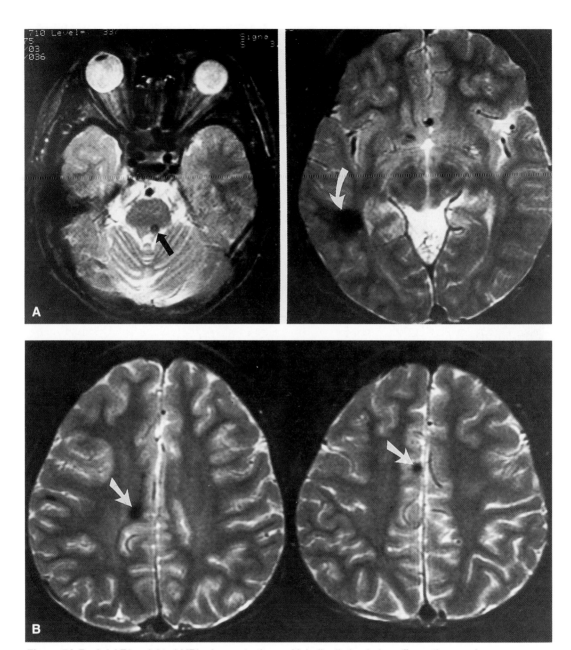

Figure 7A,B. Axial T2-weighted MRIs demonstrating multiple "radiation induced" cryptic vascular malformations (arrows) in a child successfully treated for medulloblastoma 9 years prior to this scan. The lesions were first noticed 5 years following craniospinal radiation therapy. His clinical course was uneventful for 8 years, at which time the brain stem lesion hemorrhaged (black arrow), after which he experienced a significant deterioration in IQ and social skills. The remaining lesions have appeared since the posterior fossa hemorrhage was evacuated.

rebleeding. Subtotal resection and/or staged resection has not prevented rebleeding or regrowth until the entire lesion has been removed. The postoperative MRI of a resected CM is difficult to interpret because T2-weighted images will reveal a hemosiderin ring staining the surrounding brain even after total resection of the lesion. Therefore, even in those lesions we believe

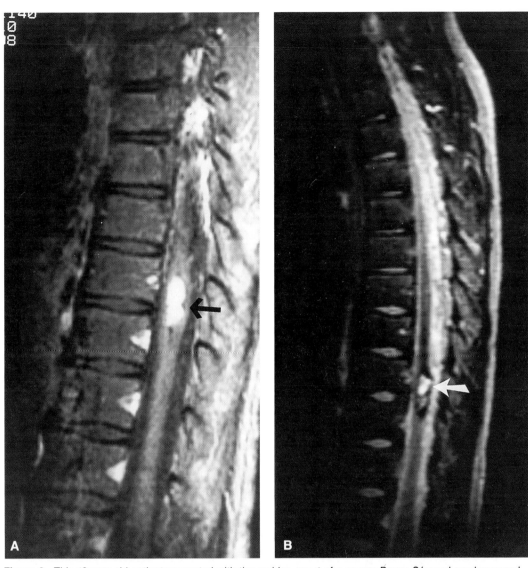

Figure 8. This 10-year-old patient presented with the sudden onset of a severe Brown-Séquard syndrome and neck pain, which resolved slowly. **(A)** T1-weighted and **(B)** T2-weighted sagittal MRIs of the spinal cord demonstrate a CM with recent hemorrhage. The lesion was totally removed. The only residual neurologic finding is a mild left lower extremity proprioceptive deficit.

we have totally removed at operation, we recommend sequential follow-up MRIs and would consider reoperation if there was evidence of repeat hemorrhage or regrowth.

Pathology

The current classification system of vascular malformations is that of McCormick[31] and Russell and Rubinstein.[47] Most authors

recognize giant cystic CMs of childhood[18,24,48] and familial CMs[20,28,41] as congenital lesions—the pathophysiology of CMs occurring later in life is controversial.[59] While each of the four subtypes (CM, occult AVM, capillary telangiectasia, and venous malformation) exist in a "pure" form, this is not always the case. The frequent occurrence of hybrid forms of cryptic vascular malformations[12,26,42,49,59,62] suggests that

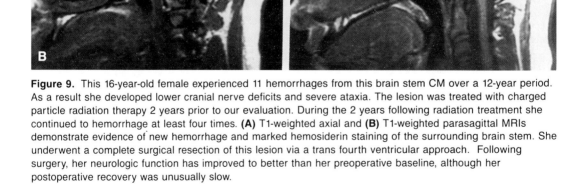

Figure 9. This 16-year-old female experienced 11 hemorrhages from this brain stem CM over a 12-year period. As a result she developed lower cranial nerve deficits and severe ataxia. The lesion was treated with charged particle radiation therapy 2 years prior to our evaluation. During the 2 years following radiation treatment she continued to hemorrhage at least four times. **(A)** T1-weighted axial and **(B)** T1-weighted parasagittal MRIs demonstrate evidence of new hemorrhage and marked hemosiderin staining of the surrounding brain stem. She underwent a complete surgical resection of this lesion via a trans fourth ventricular approach. Following surgery, her neurologic function has improved to better than her preoperative baseline, although her postoperative recovery was unusually slow.

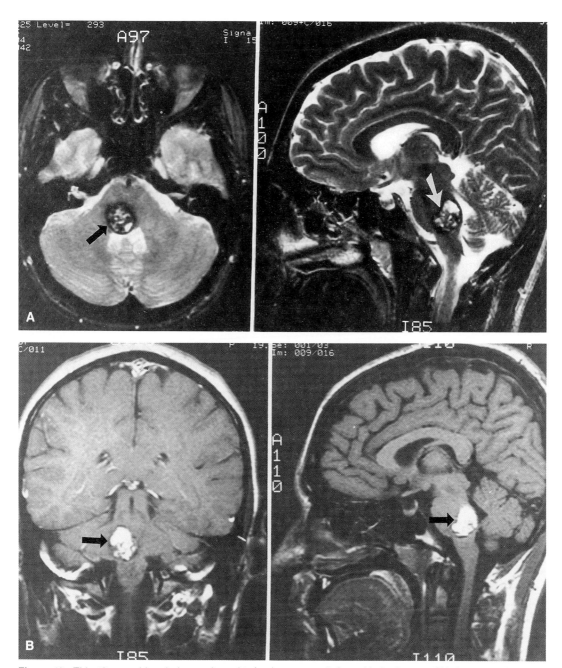

Figure 10. This 18-year-old male hemorrhaged twice in one month from this brain stem CM. It resulted in significant occular motility dysfunction and long tract sensory and motor findings. **(A)** T2-weighted axial (left) and sagittal (right); and **(B)** T1-weighted coronal (left) and sagittal (right) images of a brain stem CM that was totally resected with excellent recovery—to better than his preoperative status.

lesion subtypes may represent a pathologic continuum. The pathology literature cautions that distinguishing between the various cryptic vascular malformations may be difficult as they share many similarities.[12,42,54] In an interesting discussion, Ebeling et al present initial pathologic reports with blinded review reports that have been modified or completely changed in five out of five cases. This demonstrates the difficulty in classifying these lesions histopathologically.[12] We have recently begun a retrospective review of the pathology of our own series of pediatric cryptic vascular malformations. Although this study is still in progress, we have found it necessary to modify the original pathology reports in four of ten cases reviewed to date.

Equally troubling is the frequent assumption, in the neurosurgical and neuroradiologic literature, that MRI characteristics can accurately predict pathology. Several studies have extrapolated a limited amount of surgical pathology to a large number of MRI lesions and have drawn conclusions on the natural history of these lesions.[10,44] Great care must be taken in the classification of tissue specimens and the use of pathologic terms if the natural history of the cryptic vascular malformations is to be understood.

Outcome

If total resection of clinically significant lesions can be achieved, the outcome is good. In our experience and that of others,[52,56] subtotal resection leaves the patient with a significant risk of further neurologic insult. It is apparent that hereditary CMs may be more prone to hemorrhage than the sporadically occurring cryptic vascular malformations.[41,52] The exact incidence of hemorrhage is not yet certain, but Tung et al[56] and recent reports at the 1992 American Association of Neurological Surgeons Annual Meeting suggest an annual rate of hemorrhage of 6.5% for patients with hereditary CMs[60] and an annual rate of hemorrhage of 1% for sporadic lesions.[44] With an improved understanding of the natural history of CMs will come a better idea of their long-term prognosis.

Pathophysiology

The pathophysiology of CMs and other cryptic vascular malformations remains an enigma. Although a number of possibilities have been suggested, no one universal theory explains all the manifestations seen in association with these lesions.

In children, CMs have been diagnosed during the first year of life, confirming a congenital etiology for a proportion of these lesions.[18,24,48] In general, the symptoms of an enlarging head and ventricular obstruction seen during the first year of life are different than the symptoms seen in other age groups. In addition, a significant proportion are accompanied by a very large, hyperdense, inhomogeneous cyst, a rare occurrence in older children.

The hereditary form of this disorder has a preference for the Hispanic population, and the CMs are most frequently multiple.[20] The inheritance may be autosomal dominant.[29,41] In addition, a kindred of Jewish descent has been described as having CM of the brain in association with retinal vascular lesions and as a feature of a dysgenetic syndrome of multiple hemangiomatosis, in which hamartomas of a similar nature exist in other extracentral nervous system regions of the body.[11]

It seems apparent that many CMs are acquired. The unquestionable development of a lesion mimicking CM in the irradiated field of brain after a delay of months to years is just now becoming recognized. Their origin may be related to the delayed effects of radiation on the vascular system. Local vascular necrosis may result in pinpoint hemorrhages and/or small vessel thrombosis. These events may lead to increased capillary permeability, especially involving the small vessels within the white matter. In addition, local ischemia secondary to these events may result in the production of angiogenic factors, resulting in the development of local vascular shunts. We believe the initiating factor is the extravasation of blood—whether this occurs by diapedesis or small vessel necrosis—and that disruption of the vessel wall is open to speculation. This would explain the local accumulation of hemosiderin, which is usually the earliest manifestation seen on MRI. It is more plausible to believe that intermittent oozing of red blood cells through defective capillaries produces the deposition of hemosiderin rather than multiple episodes of frank disruption of capillaries from vessel necrosis. An ongoing process of ischemia, leakage of red blood cells, production of angiogenic factors secondary to local ischemia, ingrowth of fragile, thin-walled new vessels, recurrent bleeding, and ongoing thrombosis could account for the MRI and clinical manifestations of this disorder. It is based on this group of lesions that we feel strongly that radiosurgery not be used as a treatment option.

A relationship between venous malformations and CMs is a relatively common finding in adult patients but has been seen in our childhood patients only infrequently. It is critical to perform the MRI with and without contrast to identify these venous lesions; the association between these two entities may therefore be more common than we believed initially. This association seems to be less common in children; nevertheless it does occur and also speaks to another potential acquired mechanism. Venous malformations could contribute to the development of CMs by producing a local elevation of venous pressure. This in turn could be transmitted to the capillary bed it drains resulting in diapedetic hemorrhage and leading to similar events that occur in postradiation therapy-induced lesions. Outflow restriction of a venous malformation where it enters a central vein or venous sinus, acute rises in intracranial venous pressure that are transmitted without being clamped to the large distal radicals, or less likely, the silent thrombosis

within the axis of a venous malformation could all be considered as potential inciting causes.

If venous hypertension in venous malformations plays a role in the pathogenesis of associated CMs, the surgical removal of the associated CMs would not permanently resolve the underlying pathology. This group of patients would still be subject to the repeat development of similar lesions some time in the future. Only long-term followup of this group of children will help answer this important question.

It appears that, for the present time, there is no one uniform theory to explain the development of cavernous and other cryptic vascular malformations. It is highly likely that the etiology is multifactorial, some being hereditary, others congenital, and some acquired.

References

1. Barnwell SL, Dowd CF, Davis RL, et al. Cryptic vascular malformations of the spinal cord: diagnosis by magnetic resonance imaging and outcome of surgery. *J Neurosurg*. 1990;72:403–407.

2. Bremer L, Carson NB. A case of brain tumor (angioma cavernosum), causing spastic paralysis and attacks of tonic spasms: operation. *Am J Med Sci*. 1890;100:219–242.

3. Buckingham MJ, Crone K, Ball WS, et al. Management of cerebral cavernous angiomas in children presenting with seizures. *Child's Nerv Syst*. 1989;5:347–349.

4. Carter JE, Wymore J, Ansbacher L, et al. Sudden visual loss and a chiasmal syndrome due to an intrachiasmatic vascular malformation. *J Clin Neuro Ophthalmol*. 1982;2:163–167.

5. Chee CP, Johnston R, Doyle D, et al. Oligodendroglioma and cavernous angioma: case report. *J Neurosurg*. 1985;62:145–147.

6. Chusid JG, Kopeloff LM. Epileptogenic effects of pure metal implanted in motor cortex of monkeys. *J Appl Physiol*. 1962;17:679–700.

7. Cohen HCM, Tucker WS, Humphreys RP, et al. Angiographically cryptic histologically verified cerebrovascular malformations. *Neurosurgery*. 1982;10:704–714.

8. Cosgrove GR, Bertrand G, Fontaine S, et al. Cavernous angiomas of the spinal cord. *J Neurosurg*. 1988;68:31–36.

9. Crawford JV, Russell DS. Cryptic arteriovenous and venous hamartomas of the brain. *J Neurol Neurosurg Psychiatry*. 1956;19:1–11.

10. Curling OD Jr, Kelly DL, Elster AD, et al. An analysis of the natural history of cavernous angiomas. *J Neurosurg*. 1991;75:702–708.

11. Dobyns WB, Michels VV, Groover RV, et al. Familial cavernous malformations of the central nervous system and retina. *Ann Neurol.* 1987;21:578–583.

12. Ebeling JD, Tranmer BI, Davis KA, et al. Thrombosed arteriovenous malformations: a type of occult vascular malformation: magnetic resonance imaging and histopathological correlations. *Neurosurgery.* 1988;23:605–610.

13. Fahlbusch R, Strauss C, Huk W, et al. Surgical removal of pontomesencephalic cavernous hemangiomas. *Neurosurgery.* 1990;26:449–457.

14. Farmer J-P, Cosgrove GR, Villemure J-G, et al. Intracerebral cavernous angiomas. *Neurology.* 1988;38:1699–1704.

15. Fierstein SB, Pribram HW, Hieshima G. Angiography and computed tomography in the evaluation of cerebral venous malformations. *Neuroradiology.* 1979;17:137–148.

16. Finkelnburg R. Zue Differentialdiagnose zwischen Kleinhirntumoren und chronishen Hydrocephalus. (Zugleich ein Beitrag zur Kenntnis der Angiome des Zentralnervensystems.) *Dtsch Z Nervenheilkd.* 1905;29:135–151.

17. Fortuna A, Ferrante L, Mastronardi L, et al. Cerebral cavernous angiomas in children. *Child's Nerv Syst.* 1989;5:201–207.

18. Gangemi M, Longatti P, Maiure F, et al. Cerebral cavernous angiomas in the first year of life. *Neurosurgery.* 1989;25:465–469.

19. Goodkin R, Zaias B, Michelsen WJ. Arteriovenous malformations and glioma: coexistent or sequential? Case report. *J Neurosurg.* 1990;72:798–805.

20. Hayman LA, Evans RA, Ferrell RE, et al. Familial cavernous angiomas: natural history and genetic study over a 5-year period. *Am J Med Genet.* 1982;11:147–160.

21. Herter T, Brandt M, Szüwart U. Cavernous hemangiomas in children. *Child's Nerv Syst.* 1988;4:123–127.

22. Jellinger K. The morphology of centrally situated angiomas. In: Pia HW, Gleave JRW, Grote E, Zierski T, eds. *Cerebral Angiomas: Advances in Diagnosis and Therapy.* New York, NY: Springer-Verlag; 1975:9–20.

23. Kashiwagi S, van Loveren HR, Tew JM, et al. Diagnosis and treatment of vascular brain stem malformations. *J Neurosurg.* 1990;72:27–34.

24. Khosla VK, Banerjee AK, Mathuriya SN, et al. Giant cystic cavernoma in a child: case report. *J Neurosurg.* 1984;60:1297–1299.

25. Kondziolka D, Lunsford LD, Coffey RJ, et al. Stereotactic radiosurgery of angiographically occult vascular malformations: indications and preliminary experience. *Neurosurgery.* 1990;27:892–900.

26. Lobato RD, Perez C, Rivas JJ, et al. Clinical, radiological and pathological spectrum of angiographically occult intracranial vascular malformations: analysis of 21 cases and review of the literature. *J Neurosurg.* 1988;68:518–531.

27. Luschka H. Cavernose blutgeschwulste des gehirns. *Arch Pathol Anat.* 1853;6:458.

28. Mallory TB, ed. Case record of the Massachussetts General Hospital. Case 26051. *N Engl J Med.* 1940;222:191–195.

29. Mason I, Aase JM, Orrison WW, et al. Familial cavernous angiomas of the brain in an Hispanic family. *Neurology.* 1988;38:324–326.

30. Mazza C, Scienza R, Beltramello A, et al. Cerebral cavernous malformations (cavernomas) in the pediatric age-group. *Child's Nerv Syst.* 1991;7:139–146.

31. McCormick WF. The pathology of vascular ("arteriovenous") malformations. *J Neurosurg.* 1966;24:807–816.

32. McCormick WF, Hardman JM, Boulter TB. Vascular malformations ("angiomas") of the brain with specific reference to those occurring in the posterior fossa. *J Neurosurg.* 1968;28:241–251.

33. McCormick WF, Nofzinger JD. "Cryptic" vascular malformations of the central nervous system. *J Neurosurg.* 1966;24:865–875.

34. Nazek M, Mandybur TI, Kashiwagi S. Oligodendroglial proliferative abnormality associated with arteriovenous malformation: report of three cases with review of the literature. *Neurosurgery.* 1988;23:781–785.

35. Ogilvy CS, Heros RC, Ojemann RG, et al. Angiographically occult arteriovenous malformations. *J Neurosurg.* 1988;69:350–355.

36. Pagni C, Canavero S, Forni M. Report of a cavernous angioma of the cauda equina and review of the literature. *Surg Neurol.* 1990;3:124–131.

37. Pak H, Patel SC, Malik GM, et al. Successful evacuation of a pontine hematoma secondary to rupture of a venous angioma. *Surg Neurol.* 1980;15:164–167.

38. Pozatti E, Padovani R, Morrone B, et al. Cerebral cavernous angiomas in children. *J Neurosurg.* 1980;53:826–832.

39. Ramos F Jr, de Toffol B, Aesch B, et al. Hydrocephalus and cavernoma of the cauda equina. *Neurosurgery.* 1990;27:139–142.

40. Rigamonti D, Drayer BP, Honhson PC, et al. The MRI appearance of cavernous malformations (angiomas). *J Neurosurg.* 1987;67:518–524.

41. Rigamonti D, Hadley MN, Drayer BP, et al.: Cerebral cavernous malformations: incidence and familial occurrence. *N Engl J Med.* 1988;319:343–347.

42. Rigamonti D, Johnson PC, Spetzler RF, et al: Cavernous malformations and capillary telangietasia: a spectrum within a single pathological entity. *Neurosurgery.* 1991;28:60–64.

43. Rigamonti D, Spetzler RF, Medina M, et al. Cerebral venous malformations. *J Neurosurg.* 1990;73:560–564.

44. Robinson JR, Awad IA, Little JR. Natural history of the cavernous angioma. *J Neurosurg.* 1991;75:709–714.

45. Russell DS. Discussion on vascular tumors of the brain and spinal cord. *Proc R Soc Med.* 1931;24:383–385.

46. Russell, DS. The pathology of spontanious intracranial haemorrhage. *Proc R Soc Med.* 1954;47:689–693.

47. Russell DS, Rubinstein LJ. *Pathology of Tumours of the Central Nervous System.* 4th ed. Baltimore, Md. Williams & Wilkins. 1977: 116–145.

48. Sakai N, Yamada H, Nishimura Y, et al. Intracranial cavernous angioma in the first year of life and a review of the literature. *Child's Nerv Syst.* 1992;8:49–52.

49. Sasaki O, Tanaka R, Koike T, et al. Excision of cavernous angioma with preservation of coexisting venous angioma: case report. *J Neurosurg.* 1991;75:461–464.

50. Schneider RC, Liss L. Cavernous hemangiomas of the cerebral hemispheres. *J Neurosurg.* 1958;15:392–399.

51. Scott RM. Brain stem cavernous angiomas in children. *Pediatr Neurosurg.* 1990–91;16:281–286.

52. Scott RM, Barnes P, Kupsky W, et al. Cavernous angiomas of the central nervous system in children. *J Neurosurg.* 1992;76:38–46.

53. Scotti LN, Goldman RL, Rao GR, et al. Cerebral venous angiomas. *Neuroradiology.* 1975;9:125–128.

54. Senegor M, Dohrmann GJ, Wollmann RL. Venous angiomas of the posterior fossa should be considered anomalous venous drainage. *Surg Neurol.* 1983;19:26–32.

55. Sze G, Krol G, Olsen WL, et al. Hemorrhagic neoplasms: MR mimics of occult vascular malformations. *AJR.* 1987;149:1223–1230.

56. Tung H, Gianotta SL, Chandrasoma PT, et al. Recurrent intraparenchymal hemorrhages from angiographically occult vascular malformations. *J Neurosurg.* 1990;73:174–180.

57. Virchow R, ed. *Die krankhaften geschwülste; Dreissig vorlesungen.* Berlin, Germany: Hirschwald. 1863; 456–463.

58. Wakai S, Ueda Y, Inoh S, et al. Angiographically occult angiomas: a report of thirteen cases with analysis of the cases documented in the literature. *Neurosurgery.* 1985;17:549–556.

59. Wilson CB. Cryptic vascular malformations. *Clin Neurosurg.* 1990;38:49–84.

60. Wascher TM, Zabramski, Johnson B, et al. Natural history of familial cavernous malformations. *J Neurosurg.* 1992;76:376A.

61. Woo E, Chan Y-F, Lame K. Apoplectic intracerebral hemorrhage: an unusual complication of cerebral radiation necrosis. *Pathology.* 1987;19:95–98.

62. Yamasaki T, Handa H, Yamashita J, et al. Intractranial cavernous angioma angiographically mimicking venous angioma in an infant. *Surg Neurol.* 1984;22:461–466.

63. Yamasaki T, Handa H, Yamashita J, et al. Intracranial and orbital camernous angiomas: a review of 30 cases. *J Neurosurg.* 1986;64:197–208.

64. Yasargil MG. *Microneurosurgery IIIB.* Stuttgart, Germany: Georg Thieme; 1988:415–472.

65. Yoshimoto T, Suzuki J. Radical surgery on cavernous angioma of the brainstem. *Surg Neurol.* 1986;26:72–78.

66. Zimmerman RS, Spetzler RF, Lee KS, et al. Cavernous malformations of the brain stem. *J Neurosurg.* 1991;75:32–39.

Editorial Comment

Pediatric Lesions

Chapter 14 elegantly summarizes published literature experience with 56 cases of cavernous malformations (CMs) and another 11 cases of other types of angiographically occult vascular malformations in the pediatric age group. These published cases represent mostly case reports treated surgically, and would expectably be heavily biased toward clinically aggressive cases.

The authors chose to examine these cases and their own extensive experience within the spectrum of "cryptic vascular malformations" and strongly defend the use of this term. They rightly question the relevance of seperating subtypes of such cryptic vascular malformations and the precision and accuracy of current classification schemes of such lesions. They correctly argue that some lesions may be mixed (or transitional), containing features of more than one discrete pathologic lesion type, while other lesions frequently coexist (i.e. cavernous and venous or cavernous and capillary malformations).

These issues are addressed at great length throughout this book and are not peculiar to pediatric lesions. These controversies are further synthesized in the last chapter of the book. We agree with the authors' plea to be as specific as possible

when defining lesion types, and for this very reason urge the examination and characterization of CMs separately whenever possible. We clearly recognize the occasional lack of specificity of radiologic, clinical, and pathologic features of the CM, and the differential diagnostic considerations associated with it.

The authors present several pathophysiologic concepts regarding lesion genesis and progression. It is likely that these do not apply equally to all subtypes of "cryptic vascular malformations." Yet, some of these concepts may explain lesion progression and the association of venous and cavernous malformations.

In general, the pediatric experience with these lesions mirrors issues and controversies encountered in all age groups. It is not known why some CMs become clinically manifest at an earlier age, and what biologic features predispose to such aggressive clinical behavior. It is not known if such lesions will invariably progress or if they may later become clinically more quiescent—and what features determine this change.

Lastly, lesions mimicking "cryptic vascular malformations," which appear to be induced by radiation therapy, are highly intriguing. Such lesions have not yet been encountered by any other group, and may be related to the extensive experience with radiation therapy at UCSF. The prevalence of such lesions is clearly low, and predisposing factors including radiation dosimetry and host-related factors need to be characterized. Any relationship of such lesions to CMs (beyond the curiously similar MRI appearance of hemorrhage) must await better pathologic characterization of these "lesions." The one biopsied case revealed only hemorrhage and no underlying vascular malformation.

We are indebted to the authors for allowing us to include their perspective on these lesions in a book otherwise dedicated to CMs. Their review of published pediatric experience with this lesion and their own clinical management strategies in the pediatric age group are invaluable.

Issam A. Awad, MD

Daniel L. Barrow, MD

Radiosurgery of Cavernous Malformations and Other Angiographically Occult Vascular Malformations

Robert J. Coffey, MD, and L. Dade Lunsford, MD

Before the introduction of magnetic resonance imaging (MRI), the diagnosis of angiographically occult vascular malformations, including cavernous malformations (CMs), was most often established by surgical resection of an expanding or hemorrhagic intracranial lesion that did not exhibit arteriovenous shunting on cerebral angiography.* Modern imaging methods facilitate diagnosis of a presumed CM preoperatively.[26] Significant controversy still exists, however, regarding the ability of MRI to distinguish true CMs from other angiographically occult vascular lesions. Pathologic examination of surgically resected occult vascular malformations has revealed either a true arteriovenous malformation (AVM) (patent, partially thrombosed, or completely thrombosed), a CM, or rarely, a venous malformation or capillary malformation.[6,7,17,27,37,38,40]

A newly identified CM or angiographically occult vascular malformation can present a predicament. Many are discovered incidentally during MRI scans performed for unrelated symptoms. The natural history of these lesions is still poorly understood. While the lesions can remain quiescent in

many patients, multiple hemorrhages with recurring or incremental neurologic deficits occur in others.[36] Some individuals experience progressive symptoms due to expansion of the hematoma cavity or continued microhemorrhages. True CMs are often multiple.

CMs and angiographically occult vascular malformations in superficial or subcortical locations sometimes are associated with medically intractable seizures. Microsurgical resection can lead to gratifying seizure control.[40] Stereotaxic guidance increases the safety of surgery for superficial lesions, and makes the removal of deep malformations feasible.[6] Many patients harbor malformations in diencephalic or brain stem regions where the risks of open surgery may be unacceptable. In such patients, stereotaxic radiosurgery may represent a valuable treatment alternative.

While the treatment of angiographically apparent AVMs by radiosurgery has become widely accepted, the treatment of angiographically occult vascular malformations, including CMs, has remained controversial for several reasons.** **(1)** The lack of long-term follow-up data regarding the

*References 7,12,17,21,25,26,31,37,38,40

**References 2,4,9,11,13-16,18,19,23,32-34

natural history of the lesions complicates patient selection; **(2)** during radiosurgical treatment planning, the extent of the nidus (as opposed to the surrounding hemosiderin rim) may not be defined satisfactorily by MRI. As a corollary, no currently available imaging modality can confirm absolute obliteration of an angiographically occult vascular malformation or CM during follow-up. Until recently, no data were available regarding the safe dose-volume parameters or effective dose-response rates for radiosurgical treatment of these lesions.

Over the past 4¹/₂ years, clinical followup and serial MRI of our growing patient series has allowed a thorough evaluation of radiosurgical treatment of CMs and other angiographically occult vascular malformations. The criteria for patient selection, the method of treatment, and the results of radiosurgery using the cobalt-60 gamma knife are discussed below. These represent the authors' further experience since an initial report.[5,11] Given the nature of radiosurgery, the absence of a pathologic tissue diagnosis in these patients prevents us from differentiating the results of treatment of true CMs from other radiographically occult vascular malformations.

Patient Selection and Clinical Material

Among well over 200 patients with angiographically occult vascular malformations and CMs referred for radiosurgery, those selected for radiosurgical treatment all had experienced two or more clinically and/or radiographically defined hemorrhages. At the Mayo Clinic, all patients were evaluated by a neurosurgeon, a neurologist with expertise in cerebrovascular disease, and a radiation oncologist before final acceptance for treatment. At the University of Pittsburgh, patients were evaluated for treatment by a multidisciplinary team consisting of neurosurgeons, neuroradiologists, radiation oncologists, and medical physicists.

At both institutions, all radiosurgically treated patients had clinical and imaging confirmation of two or more events indicating hemorrhage and rehemorrhage. When clinically warranted, additional neurophysiologic studies (somatosensory or brain stem evoked potentials) or specialized examinations (neuro-ophthalmologic) were performed.

The imaging characteristics of the lesions in our patients included: **(1)** a mixed signal lesion with MRI characteristics consistent with recent and remote hemorrhage—these included mixed internal density and a halo of hemosiderin defined on T1- and T2-weighted images; **(2)** absence of prominent enhancement after the administration of paramagnetic contrast material; **(3)** lack of progression on serial imaging studies that might suggest a neoplastic or infectious process; **(4)** no angiographically visible arteriovenous or venous malformation on good quality cerebral angiography that included films into the late venous phase. Superficial lesions easily accessible for microsurgical removal were not treated with radiosurgery. If multiple CMs were present, only the one documented to have bled repeatedly or known to be responsible for increasing neurologic symptoms was treated using radiosurgery.

The clinical features of 36 patients treated to date at the University of Pittsburgh (n = 33) or Mayo Medical Center (n = 3) appear in Table 1. Most patients were young (mean age, 38) and female (60%). Patients had suffered as many as 5 hemorrhages before referral for treatment. A fixed neurologic deficit was present in 23 patients (63.8%) preoperatively, although most patients were capable of independent self-care or employment (mean Karnofsky rating, 85).

The majority of radiosurgically treated lesions were located in the brain stem (n = 24, 66.7%), thalamus (n = 5, 13.9%), or basal ganglia (n = 2, 5.5%). Only 5 lesions (13.9%) were located in the deep white matter of the cerebral hemispheres (Table

Table 1. Clinical Features of 36 Patients with Angiographically Occult Vascular Malformations Treated Using Radiosurgery

Age		Sex		Number of Hemorrhages		Neurologic Deficit		Karnofsky Rating		Prior Operation	
Mean	(Range)	Male	Female	Mean	(Range)	No.	(Percent)	Mean	(Range)	No.	(Percent)
38	(8–70)	15	21	2	(1–5)	23	63.8	85	(50–100)	6	17

Table 2. Location of 36 Angiographically Occult Vascular Malformations Treated Using Radiosurgery

	Number	(Percent)
Lobar	5	13.9
Thalmus	5	13.9
Basal ganglia	2	5.5
Brain stem	24	66.7

2). Six patients (16.7%) had undergone neurosurgical operations before referral for treatment. These consisted of craniotomy and partial resection of the lesion and associated hematoma in 4 patients, stereotaxic aspiration of a brain stem hematoma in 1 patient, and exposure of a pontine vascular malformation without attempted resection in 1 patient.

Radiosurgical Technique

All patients were admitted to the hospital on the day of or one day before radiosurgery. Those with a known or suspected seizure disorder received anticonvulsant medication preoperatively. Patients underwent application of the Leksell Model-G stereotaxic frame (Elekta Instruments, Tucker, Ga.) under local anesthesia with intravenous sedation. Electrocardiographic and pulse-oximeter monitoring were performed continuously.

MRI and computed tomographic (CT) scans with contrast enhancement were performed in all patients for target localization. Either the T1 spin-echo MRI sequence with gadolinium enhancement or a delayed TR (T2-weighted) scan was used to define the treatment volume. MRI-derived target coordinates correlated well with corresponding stereotaxic CT images. Measurements of the angle of the stereotaxic frame with respect to the central beam of the gamma unit, and radial measurements of the patient's head surface in relation to the stereotaxic frame were also performed.

These data, plus the target coordinates, collimator size, and relative contribution of each shot (weighting, for multiple isocenter treatments) were entered into the dose-planning computer. The three-dimensional series of isodose plots were viewed on a color video monitor and superimposed on the stereotaxic CT scans and MRIs. Adjustments in the number, position, collimator size, or relative weighting of the isocenters were made until optimal isodose contours were achieved. All lesions were enclosed within the 50% or higher isodose shell. Due to the rapid fall off of the radiation dose outside the 50% isodose line, surrounding structures received minimal radiation. Additionally, individual beam channels within each collimator helmet were plugged to prevent irradiation of the lens of the eye. The surgeon, radiation oncologist, and radiation physicist then determined the dose to be delivered to the center and margins of the lesion.

In our initial 24 patients, radiosurgical dosimetry was based upon published experience in the treatment of angiographically overt AVMs.[3,14,16,33] Subsequent experience led us to reduce the dose in order to minimize the occurrence of delayed, temporary radiation-induced complications. For small malformations located within the brain

Table 3. **Volume of 36 Angiographically Occult Vascular Malformations Treated Using Radiosurgery**

Lesion Volume (mm³)	Number	(Percent)
< 1,000	10	21.8
1,000–10,000	23	63.9
> 10,000	3	8.3

Table 4. **Radiosurgical Dosimetry for 36 Angiographically Occult Vascular Malformations**

Treatment Isodose (%)		Dose to Margin (Gy)		Central Dose (Gy)	
Mean	(Range)	Mean	(Range)	Mean	(Range)
57.7	(50–90)	17.5	(16–20)	31	(20–40)

stem (diameter 16 mm; volume 2,100 mm³), patients now receive a maximum marginal dose of 18–20 Gy (maximum central dose of 36–40 Gy).

The size of the treated lesions and radiosurgical dosimetry are summarized in Tables 3 and 4. Ten lesions (27.8%) had a volume less than 1,000 mm³, equivalent to an average lesion diameter $\leq$12.4 mm. Twenty-three had a volume between 1,000 and 10,000 mm³ (average lesion diameter $\leq$26.8 mm). Forty-three isocenters were employed to treat these 36 patients (average 1.19 isocenters/patient). The mean treatment isodose at the lesion margin was 57.7% (range, 50% to 90%). The mean dose to the margin was 17.5 Gy (range, 16–20 Gy), and the mean central dose was 31 Gy (range, 20–40 Gy).

After completion of dose planning, the patient was set to the proper coordinates for each isocenter, and the irradiations were performed sequentially. The head frame was then removed and a sterile dressing applied. Afterwards, a single dose of 40 mg of methylprednisolone was administered intravenously. The entire procedure from frame application to removal lasted 3–5 hours, depending upon the number of isocenters and complexity of dose planning.

Most patients were discharged from the hospital the day after treatment.

Clinical followup and imaging studies were scheduled at 3–6 months, and 12, 18, and 24 months after radiosurgery. Annual followup was planned for these patients for several years in order to detect long-delayed clinical deterioration or recurrence of the lesion. All imaging studies were reviewed by a neuroradiologist and compared to the studies performed at the time of treatment.

Results and Complications

All 24 patients in our initial report have been followed for longer than 2 years, and 12 have been followed for longer than 3 years after radiosurgery. An additional 9 patients have been treated at the University of Pittsburgh and 3 patients have been treated at the Mayo Clinic where identical selection criteria and treatment planning protocols were utilized. No acute postoperative morbidity or mortality occurred. The results of follow-up clinical and imaging examinations are listed in Tables 5 and 6.

The majority of patients remained neurologically stable after radiosurgery and did not suffer repeated episodes of hemorrhage or neurologic deterioration. To date, no malformation has rebled if more than 18

Table 5. **Outcome in Patients with CMs and Other Deep-Seated Angiographically Occult Vascular Malformations Treated Using Radiosurgery (n = 36) Versus Microsurgical Resection (n = 37)***

	Improved or Good	Stable or Unchanged	**Worse or Poor**		Dead
			Temporary	Permanent	
Radiosurgery (n = 36)	3	27	3	2	1
Microsurgical resection (n = 37)	21	6	—	4	6

*References 6, 7, 10, 12, 21, 22, 24, 28–31, 35, 37, 38, 40, 42

Table 6. **Followup Imaging of Angiographically Occult Vascular Malformations Treated Using Radiosurgery**

Lesion Size			
Decreased	Stable	Enlarged	Repeat Hemorrhage
5	28	0	2

months have elapsed after radiosurgery. Three patients had clinical improvement between 6 and 36 months after radiosurgery. On follow-up imaging studies, no lesion enlarged after radiosurgery. Five lesions decreased in size and MRI signal intensity (14.3%, Figures 1 and 2) and 28 lesions remained stable (80%).

Complications occurred in 7 patients (19.4%) after radiosurgery. These included repeat hemorrhage in 2 patients (5.5%) with brain stem lesions (both bled within 18 months of treatment). One patient recovered completely and the other patient had mild residual disability. One additional patient, whose early post-treatment course was described in previous publications,[4,11] experienced 2 episodes of edema surrounding a left thalamic and midbrain lesion 4 and 12 months after radiosurgery (Figure 3). Each time, she developed worsening of right hemiparesis, ataxia, and diplopia. The first episode was treated successfully by a brief course of corticosteroids. The patient refused to take medication during the second episode, and was left with a moderate increase in her pre-existing deficits.

Delayed temporary deficits that resolved completely occurred in 4 patients. These were associated with perilesional edema seen on T2-weighted MRIs as early as 1 month after treatment. The resolution of imaging changes paralleled clinical improvement in these patients—all of whom were treated with a brief course of corticosteroids.

Discussion

Although modern imaging technology permits the clinical and radiographic diagnosis of CMs and angiographically occult vascular malformations, widely accepted guidelines for patient treatment and followup remain to be established. Important issues and questions still surround the accuracy of diagnosis, the natural history of the disorder, patient selection for surgical resection or expectant management (observation), the role of radiosurgery, and methods to measure and report results so that meaningful comparisons between series can be made.

While histologic examination of tissue removed at surgery or postmortem examination is the gold standard for diagnostic accuracy, much confusion still exists in the

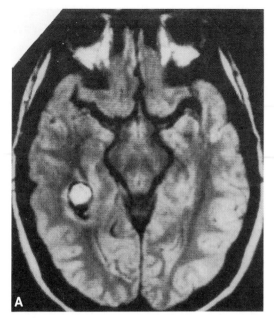 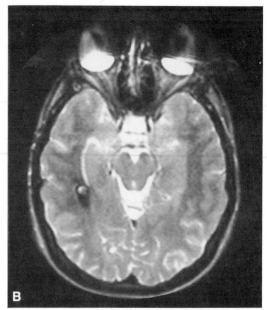

Figure 1. (A) T2-weighted MRI (spin-echo) before radiosurgical treatment of a deep, right, temporal/periventricular, angiographically occult, vascular malformation. **(B)** Follow-up MRI (T2, late spin-echo) in the same phase as Figure 1A, 27 months after radiosurgery. (A 6-month follow-up MRI of this patient was published previously.) The lesion continued to shrink and lose signal intensity, leaving only hemosiderin staining from her prior hemorrhages. The patient remained neurologically normal.

terminology used to describe patient series of angiographically occult or even angiographically visible vascular malformations of the brain.[1,15,20,25-27,31,38] Reports often confuse cavernous and arteriovenous malformations with highly vascularized neoplastic processes (hemangiomas) and venous malformations, or with capillary malformations. The natural history of CMs, discussed elsewhere in this volume, is still difficult to sort out because of the lack of uniformity in identifying and reporting cases, and the lack of pathologic corroboration in many reports.

Interestingly, in several recently reported surgical series a fraction of resected angiographically occult vascular malformations proved to be true AVMs on pathologic examination.[6,7,10,17,24] Thus, the practice of calling an unoperated angiographically occult hemorrhagic lesion in the brain a CM may be incorrect. In any study of the natural history of CMs and other angiographically

occult vascular malformations, we believe that the most precise diagnostic criteria are those set forth earlier in this report: a characteristic appearance on MRI and no angiographically demonstrable arteriovenous nidus or venous malformation on high-quality magnification-subtraction angiographic studies.

Since the performance of surgery on patients with suspected CMs has been sporadic, statements regarding natural history represent, at best, an educated guess. In aggregate, angiographically occult vascular malformations are suspected to rebleed at a rate similar to arteriovenous malformations—between 0.5% to 4% per year.[3,24,35,41] In individual patients the clinical course and rebleeding rate vary widely. From our own referral base that includes nearly 200 patients with such lesions, only a minority of patients (approximately 25%) had sustained multiple hemorrhages or clinical deterioration which we felt warranted therapeutic intervention. The remainder were

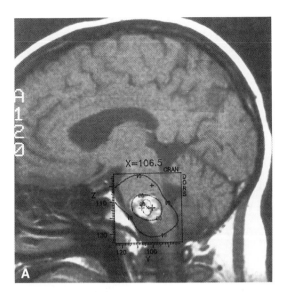

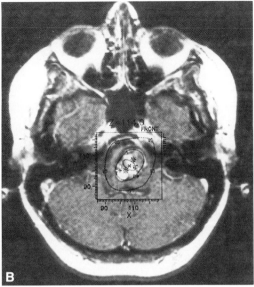

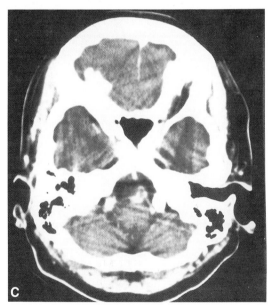

Figure 2. Stereotaxic MRIs (T1 spin-echo, with gadolinium enhancement) in the sagittal **(A)** and axial **(B)** planes during radiosurgical treatment of a ponto-medullary angiographically occult vascular malformation in a 36-year-old woman. Radiosurgical dosimetry: 16 Gy margin dose at 50% isodose line using two 14 mm isocenters (central dose, 32 Gy). The patient was bedridden at the time of treatment and deteriorated temporarily two months after radiosurgery. **(C)** CT scan with contrast enhancement 9 months after radiosurgery showing dramatic shrinkage of the lesion. MRI was not possible because of interval placement of an inferior vena cava filter. The patient had improved beyond her pretreatment status and resumed normal household activities.

discovered after a single neurologic event, or were incidental findings on imaging studies performed for other purposes (unrelated headache disorder, trauma, unrelated intracranial lesion).

In cases where a single event has occurred, imaging often cannot distinguish a vascular malformation that may rebleed from a vascular malformation that has obliterated itself during the hemorrhagic process. Thus, when advising patients regarding surgery, radiosurgery, or expectant observa-

tion, one must base recommendations upon the expected outcome for treatment of lesions of comparable size and location in patients in comparable neurologic condition. Dogmatic statements regarding whether or not one particular treatment strategy is best or "recommended" for all patients cannot be supported by the available evidence.

Fortunately, many patients who have malformations located in superficial or subcortical regions of the cerebral hemispheres can undergo microsurgical resection using conventional or stereotaxic approaches. In patients with fixed or fluctuating neurologic deficits and/or seizures, the results of open surgery are often gratifying. The re-

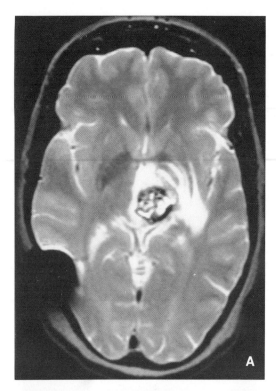

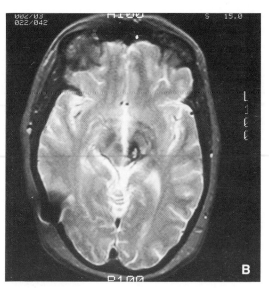

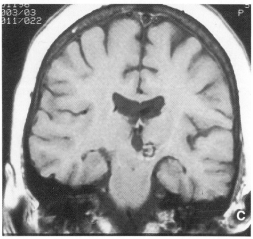

Figure 3. (A) Axial T2-weighted spin-echo MRI showing perilesional edema 4 months after radiosurgical treatment of a left-sided, thalamic and midbrain, angiographically occult, vascular malformation. The patient had sustained 4 hemorrhages approximately 10 months apart before treatment. Radiosurgical dosimetry: single 14 mm isocenter, 18 Gy marginal dose at 70% isodose line, 25.7 Gy central dose. **(B)** axial T2-weighted and **(C)** coronal T1-weighted MRIs 26 months after radiosurgery showing considerable shrinkage of the lesion and complete resolution of edema. The patient stabilized neurologically and has not rebled in over 33 months since radiosurgical treatment.

ported results of surgical resection for deeply situated lesions are less favorable.

In collected surgical series of angiographically occult vascular malformations operated during the microsurgical era, 44 patients with lesions in the thalamus, basal ganglia, brain stem, third or fourth ventricle were identified.* The reports allowed

---

*References 6,7,10,12,21,22,24,28-31,35,37,38,40,42

correlation of location with pathology (venous malformation, CM, or AVM) and clinical outcome in 37 patients (Table 5). Postoperatively, 10 patients (27%) were either dead (n = 6, 16.2%) or significantly worse (n = 4, 10.8%) as a result of surgery. Six patients (16.2%) had lasting, but not debilitating, deficits after surgery. Twenty-one patients (56.8%) had a good or excellent outcome as judged by the authors and surgeons in the original reports.

While the above figures represent the best available surgical standard against which to compare the results of radiosurgery, even these numbers may be a bit optimistic for a number of reasons: **(1)** because poor results tend to go unreported, it is likely that the results reported by experienced neurosurgeons are among the best that can be expected; and **(2)** many patients

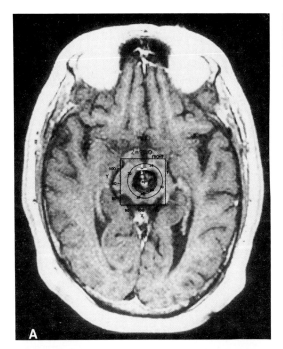

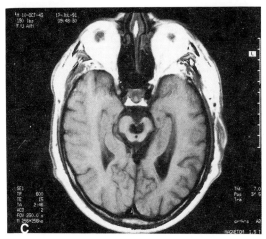

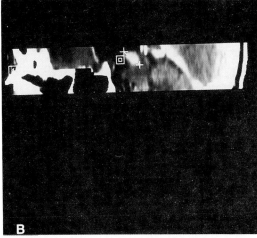

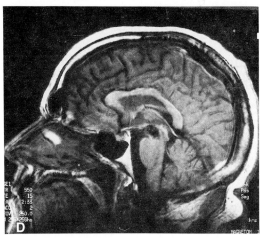

Figure 4. (A) Stereotaxic axial MRI (T1-weighted) and **(B)** reconstructed sagittal CT image (with contrast enhancement) during radiosurgical treatment of a midbrain, angiographically occult, vascular malformation that had hemorrhaged twice causing diplopia, dysarthria, ataxia, and spastic quadriparesis. The patient had undergone a stereotaxic biopsy of the lesion 3¹/₂ years before radiosurgery and stereotaxic aspiration of his second brain stem hematoma 9 months before radiosurgery. Radiosurgical dosimetry: single 14 mm isocenter, 60% isodose line, 18 Gy margin dose, and 30 Gy central dose. **(C)** and **(D)** MRIs (T1-weighted) in the same imaging planes as A and B four months after treatment. The lesion appeared slightly smaller, had diminished signal intensity, and caused less deformation of the midbrain.

operated for deep lesions underwent surgery during the acute or subacute phase of their illness when significant, often progressive, neurologic deficits were present.

As Fahlbusch et al emphasized, "Performing surgery soon after the hemorrhage minimizes the risk of additional postoperative neurologic deficit, since surgical excision is facilitated when the hematoma is not completely organized."[8] Urgent surgery sometimes is required to remove a brain stem hematoma in an unstable or deteriorating patient. Both open and stereotaxic methods have been employed with good results. However, when patients are operated early after a first hemorrhage, while deficits are still present, persistence of those deficits postoperatively is counted as a "stable patient" or "good" result.

Given the nature of patient referrals and selection for radiosurgery, the acute neurologic symptoms and deficits almost always have subsided considerably by the time of treatment, at which time the patient's baseline condition is recorded. Although the majority of our patients (63.8%) had detectable neurologic deficits at the time of treatment, the mean Karnofsky rating in our series was 85. All but 2 patients were independent in self-care and/or working at the time of initial evaluation. Thus, our radiosurgical patient series was skewed towards patients with difficult lesions who had more to lose than those reported in the microsurgical series.

While six of our patients had undergone one or more operations before radiosurgery, most had lesions for which the risks of open surgery were judged unacceptable by multiple neurosurgeons and the patient. In surgical series, the operated brain stem CMs presented on or just below a pial or ependymal surface, and were surgically accessible. In contrast, most of our radiosurgically treated brain stem lesions presented no such corridor of accessibility (Figure 4). While surgical resection of deep, midline, or brain stem CMs is sometimes necessary to relieve acute or progressive symptoms due to mass effect, many patients stabilize and recover completely or significantly, even after multiple hemorrhages. In this group of patients, especially when the residual MRI-defined lesion is small (volume $\leq 10,000$ mm^3, diameter < 26.8 mm) radiosurgery should be considered.

The mortality and morbidity of patients with comparable lesions appears to be lower after radiosurgery than after microsurgery. Even so, the incidence of delayed (presumably) radiation-induced side effects was 20% in our experience. Most symptoms were temporary and responded to a limited course of oral corticosteroid medication. The reason for this apparent difference between the radiation dose-volume tolerance of brain for similarly located and similarly sized CMs and other angiographically occult vascular malformations compared to AVMs remains unclear.

As discussed in the methods section and in an earlier publication, we have adjusted our dosimetry for these lesions in accordance with our empirical observations.[11] We believe these guidelines are valid for gamma knife radiosurgery at dose rates corresponding to relatively fresh cobalt-60, within one half-life of loading (≤ 5.2 years old). Virtually no interpretable data are available regarding the results of radiosurgery using linear accelerator-based or particle-beam techniques.[2]

Angiographically occult lesions, including CMs, were specifically excluded from the report by Steinberg et al that described the results of helium-ion radiosurgery for AVMs.[31] Levy et al and Marks et al mentioned a few cases of deep-seated angiographically occult vascular malformations (n = 3) or "slow flow" vascular malformations (n = 4), respectively, treated with heavy-charged-particle radiosurgery at the Lawrence Berkeley Laboratory.[15,20] In the Levy et al report, 1 patient was normal, 1 was unchanged, and 1 developed progressive neurologic deficit after treatment.[15] Among Marks' 4 patients, 2 had "venous angiomas."[20] The clinical outcome in these and the two patients with possible CMs was not specifically addressed in the article.

Weil et al stated in a recent abstract and presentation that "six cavernous-type vascular malformations treated with gamma stereotaxic radiosurgery (doses of 27–50 Gy) remained unchanged in size and in appearance after two years of follow-up..."[39] Reportedly, 2 patients rebled and 3 patients deteriorated, due to what the authors believed was radiation-induced injury. The authors concluded that "stereotaxic radiosurgery is not recom-

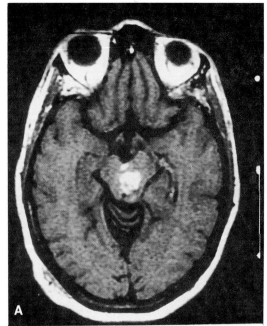

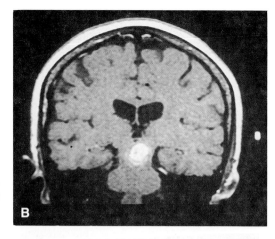

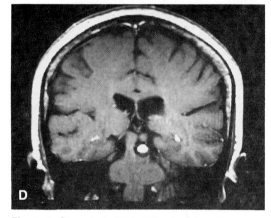

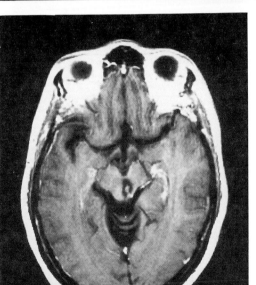

Figure 5. Stereotaxic MRIs (T1 spin-echo with gadolinium enhancement) in the **(A)** axial and **(B)** coronal planes during radiosurgery of a left-sided, midbrain, angiographically occult vascular malformation. This patient had fluctuating, but progressive ptosis and diplopia after two radiographically documented hemorrhages. Radiosurgical dosimetry: 20 Gy margin dose at 90% isodose line (central dose, 22.2 Gy), single 14 mm isocenter. **(C and D)** Follow-up MRIs (T1, gadolinium enhanced) in comparable imaging planes to A and B 18 months after treatment. The lesion had decreased significantly in size and signal intensity. The patient remained clinically stable.

mended for the treatment of cavernous brain stem malformations." Since no imaging studies or other essential data were presented, it is impossible to know what kind of lesions were treated, or even whether MRI was utilized as a diagnostic or treatment-planning tool. That 2 patients

rebled, yet the lesions "remained unchanged in size and appearance," seems inconsistent. Similarly, that 3 patients developed radiation-induced injury without corresponding imaging changes is also inconsistent with our own experience. We do

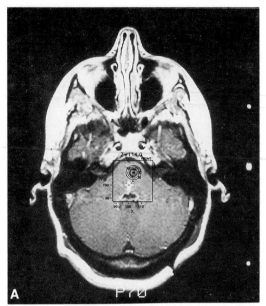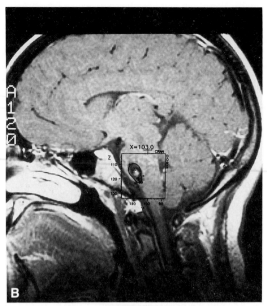

Figure 6. Stereotaxic **(A)** axial and **(B)** sagittal MRIs (T1 spin-echo with gadolinium enhancement) during radiosurgical treatment of a small, left pontine, angiographically occult vascular malformation (lesion volume: 500 mm³). This 20-year-old woman had suffered two hemorrhages accompanied by a right hemiparesis that resolved each time. Note the tight shaping of the 50% isodose line to the lesion margin. Radiosurgical dosimetry: one 8 mm and one 4 mm isocenter, 18 Gy margin dose, 36 Gy central dose. The patient remains neurologically normal.

not believe that the data presented in this anecdotal report justified the authors' conclusions.

Summary

We believe that the results of stereotaxic radiosurgery in the treatment of small, deeply situated CMs and other angiographically occult vascular malformations may be superior to the published results of microsurgical resection for comparable lesions. Strict patient selection criteria, the use of stereotaxic MRI for treatment planning, and adherence to lower dose-volume parameters than for angiographically visible AVMs seem essential to minimize complications. Radiosurgery can be undertaken with acceptable risk in patients who have recovered neurologic function after previous hemorrhages (Figures 5 and 6).

From the data currently available, we cannot determine whether comparable results can be expected with other stereo-taxic irradiation techniques (linear accelerator, particle beam, etc.). Even less information is available regarding the use of conventional fractionated radiation therapy to treat such lesions. Modern imaging, microsurgical, and stereotaxic radiosurgical techniques have virtually eliminated conventional radiation therapy as a treatment for angiographically visible and angiographically occult vascular malformations.

Since gamma knife radiosurgery is efficacious in carefully selected patients, we believe that its continued use to treat difficult CMs is justified. Careful clinical and imaging followup of patients will establish the role of radiosurgery more clearly in the treatment of this challenging group of patients.

References

1. Abe M, Tabuchi K, Takagi M, et al. Spontaneous resolution of multiple hemangiomas of the brain: case report. *J Neurosurg.* 1990;73:448–452.

2. Alexander EA III. Comment on Kondziolka D, Lunsford LD, Coffey RJ, et al. Stereotactic radiosurgery of angiographically occult vascular malformations: indications and preliminary experience. *Neurosurgery.* 1990;27:900.

3. Brown RD, Wiebers DO, Forbes G, et al. The natural history of unruptured intracranial arteriovenous malformations. *J Neurosurg.* 1988;68:352–357.

4. Coffey RJ, Lunsford LD. Stereotactic radiosurgery using the 201 cobalt-60 source gamma knife. In: Friedman WA, ed. *Stereotactic Neurosurgery (Neurosurg Clin of North Am*, Vol. 1, No. 4.), Philadelphia, Pa: WB Saunders; 1990:933–954.

5. Coffey RJ, Lunsford LD. Stereotactic gamma radiosurgery for brain stem AVM. *Neurosurgeons. Vol. 10. Proceedings of the 10th Annual Meeting of the Japanese Congress of Neurological Surgeons.* Toyko, Japan: SciMed Publications; 1991:238–246.

6. Davis DH, Kelly PJ. Stereotactic resection of occult vascular malformations. *J Neurosurg.* 1990;72:698–702.

7. Ebeling JD, Tranmer BL, Davis HA, et al. Thrombosed arteriovenous malformations: a type of occult vascular malformation. Magnetic resonance imaging and histopathological correlations. *Neurosurgery.* 1988;23:605–610.

8. Fahlbusch R, Strauss C, Huk W, et al. Surgical removal of pontomesencephalic cavernous hemangiomas. *Neurosurgery.* 1990;26:449–457.

9. Hosobuchi Y. Stereotactic heavy-particle irradiation of brain stem arteriovenous malformations. *Neurosurgeons. Vol. 10. Proceedings of the 10th Annual Meeting of the Japanese Congress of Neurological Surgeons.* Tokyo, Japan: SciMed Publications; 1991;230–233.

10. Kashiwagi S, van Loveren HR, Tew JM, et al. Diagnosis and treatment of brain stem malformations. *J Neurosurg.* 1990;72:27–34.

11. Kondziolka D, Lunsford LD, Coffey RJ, et al. Stereotactic radiosurgery of angiographically occult vascular malformations: indications and preliminary experience. *Neurosurgery.* 1990;27:892–900.

12. Le Doux MS, Aronin PA, Odrezin GT. Surgically treated cavernous angiomas of the brain stem: report of two cases and review of the literature. *Surg Neurol.* 1991;35:395–399.

13. Leksell DG. Stereotactic radiosurgery: present status and future trends. *Neurological Research.* 1987;9:60–68.

14. Leksell L. Stereotactic radiosurgery. *J Neurol Neurosurg Psychiatry.* 1983;46:797–803.

15. Levy RP, Fabrikant JI, Frankel HA, et al. Stereotactic heavy-charged-particle Bragg peak radiosurgery for the treatment of intracranial arteriovenous malformations in childhood and adolescence. *Neurosurgery.* 1989; 24:841–852.

16. Lindquist C, Steiner L. Stereotactic radiosurgical treatment of malformations of the brain. In: Lunsford LD, ed. *Modern Stereotactic Neurosurgery.* Boston, Ma: Martinus Nijhoff Publishing; 1988:491–505.

17. Lobato RD, Perez C, Rivas JJ, et al. Clinical, radiological and pathological spectrum of angiographically occult intracranial vascular malformations: analysis of 21 cases and review of the literature. *J Neurosurg.* 1988;68:518–53l.

18. Lunsford LD, Flickinger J, Coffey RJ. Stereotactic gamma knife radiosurgery: initial North American experience in 207 patients. *Arch Neurol.* 1990;47:169–175.

19. Lunsford LD, Kondziolka D, Flickinger JC, et al. Stereotactic radiosurgery for arteriovenous malformations of the brain. *J Neurosurg.* 1991;75:512–524.

20. Marks MP, Delapaz RL, Fabrikant JI, et al. Intracranial vascular malformations: imaging of charged-particle radiosurgery: I. Results of therapy. *Radiology.* 1988;168:447–455.

21. McFerran DJ, Marks PV, Garvan NJ. Angiographically occult arteriovenous malformations of the brainstem. *Surg Neurol.* 1987;28:221–224.

22. Ogawa A, Katakura R, Yoshimoto T. Third ventricle cavernous angioma: report of two cases. *Surg Neurol.* 1990;34:414–420.

23. Ogilvy CS. Radiation therapy for arteriovenous malformations: a review. *Neurosurgery.* 1990;26:725–735.

24. Ogilvy CS, Heros RC, Ojemann RG, et al. Angiographically occult arteriovenous malformations. *J Neurosurg.* 1988;69:350–355.

25. Rigamonti D, Hadley MN, Drayer BP, et al. Cerebral cavernous malformations: incidence and familial occurrence. *N Engl J Med.* 1988;319:343–347.

26. Rigamonti D, Drayer OP, Johnson PC, et al. The MRI appearance of cavernous malformations (angiomas). *J Neurosurg.* 1987;67:518–524.

27. Rigamonti D, Johnson PC, Hadley MN, et al. Cavernous malformations and capillary telangiectasia: a spectrum within a single pathological entity. *Neurosurgery.* 1991;28:60–64.

28. Roda JM, Alvarez F, Isla A, et al. Thalamic cavernous malformation: case report. *J Neurosurg.* 1990;72:647–649.

29. Seifert V, Gaab MR. Laser-assisted microsurgical extirpation of a brain stem cavernoma: case report. *Neurosurgery.* 1989;25:986–990.

30. Shuey NM Jr, Day AL, Quisling RB, et al. Angiographically cryptic cerebrovascular malformations. *Neurosurgery.* 1979;5:476–479.

31. Simard JM, Garcia-Bengochea F, Ballinger WE Jr, et al. Cavernous angioma: a review of 126 collected and 12 new clinical cases. *Neurosugery.* 1986;18:162–172.

32. Steinberg GK, Fabrikant JI, Marks MP, et al. Stereotactic heavy-charged-particle Bragg-peak radiation for intracranial arteriovenous malformations. *N Engl J Med.* 1990;323:96–101.

33. Steiner L, Lindquist CH. Radiosurgery in cerebral arteriovenous malformations. In: Tasker RR, ed. *Neurosurgery: State of the Art Reviews. Stereotactic Surgery.* Philadelphia, Pa: Hanley and Belfus; 1987:329–336.

34. Sturm V, Schlegel W, Pastyr O, et al. Stereotactic linac-radiosurgery for brain stem and peribrainstem arteriovenous malformations. *Neurosurgeons. Vol. 10. Proceedings of the 10th Annual Meeting of the Japanese Congress of Neurological Surgeons.* Tokyo, Japan: SciMed Publications; 1991;234–237.

35. Tagle P, Huete I, Mendez J, et al. Intracranial cavernous angioma: presentation and management. *J Neurosurg.* 1986;64:720–723.

36. Tung H, Giannotta SL, Chandrasoma PT, Zee C-H. Recurrent intraparenchymal hemorrhages from angiographically occult vascular malformations. *J Neurosurg.* 1990;73:174–180.

37. Vaquero J, Salazar J, Martinez R. Cavernomas of the central nervous system: clinical syndromes, CT scan diagnosis, and prognosis after surgical treatment in 25 cases. *Acta Neurochir (Wien).* 1987;85:29–33.

38. Wakai S, Ueda Y, Inoh S, et al. Angiographically occult angiomas: a report of thirteen cases with analysis of the cases documented in the literature. *Neurosurgery.* 1985;17:549–556.

39. Weil S, Tew JM Jr, Steiner L. Comparison of radiosurgery and microsurgery for treatment of cavernous malformations of the brain stem. *J Neurosurg.* 1990;72:336A. Abstract.

40. Wharen RE Jr, Scheithauer BW, Laws ER Jr. Thrombosed arteriovenous malformations of the brain: an important entity in the differential diagnosis of intractable focal seizure disorders. *J Neurosurg.* 1982;57:520–526.

41. Wharen RE. Comments on Ebeling JD, Tranmer BI, Davis HA, et al. Thrombosed arteriovenous malformations: a type of occult vascular malformation. *Neurosurgery.* 1988;23:610.

42. Yoshimoto T, Suzuki J. Radical surgery on cavernous angioma of the brain stem. *Surg Neurol.* 1986;26:72–78.

Editorial Comment

Radiosurgery

Drs. Coffey and Lunsford have carefully analyzed the most comprehensive series of angiographically occult vascular malformations treated with stereotaxic radiosurgery. They are careful to point out that they cannot differentiate, without pathologic confirmation, the CMs in this series from other pathologic subtypes of angiographically occult lesions. It appears from their radiologic definitions and from illustrated cases that the majority of lesions represent presumed CMs.

The authors carefully point out the difficulty in evaluating the "effectiveness" of radiosurgery in such lesions. On the one hand, there is no radiographic or other criterion of therapeutic success since the lesion does not disappear following radiosurgery. Furthermore, fluctuations in lesion size and in clinical behavior are commonly observed during the natural course of such lesions. Any "stabilization" of lesion size or clinical course cannot be necessarily attributed to therapeutic benefit.

The above points are most obviously illustrated in Figure 1 in the previous chapter, where the expected shrinkage of an intralesional hematoma was attributed by the authors to the benefits of radiotherapy.

Similarly, another lesion shrinkage is claimed in Figure 2 by comparing a post-treatment CT scan to a pretreatment MRI despite the well-known shortcomings of CT in visualizing the true size of such lesions. These cases demonstrate the difficulties and potential pitfalls of claiming therapeutic success in the absence of complete lesion elimination.

It appears that the effects of radiosurgery on these lesions may be best characterized as palliative, and cannot clearly be shown to be superior to expectant therapy alone outside the setting of carefully controlled prospective randomized studies. Uncontrolled comparison to historical series of operated and unoperated cases cannot prove therapeutic benefit. In the absence of lesion elimination, controlled data and long-term followup of treated and untreated lesions are necessary to substantiate any claim of therapeutic benefit.

The authors' experience can best be viewed as phase I information about therapeutic safety, toxicity, and possible benefit. By the authors' own conclusions, it appears that complications of radiosurgery in or near eloquent brain regions may be prohibitive unless substantially reduced radiation dosimetry is planned. Any therapeutic benefit of such empirically reduced dosimetry (as compared to placebo) is difficult to demonstrate, especially in view of the variable natural history of the lesions and absence of true cure by the modality. Clearly, the biologic response of CMs to radiation may be very different from angiographically overt arteriovenous malformations, and parameters of therapeutic success or failure may be equally different.

Any comparison of therapeutic benefit and morbidity of radiosurgery and microsurgical resection of CMs may be misleading. Clearly, lesions treated by these modalities are not necessarily comparable in location, size, or neurologic status at the time of treatment. Objectives of open surgery are to totally excise a lesion which abuts a pial surface. The presumed objectives of radiosurgery are to stabilize and palliate the clinical course of a lesion without excising it. Relative morbidities of the two therapeutic modalities cannot be rationally compared without any convincing measure of therapeutic effectiveness of radiosurgery on identical lesions.

As per the authors' own recommendations, consideration of radiosurgery for presumed CMs should be reserved for progressively symptomatic lesions in truly inoperable locations. Whether the benefit of such therapy justifies the potential radiation toxicity in these locations remains to be proven. Any generalization of possible indications to other lesions or other locations cannot be supported by any published data at the present time.

Issam A. Awad, MD
Daniel L. Barrow, MD

Chapter 16

Conceptual Overview and Management Strategies

Daniel L. Barrow, MD, and Issam A. Awad, MD

Appropriate clinical decision making for the management of any medical problem requires an accurate assessment of the natural history of the disorder and the risks inherent in the treatment of the condition. As further knowledge of natural history accumulates and safer treatments are developed, clinical decision making evolves. Such is the case for cavernous malformations (CMs) of the brain and spinal cord. Prior to the advent of magnetic resonance imaging (MRI), CMs were rarely diagnosed in the absence of clinically significant symptoms, particularly extensive mass effect, or devastating hemorrhage. Most CMs are not visualized on angiography or they demonstrate only subtle abnormalities in the capillary phase of the study. Even computed tomography (CT) poorly images the lesions in the absence of significant acute or subacute hemorrhage or calcifications. Prior to the availability of MRI, lesions were rarely diagnosed unless they reached a large size or presented with serious clinical sequelae. This led to the erroneous perception that these are rare lesions and that they carry a uniformly poor prognosis. On the other hand, many smaller lesions in the infratentorial compartment were not clearly visualized, despite overt symptomatology, and were erroneously diagnosed as multiple sclerosis or brain stem tumors.

The routine use of MRI in clinical practice has made the diagnosis of asymptomatic and minimally symptomatic CMs commonplace. Overall, this more recent experience has shown that CMs are more common than estimated in the pre-MRI era, and that the natural history of the lesion is more benign.

Several chapters in this book provide a synthesis of the extensive information accumulated in the past decade with improved detection and followup of these lesions and the spectrum of therapeutic strategies available for their management. In this chapter, we attempt to place this information in perspective while highlighting areas of general consensus and remaining controversies. The reader is referred to individual chapters of the book and their respective bibliographies for additional detail and substantiation of these concepts.

Lesion Nomenclature

As discussed in Chapter 1, CMs have a specific pathologic appearance, which allows these lesions to be differentiated from other vascular malformations. In the absence of pathologic verification, the precise diagnosis of a lesion may remain in doubt, but every attempt should be made to describe the lesion precisely and avoid confounding terminologies.

Throughout this volume and particularly in Chapter 4, the typical MRI appearance of CMs is discussed and illustrated. While this appearance is not pathognomonic, it is sufficiently representative to permit a confident diagnosis in the majority of cases within the appropriate clinical context and with corroborative ancillary diagnostic tests.

The nomenclature of the CM has evoked many controversies, especially with regard to precise lesion definition and to the choice of naming terminology. As indicated above, the clinical behavior of the lesion and its radiologic appearance are quite typical but not absolutely specific. Clinically, the lesion may cause seizures, focal neurologic deficits, or nonspecific neurologic symptoms. It is associated with calcifications and focal hemorrhages. Certainly, numerous other pathologic conditions can present these same features, although with variable differential diagnostic subtleties.

The CM is an angiographically occult vascular lesion. There has been dispute as to the relevance of differentiating this particular lesion from other angiographically occult vascular malformations. It may be argued that the clinician has no access to a detailed histopathologic diagnosis at the time of management decisions, and therefore will manage the lesion essentially as an "angiographically occult vascular malformation." The post facto pathologic characterization of a "cavernous malformation" may only be of academic interest, without substantial contribution to prognostication or specific management of such cases. In patients who undergo nonsurgical management (medical therapy, expectant therapy, radiosurgery, etc.), the pathologic diagnosis is never known, and the cases remain essentially as "angiographically occult vascular malformations" without further subclassification.

The morphologic and histopathologic appearance of the CM is highly characteristic. When presented with a specimen in toto, the pathologist can provide an accurate and highly specific diagnosis of this lesion as distinct from other angiographically overt or occult vascular malformations. Furthermore, the lesion diagnosed as such by the pathologist has a distinct radiologic appearance, clinical profile, and unique associated multiplicity and familial transmission. These are the most powerful arguments for considering this lesion as distinct from other angiographically occult vascular malformations.

Yet, the pathologic criteria do not represent an absolute gold standard. There are numerous transitional and mixed lesions with features of CMs mixed with arteriovenous, venous, or capillary malformations in different regions of the same lesion. Such mixed and transitional lesions raise important questions about etiology, pathophysiology, and lesion evolution. Also, there is no evidence that such mixed lesions behave any differently than pure CMs. Furthermore, the pathologist is often at a significant disadvantage, receiving a fragmented, highly coagulated specimen without global morphology or orientation. The fragment is often mixed with hematoma or surrounding brain tissue. These considerations introduce additional limitations and imprecisions to the pathologic diagnosis in the clinical setting.

The above issues notwithstanding, Chapters 1–3 set forth powerful arguments that the CM represents a unique clinical-radiologic-pathologic entity with a predictable incidence, clinical behavior, and other associations. As with other medical conditions, there remains a problem with absolute specificity of any features of this lesion. This calls for astute differential diagnosis, but does not call into question the actual existence of the lesion.

Issues of specific lesion nomenclature are more complex. Having made the argument to separate the CM from the broader category of "angiographically occult vascular malformation," we wish to make a strong plea for a uniform designation. Some authors have referred to the lesion as *cavernoma, cavernous angioma,* or *cavernous hemangioma*—thereby emphasizing its "tumor-like behavior" and its frequent presentation as a "mass lesion." We disagree with this concept, as there is no evidence that the lesion represents a growing tumor of blood vessels. With the exception of extradural lesions (which actually do behave as vascular neoplasms), CMs more often behave as hamartomas with "hemorrhagic tendencies." It is the hemorrhage into the lesion and into surrounding brain with subsequent reactive angioblastic proliferation that most often characterize CMs pathologically. While some cases may not be congenital or familial, there is firm evidence among familial and multiple cases of a congenital predisposition to this lesion. The term *cavernous malformation* appears to be the most accurate among the widely used terminologies for this lesion. This name should not be construed as evidence that the lesion is an ectatic congenital malformation of blood vessels. Yet, the term CM illustrates the presence of truly dysmorphic vessels forming cavernous cavities. These are associated with pathologic phenomena, including hemorrhage and subsequent angiogenesis. The term *hemorrhagic proliferative cavernous vascular malformation* would appear to be the most descriptive, although it is not likely to be widely used or accepted. At the present time, we propose uniform utilization of the term *cavernous malformation (CM)* despite clearly articulated limitations and possible lack of specificity of these simple words.

Etiology and Pathophysiology

Several hypotheses about the etiology and pathophysiology of CMs are emerging. On the one hand, the presence of the lesion in the pediatric age group, familial incidence with autosomal dominant transmission, and cases with multiple focal lesions all argue for a congenital pathology akin to a phakomatosis. Cases with single lesions and without familial association could represent possible *formes frustes* of the same disease. Yet, there are lines of evidence that suggest an acquired and/or progressive phenomenology. There have been well-documented reports of the sporadic appearance of new CMs spontaneously or following trauma or radiotherapy. Admittedly, "normal" antecedent imaging does not preclude an underlying microscopic vascular abnormality in the same area. Also, etiologic associations with trauma or radiotherapy are very uncommon and certainly do not prove causation. Indeed, they may be purely incidental.

Lesions have been shown to enlarge over time, mostly through the expansion of one or more caverns within the lesion itself or into surrounding brain. The surrounding hemosiderin ring can darken substantially on serial imaging, and the reticulated core of the lesion on serial MRI has been shown to enlarge in many instances. There has not been to date any direct molecular, cellular, immunohistochemical, or other evidence of true angiogenic proliferation within the lesion. Yet, such angiogenic proliferation is strongly suspected on the basis of lesion appearance, and the reported association of CM in or near regions of capillary malformations, venous malformations, or within true arteriovenous malformations (AVMs) (Figure 1).

Hemorrhage is a constant accompanying feature of the CM. It has become obvious that the pathologic entity of the CM cannot exist without at least microscopic evidence of hemorrhage. It is not known, however, if hemorrhage is a necessary result of the lesion or an etiologic prerequisite of this pathologic entity.

The above concepts can be synthesized into a schema outlining hypotheses about the etiology and pathophysiology of this

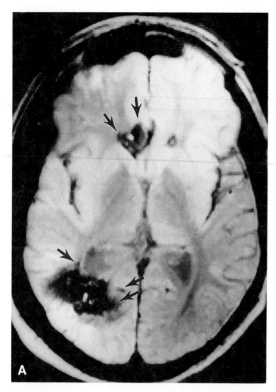

Figure 1. (A) Cases with multiple CMs frequently reveal apparent coalescence of smaller lesions in or near larger hemorrhagic lesions (arrows). Histologically, many of the smaller lesions represent zones of capillary malformation (telangiectasia). **(B)** A photomicrograph of such an area reveals coalescence of capillary malformation in the presence of microhemorrhage (arrow), within a wider area of the malformation and otherwise normal brain parenchyma. The coalesced abnormal capillaries mimic the appearance of a "baby cavernous malformation" and may represent *de novo* genesis of a CM in an area of capillary malformation. We have not seen such coalescence of capillary malformation in the absence of microhemorrhage.

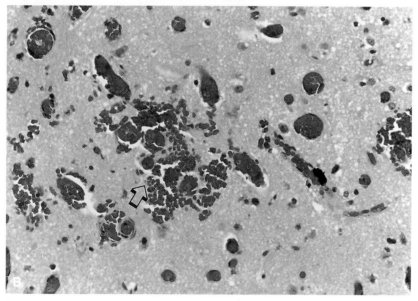

lesion (Figure 2). Such a schema is purely speculative at the present time and is based on empiric observations and clinical associations. It allows the formulation of specific hypotheses amenable to scientific investigation using a variety of tools. Several aspects of these hypotheses can best be studied using the resected specimen of CMs from surgery or autopsy. Immunohistochemical and other cellular markers coupled with molecular biologic and cell culture tech-

HYPOTHETICAL SCHEMA REGARDING THE GENESIS AND PROLIFERATION OF THE CAVERNOUS MALFORMATION

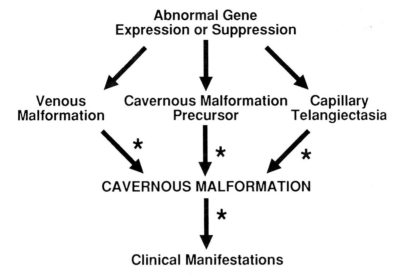

Abnormal Gene Expression or Suppression

Venous Malformation   **Cavernous Malformation Precursor**   **Capillary Telangiectasia**

CAVERNOUS MALFORMATION

Clinical Manifestations

* Hemorrhagic Angiogenic Proliferation (may be affected by host-related or environmental factors)

Figure 2. Hypothetical schema regarding the genesis and proliferation of the CM. It is postulated that venous malformations and capillary malformations (telangiectasia) may be the result of mutation and abnormal gene expression or suppression. These lesions may subsequently predispose to the development of associated CMs. An inherited gene may also predispose to the development of CMs in the absence of venous or capillary malformations. Development and progression of the CM is invariably associated with microhemorrhages, and can best be characterized as "hemorrhagic angiogenic proliferation." This may be influenced by host-related factors, including age, hormonal influences, previous hemorrhage, and/or disinhibition of a suppressor gene, or activation of an angiogenic gene. The process can also be affected by environmental factors, including trauma or radiation, perhaps also via gene activation or suppression. Such schema is purely speculative at the present time, and is based on empiric observations of angiogenic proliferation within CMs, and also on the association of CM in or near venous and capillary malformations.

niques may prove or disprove specific hypotheses about angiogenesis and the role of hemorrhage in lesion progression. Other aspects of this schema cannot be investigated without a laboratory model of the lesion, preferably in animals. Undoubtedly, these many mysteries will be clarified by rigorous scientific investigation in the coming years.

In our opinion, this lesion is best viewed as a vascular hamartoma with progressive tendencies related to hemorrhage and possible reactive angiogenesis. These features appear to be highly consistent with the morphology and clinical behavior of the lesion. It is not known whether the lesion can evolve totally de novo with one or

more inciting factors, or whether it always evolves from a pre-existing structural anomaly.

Therapeutic Options

Following the diagnosis of one or more suspected CMs, the clinician faces a wide variety of options for treatment. An expectant therapeutic approach is possible in many cases and may be safer than any attempt at lesion excision. In other instances, medical treatment of seizures, headaches, or other associated symptoms is indicated. Physical excision of the lesion may be entertained as a definitive treatment. Lastly, therapy may be aimed at preventing lesion progression, perhaps through radiosurgery or other yet undiscovered modalities.

Each of the above options raises particular questions about safety, efficacy, and global outcome. A given therapeutic approach may be more appropriate for a lesion of a particular size, location, or at a particular point in the natural history of the lesion. A given therapeutic attitude may be most appropriate only when a lesion has caused a specific set of symptoms.

These numerous variables have not yet been subjected to rigorous scientific investigations. Yet, there are emerging areas of consensus and well-defined questions undergoing intense clinical investigations.

Lesion Excision

When considering the issue of definitive lesion excision, the criteria for patient selection include lesion size, location, and symptomatology. The timing of surgery is another important consideration. An accessible lesion does not necessarily imply a need for excision in every instance. Similarly, a so-called "deep, inaccessible lesion" in eloquent brain may enlarge sufficiently or approach a pial surface making it more accessible. Symptom progression may be so advanced that surgical excision may be less likely to cause further significant harm. The same lesion would be associated with significant added morbidity if excised when smaller, less symptomatic, or slightly more distant from a pial surface.

The morbidity of lesion excision should be weighed against the likelihood of further symptomatology from the same lesion during a patient's lifetime. It has now become evident that symptomatic CMs within the brain stem will likely remain symptomatic with slow progressive and stepwise exacerbation of disability related to the lesion. A slight worsening in clinical symptoms immediately following surgical excision may be worthwhile in relation to expected accumulated morbidity over time if the lesion is not excised.

These issues may not be easy to elucidate from retrospective reports published in the literature or from anecdotal clinical series. Only careful prospective registries and well-designed clinical trials will help provide scientifically valid answers. Other subtle issues vary slightly from patient to patient and call for astute clinical judgment coupled with an honest estimate of the surgeon's own abilities, particularly in the setting of certain deep or inaccessible lesions.

Furthermore, there is the possibility of lesion recurrence following an apparently successful surgical excision. While this phenomenon has not been commonly reported, it does appear to be more prevalent following lesion excision in deep and infratentorial locations. In some cases, lesion recurrence may be due to incomplete lesion excision at first operation (whether or not this was appreciated by the surgeon). *De novo* lesion recurrence may be the result of microscopic remnants of the previous CM or pre-existing microstructural pathology predisposing to the genesis of a CM. We have encountered a case of lesion recurrence in a pediatric patient in which a right temporal lobe CM was grossly removed with a good histologic margin and documented by postoperative imaging. The lesion recurred within 2 years in this 5-year-old child. A host-related tendency toward lesion recurrence is highly suspect in such a case. Followup of patients with CMs should proceed beyond documented lesion excision. The aspects of this disease that results in lesion recurrence or the appearance of new lesions are unknown.

Nevertheless, lesion recurrence following excision of a CM appears to be uncommon. Excision of a symptomatic lesion appears to be the most effective and definitive therapeutic option, and is probably curative in the vast majority of instances. Such a radical and effective intervention is nevertheless associated with a limited risk of morbidity, which is not justified in many lesions without aggressive clinical behavior.

Single Supratentorial Lesions

A number of CMs will be discovered as incidental findings or associated with minimal symptomatology. One should be extremely careful in attributing headaches to a CM. Headache is an extremely common neurologic symptom; and, the majority of patients with headaches do not harbor a structural abnormality. If a supratentorial CM is associated with headaches that are medically intractable and can be related to the malformation, surgical removal is reasonable if the lesion can be safely removed without significant risk of neurologic deficit. However, lesion accessibility alone should not justify the surgical removal of a CM.

In a patient with a single supratentorial lesion presenting with a seizure disorder, again one should be fastidious in ascribing the seizure disorder to the CM. Not all CMs associated with seizures require surgical removal. Medical management of the seizure disorder is an excellent option in many cases. If the lesion can be removed with a very low prospect of neurologic deficit, this may be the most reasonable treatment. Certainly, for medically intractable seizures related to a CM, surgery provides an excellent chance for elimination or better control of the seizures. For most CMs associated with a seizure disorder, we would recommend surgery with the initial objective of resection of the CM. If the lesion resides in a functionally noneloquent area, it is advisable to resect the surrounding hemosiderin-stained brain parenchyma to further ensure a seizurefree postoperative course. Formal epilepsy surgery (including resection of hippocampus or other brain epileptogenic zones) is reserved for cases with truly intractable seizures or cases that have failed previous lesion excision (Chapter 5).

A clinically significant hemorrhage from a CM provides a much clearer indication for surgery. Again, after considering the likelihood of neurologic deficit, surgical removal will generally eliminate the risk of future hemorrhage and, in the majority of cases, this is the approach we would favor. As discussed in Chapter 6, the pathologic and MRI appearance of CMs is such that virtually all of these lesions are associated with some degree of microscopic hemorrhage. Such radiographic evidence of previous hemorrhage alone does not represent sufficient indication for surgery.

The clearest indication for surgery of a supratentorial CM is the presence of a progressive neurologic deficit. This clinical situation is usually due to recurrent hemorrhage; and those lesions presenting in such a manner tend to have a more aggressive clinical course. Surgical removal of the malformation and surrounding hemorrhage seems to offer these patients the best opportunity for reversal of the deficit and prevention of further neurologic injury.

Single Infratentorial Lesions

Even CMs residing within brain stem can be removed with minimal neurologic sequelae. The excellent results outlined in Chapter 10 illustrate this point. However, complete surgical removal of brain stem CMs is significantly more difficult than the removal of their supratentorial counterparts. Not only do these lesions lie within critical and functionally important locations, but they also tend to be more tenacious and technically more difficult to remove. This may be due to the compact nature of critical nuclei and fiber tracts within the brain stem.

Although minor hemorrhages within the brain stem may produce significant neurologic findings, these deficits will generally improve; the clinical course often resembles that of demyelinating disease. Therefore, not all symptomatic brain stem CMs require surgery. We recommend surgical removal only for those lesions presenting with a progressive neurologic deficit or with a significant hemorrhage accessible to a surface of the brain stem. If the planned surgical approach requires dissection through any uninvolved and intact brain stem structure, one must expect significant neurologic deficits from the operation. Notwithstanding these words of caution, we believe that surgical removal of brain stem CMs is at the present time the best treatment of those lesions presenting with multiple hemorrhages or progressive neurologic deficit and which are accessible via a pial or ventricular surface.

Multiple and Familial Cases

In the past, CMs were thought to be mostly sporadic and rarely familial. As discussed in Chapter 2, broader experience has revealed that a familial form of CM is almost as common as the sporadic form. Genetically, the familial form of CM appears to exhibit an autosomal dominant inheritance with high penetrance. Therefore, 50% of an affected patient's siblings and offspring are likely to harbor similar lesions. To further complicate these clinical scenarios, patients with a familial form of CMs have a high incidence of multiplicity. As asymptomatic CMs do not usually require surgery, we do not advise routine MRI screening for asymptomatic relatives of patients with a known CM. Although the family should be informed of the possibility of inheritance, the financial and psychological hardships associated with routine screening seem unjustified.

For patients with multiple CMs, we believe the decision making should be the same as for single lesions. Treatment is warranted only for those lesions with presenting symptoms that justify surgical intervention. If a second malformation can be safely removed through the same operative exposure, consideration should be given to the removal of that lesion. There is no evidence, however, that asymptomatic lesions in the same individual with a single, symp-tomatic lesion have a more aggressive natural course; we also do not believe that routine removal of the asymptomatic lesions through separate operative exposures is usually indicated.

The Role of Radiosurgery

Treatment of CMs with radiation therapy and more recently, with radiosurgery is conceptually appealing. If these modalities are shown to favorably alter the natural history of the lesion, they may be used with acceptable morbidity limited to the effects of radiation on nearby brain. The vast majority of symptomatic CMs requiring treatment are easily accessible to direct microsurgical removal. Those that are most ideally suited for radiosurgery are the same lesions that are most ideally suited for microsurgery, i.e. small and symptomatic lesions. Surgical removal, if complete, eliminates the lesion without exposing the patient to the potentially harmful effects of radiation. Furthermore, there is some evidence that the risks of radiation necrosis are greater in the treatment of CMs than in the treatment of AVMs with the same dosimetry. This has led to recent recommendations of decreased radiation dosimetry for these lesions, as outlined in Chapter 15. The potential risks and unproven efficacy of radiosurgery render this form of treatment investigational at the present time.

Although the editors do not recommend radiosurgery for CMs, we do recognize the importance of limited academic centers carrying out investigational protocols, which are also discussed in Chapter 15. Patients entering such protocols should meet rigorous entrance criteria, including inoperability of the lesion as determined by an experienced vascular neurosurgeon; and, these procedures should be reserved only for lesions that are progressively symptomatic. Centers engaged in such trials should strive toward rigorous scientific documentation of the natural course of treated and untreated lesions, using prospective methodology of registries or clinical trials. Ideally, the limited cases meeting stringent criteria of inoperability and symptom progression should be randomized to expectant versus radiosurgical therapy within the context of a prospective randomized study. If radiosurgery is demonstrated to be efficacious for such inoperable lesions, it should be explored further in comparison with open surgical excision for more accessible lesions.

Summary

Neurosurgeons have found that the surgical removal of CMs is technically less demanding and safer than removal of their arteriovenous counterparts. Indeed, however, the ease of removal and accessibility should not be the only criteria for the recommendation of surgery. Importantly, neurosurgeons should be precise in the diagnosis of CMs, accurate and in agreement as to the nomenclature of these entities, and remain forthright in recommending intervention. Finally, we must continue to strive for a better understanding of the biologic behavior and natural history of CMs to provide the best care for patients harboring these lesions.

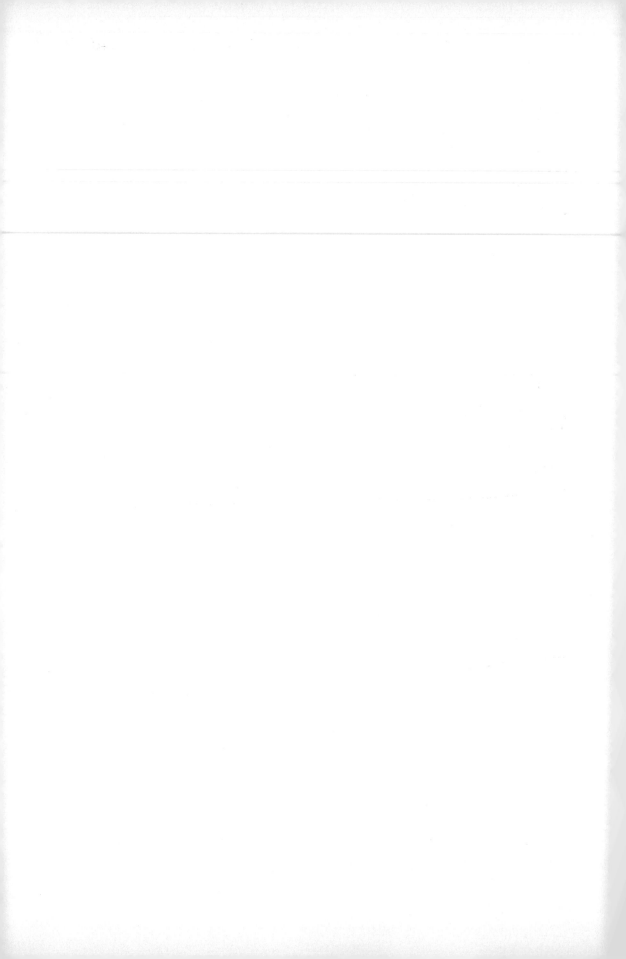

Index

Page numbers for figures, tables, and illustrations are in boldface italics.